Structured Clinical Management (SCM) for Personality Disorder

Advance Praise

'Structured Clinical Management is a practical, compassionate, and highly valued approach to helping people with personality disorder. This book provides an excellent guide for all those working in mental health services, whether they are delivering SCM or just want to provide better care to people with complex emotional health needs.'

Mike Crawford,
Professor of Mental Health Research,
Imperial College London, UK

'The beauty of this book is that it not only provides a simple and comprehensive set of evidence-based ingredients of quality treatment for personality disordered patients, but it also illustrates how to implement SCM in regular clinical services. A powerful resource for any service with an interest in providing high-quality generalist treatment.'

Joost Hutsebaut,
de Viersprong, Tilburg University and
Centre of Expertise on Personality Disorders,
The Netherlands

'Adult mental health services often struggle to respond to the complex needs of people with personality difficulties and their care often falls woefully short. Yet the provision of well-structured care can lead to tangible health benefits. Structured Clinical Management (SCM) provides a pragmatic approach to delivering such care and this comprehensive textbook tells us exactly how to do this. It is essential reading for anyone involved in the delivery, management and commissioning of adult mental health services.'

Paul Moran,
Professor of Psychiatry,
University of Bristol, UK

Structured Clinical Management (SCM) for Personality Disorder

An Implementation Guide

Edited by

STUART MITCHELL

Consultant Clinical Psychologist & Trust Lead for Personality Disorder, Cumbria, Northumberland, Tyne & Wear NHS Foundation Trust, Newcastle-upon-Tyne, UK

MARK SAMPSON

Consultant Clinical Psychologist, Professional Lead for Psychology and Psychological Therapies, Lead Clinician in Personality Disorder, Mersey Care, St Helens, UK

ANTHONY BATEMAN

Visiting Professor, University College London, UK; Honorary Professor University of Copenhagen, Denmark

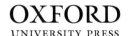

OXFORD

UNIVERSITY PRESS

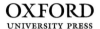

Great Clarendon Street, Oxford, OX2 6DP,
United Kingdom

Oxford University Press is a department of the University of Oxford.
It furthers the University's objective of excellence in research, scholarship,
and education by publishing worldwide. Oxford is a registered trade mark of
Oxford University Press in the UK and in certain other countries

Published in the United States of America by Oxford University Press
198 Madison Avenue, New York, NY 10016, United States of America

British Library Cataloguing in Publication Data

Data available

Library of Congress Control Number: 2021945529

ISBN 978–0–19–885152–3

DOI: 10.1093/med-psych/9780198851523.001.0001

Printed and bound by
CPI Group (UK) Ltd, Croydon, CR0 4YY

Preface

The original manual for structured clinical management (SCM) was first published 8 years ago (Bateman & Krawitz, 2013). Since then, there have been changes in classification, understanding and treatment of borderline personality disorder (BPD).[1] In parallel to these changes, generalist treatments for BPD such as SCM have been fully implemented in many organizations across the United Kingdom, Europe, and elsewhere. However, implementation of treatments and treatment approaches in clinical services are fraught with difficulties and clinical leads, operational managers, and practitioners alike grapple with how to implement SCM across complex mental health systems. The aim of this book is to provide guidance on how clinical teams, services, and organizations may implement SCM in clinical services. A range of clinical experts, researchers, service users, carers, and practitioners of SCM have contributed chapters from across the United Kingdom and Europe. Each chapter outlines a core aspect of the SCM model or its adaptation and delivery in clinical services. Key principles are highlighted in each chapter with clinical examples of application. A core theme throughout all chapters is a focus on the problem-solving structure of SCM and the clinical interventions for the core problem domains experienced by service users diagnosed with BPD or complex emotional and relational needs.

Generalist practitioners with relatively short additional training, combined with regular clinical supervision and support, can effectively implement SCM treatment. It is for this reason that the approach has become increasingly popular within general mental health services. SCM is a pluralistic and pragmatic approach that may be delivered and organized in a flexible way without rigid rules on application and implementation. SCM is an approach in terms of how a service is organized, how practitioners focus on the specific problems of service users diagnosed with personality disorder, how they are supported to deliver the clinical interventions, and how they work with other services available to the service user to effect optimal outcomes. The in-built flexibility is important because within generalist mental health services there are often competing demands, variations

---

[1] We recognize that not all service users will have received a diagnosis but may still present to mental health services. The ICD/DSM classification schemes have moved towards dimensional trait-based approaches, making the personality disorder types less relevant. It is likely that in future, trait-domain based schemes will be used more widely as they become adopted into clinical services. For the purposes of this book, we will write 'diagnosed with borderline personality disorder/personality disorder' whilst recognizing this may not always be the case.

in cultures around care, as well as significant capacity issues related to both staffing and demand that affects their state of 'readiness' to embrace change. It is worth highlighting that although SCM is permissive and flexible this does not equate to a drop in quality of the care delivered. Any SCM programme should have high levels of coherency, consistency, continuity, and collaboration, the four Cs underpinning SCM as outlined in Chapter 1.

Part 1 of the book orients the reader to the model and describes with detail the 'what' of SCM, including detailed clinical examples of 'how' to implement the model clinically. There are contributions from various authors, including the model originator, Anthony Bateman. In Chapter 1, Bateman resets the SCM scene and provides an updated model overview. In Chapter 2, Lester and Sampson go through assessment, diagnosis, and formulation. In Chapter 3, Sampson and Kayes then provide an overview of the clinical stance and individual interactions/sessions in SCM. Chapter 4 by Bevington and colleagues, provides an overview on SCM informed safety planning. Finally, in Chapter 5, Mitchell provides a detailed overview of the group component in SCM including what can be covered in the content and troubleshooting particular group-related problems.

These aspects of good-quality structured care will be familiar to most generalist practitioners working clinically with people with needs consistent with the descriptive diagnosis of borderline personality disorder. In SCM, an emphasis is strongly placed on continuity and structure along with highlighting the importance of developing a therapeutic relationship that builds the self-agency of the service user.

Part 2 of the book, different service models for implementing SCM in the United Kingdom and Europe are comprehensively described and reviewed (Chapters 6 and 7). The authors detail how they adapted and implemented the SCM model, or a variant of it, within their organizational settings, and the strategic, operational, and clinical processes involved. In the United Kingdom, Sampson and colleagues outline the ways in which they have adapted and implemented SCM in three large NHS Trusts, each with considerable success (Chapter 6). In Chapter 7, Aalders and colleagues outline the organizational processes in developing and implementing a variant of SCM in Sweden and the Netherlands, the latter they call Guideline Informed Treatment–Personality Disorders (GIT–PD). In Chapter 8, Mitchell and Harrison outline the importance of teamworking and the arrangements between SCM and the services with which it interfaces if a system to support service users diagnosed with BPD is to be developed effectively. Nair and colleagues in Chapter 9 describe a thorough review of the evidence around medication and guidance on prescribing for people diagnosed with BPD. Finally, in Chapter 10 Swift and colleagues provide a comprehensive illustration how SCM principles can provide a supporting framework to help make in-patient environments more therapeutic for service users diagnosed with BPD and/or complex trauma.

In Part 3, guidance is provided on special adaptations to SCM. In Chapter 11, Quayle and Mitchell provide a model for thinking about the meaning and processes of transitions at key points in the service user's pathway (illustrating this with clinical examples). In Chapter 12, Chiocchi and colleagues provide examples of structured family and carer programmes, illustrating how and why these should link into SCM pathways. In this chapter, John Chiocchi shares his rich, lived experience from the standpoint of a carer. This illustrates the importance of co-production and co-delivery of the family programme. In fact, co-production is a central theme to effective implementation of SCM programmes, as illustrated in Chapters 6 and 7.

Chapters 13, 14, and 15 of the book explore adapting the SCM model for service user groups who have additional problems, such as autistic spectrum disorders, complex trauma, or learning disability. Coexisting needs and complex psychopathology can make it difficult to formulate and determine with the service user what to prioritize in the treatment. Here, complexity and 'coexisting' or 'co-occurring' or 'comorbid' conditions may become problematic for clinical teams, with conflict and disagreement over the best fit of diagnosis and/or formulation. In Chapter 13, Everett and colleagues provide a rich and thoughtful account of how SCM may be developed and adapted for people with intellectual (learning) disabilities. They show, through careful reflection, how SCM may be adapted and delivered in a different way so that people with learning impairments may benefit. The adaptations extend to training and scaffolding (supervising) the care team staff who support such service users in residential settings. Graham and colleagues in Chapter 14 describe how services may use the principles of SCM to 'case manage' the service user in order to repatriate them from out of area treatments, and how SCM can provide a therapeutic model to help a dedicated 'linkworker' support people who struggle to engage in a structured therapy programme. In the final chapter in this part (Chapter 15), Mitchell looks at how SCM practitioners can work with service users with BPD who are experiencing problems related to childhood and adult adversity and trauma. The effects of such experiences may frequently be overlooked or left untreated but may nevertheless exert great impact on the person's mental and physical health and daily-life functioning. Mitchell describes with clinical examples how SCM may be adapted for people with additional problems related to complex trauma and dissociation in order help them increase their mental and behavioural stability.

Part 4 provides qualitative reflective accounts of how services users and practitioners have experienced being in or delivering an SCM programme and how clinical supervision may be organized. SCM is described as being collaborative and democratic in giving the service user as much autonomy and control of treatment as possible. But this clinical aim is not the same as reality for the service user or practitioner perspective. In Chapter 16, Watts and colleagues provide rich qualitative accounts of how service users have experienced SCM in UK clinical services and the implications of this for service development, suggesting that the appeal for democracy between service user and practitioner in SCM is only partially realized. In Chapter 17, Hanmer and colleagues provide qualitative accounts of practitioners' experiences of implementing SCM, and the implications SCM has had on their development as practitioners. In many respects, SCM has given practitioners confidence to work with people diagnosed with BPD, providing them with a structure for intervention. In Chapter 18, Harrison and colleagues look at supervision in SCM. They describe how the organization and principles of supervision may be implemented in services outlining well-known models of clinical supervision. They relate survey data from supervisors and supervisees to the model, including the use of a specific SCM implementation checklist to facilitate the areas of focus in supervision sessions. The final chapter of the book is a reflective account from the book editors summarizing and synthesizing the key aspects for practitioners and services to remember when they are implementing the model in clinical services. We also look forward to further research and changes to clinical services where SCM may be implemented as a generalist approach to treatment.

SCM is well on the way to becoming an evidence-based generalist approach for treating service users diagnosed with BPD or complex emotional or relational needs and/or associated problems. We hope this book is a useful guide for you to implement SCM within your service and organization, and that together we can help improve the lives of the many people who come forward seeking help with interpersonal problems, managing emotions, and controlling impulses. It is a privilege to be able to work with service users and practitioners with the singular aim of improving the lives of those who have been underserved by clinical services and society for many years. Good luck with your endeavours.

Stuart Mitchell

Mark Sampson

Anthony Bateman

Reference

Bateman, A., & Krawitz, R. (2013). *Borderline personality disorder: an evidence-based guide for generalist mental health professionals.* Oxford: Oxford University Press.

Contents

PART 3 SPECIAL ADAPTATIONS

PART 4 SYNTHESIS AND FUTURE DIRECTIONS

Contributors

Helga Aalders Clinical Psychologist and Medical Director, Department of Personality Disorders, Altrecht, the Netherlands

Muhammad Abdul-Rahman Specialty Doctor, Sunderland, Cumbria, Northumberland, Tyne & Wear NHS Foundation Trust, Newcastle, United Kingdom

Kristine Allam Community Practitioner, Cumbria, Northumberland, Tyne & Wear NHS Foundation Trust, Newcastle, United Kingdom

Kerry Anderson Psychological Therapist, Cumbria, Northumberland, Tyne & Wear NHS Foundation Trust, Newcastle, United Kingdom

Nicola Armstrong Patient and Carer Involvement Facilitator, Cumbria, Northumberland, Tyne & Wear NHS Foundation Trust, Newcastle, United Kingdom

Anthony Bateman Consultant to the Anna Freud Centre, London; Visiting Professor University College, London; Honorary Professor in Psychotherapy University of Copenhagen, Copenhagen

Christopher Berry Consultant Clinical Psychologist, Northamptonshire Healthcare NHS Foundation Trust, Northampton, United Kingdom

Rebecca Bevington Assistant Psychologist, Mersey Care NHS Trust (formerly North West Boroughs NHS Foundation Trust), St Helens, United Kingdom

Peder Björling Psychiatrist, Psychotherapist, Medical Director, The Program for Personality Program, Karolinska University Hospital, Huddinge, Sweden

John Chiocchi Highly Specialist Peer Support Worker, Mersey Care NHS Trust (formerly North West Boroughs NHS Foundation Trust), Warrington, United Kingdom

Katie Cummings Assistant Psychologist, Cumbria, Northumberland, Tyne & Wear NHS Foundation Trust, Newcastle upon Tyne, United Kingdom

Darren Ellis Personality Disorder Link Worker, Mersey Care NHS Trust (formerly North West Boroughs NHS Foundation Trust), Warrington, United Kingdom

Lisa Evans Psychological Therapist, Cumbria, Northumberland, Tyne & Wear NHS Foundation Trust, Newcastle, United Kingdom

Jill Everett Consultant Clinical Psychologist, Cumbria, Northumberland, Tyne & Wear NHS Foundation Trust, Newcastle upon Tyne, United Kingdom

Karen Finch SCM Practitioner, Mersey Care NHS Trust (formerly North West Boroughs NHS Foundation Trust), Knowsley, United Kingdom

Simon Graham Consultant Medical Psychotherapist, Mersey Care NHS Trust, Liverpool, United Kingdom

Catriona Gray Consultant Clinical Psychologist, Cumbria, Northumberland, Tyne & Wear NHS Foundation Trust, Newcastle upon Tyne, United Kingdom

Sarah Hanmer Principal Clinical Psychologist, Greater Manchester Mental Health NHS Foundation Trust (formerly North West Boroughs NHS Foundation Trust), Wigan, United Kingdom

Julia Harrison Senior Psychological Therapist, Cumbria, Northumberland, Tyne & Wear NHS Foundation Trust, Newcastle, United Kingdom

Allyson Jerry Principal Clinical Psychologist, Cumbria, Northumberland, Tyne & Wear NHS Foundation Trust, Newcastle upon Tyne, United Kingdom

Melanie Jones Clinical Lead Adult Mental Health Team Chester, Cheshire and Wirral Partnership, Chester, United Kingdom

Rachael Juma-Smith Personality Disorder Linkworker and DBT Therapist, Greater Manchester Mental Health NHS Foundation Trust (formerly North West Boroughs NHS Foundation Trust), Wigan, United Kingdom

Sharron Kayes Personality Disorder Link Worker, SCM Trainer, Mersey Care NHS Trust (formerly North West Boroughs NHS Foundation Trust), St Helens, United Kingdom

Rachael Lester Assistant Psychologist, Mersey Care NHS Trust (formerly North West Boroughs NHS Foundation Trust), St Helens, United Kingdom

Rachael Line Clinical Psychologist, Mersey Care NHS Trust, Liverpool United Kingdom

John Ludden SCM Practitioner, Mersey Care NHS Trust (formerly North West Boroughs NHS Foundation Trust), St Helens, United Kingdom

Louise MacDonald Psychological Therapist, Cumbria, Northumberland, Tyne & Wear NHS Foundation Trust, Newcastle, United Kingdom

Amy Maher Assistant Psychologist, Cumbria, Northumberland, Tyne & Wear NHS Foundation Trust, Newcastle upon Tyne, United Kingdom

Isaac McCann Assistant Psychologist and Support Staff, Formerly North West Boroughs, now employed by My Life Charity, Wigan, United Kingdom

Ashleigh McGuinness Assistant Psychologist, Mersey Care NHS Foundation Trust, Southport, United Kingdom

Stuart Mitchell Consultant Clinical Psychologist & Trust Lead for Personality Disorder, Cumbria, Northumberland, Tyne & Wear NHS Foundation Trust, Newcastle upon Tyne, United Kingdom

Rajesh Nair Consultant Psychiatrist and Associate Clinical Researcher, Northumberland, Cumbria, Tyne & Wear NHS Foundation Trust, Newcastle, United Kingdom

Mark Oliver Principal and Senior Clinical Psychologist, Cumbria, Northumberland, Tyne & Wear NHS Foundation Trust, Newcastle upon Tyne, United Kingdom

Donna Potts Community Practitioner, Cumbria, Northumberland, Tyne & Wear NHS Foundation Trust, Newcastle, United Kingdom

Genevieve Quayle Consultant Clinical Psychologist, Cumbria, Northumberland, Tyne & Wear NHS Foundation Trust, Newcastle upon Tyne, United Kingdom

Jon Robinson Personality Disorder Link Worker, Greater Manchester Mental Health NHS Foundation Trust (formerly North West Boroughs NHS Foundation Trust), Wigan, United Kingdom

Louise Roper Principal and Consultant Clinical Psychologist, Mersey Care NHS Trust (formerly North West Boroughs NHS Foundation Trust), Warrington, United Kingdom

Mark Sampson Consultant Clinical Psychologist Mersey Care NHS Trust (formerly North West Boroughs NHS Foundation Trust), St Helens, United Kingdom

Paula Slevin Advanced Practitioner in Personality Disorder (Strategy Lead), Greater Manchester Mental Health NHS Foundation Trust (formerly North West Boroughs NHS Foundation Trust), Wigan, United Kingdom

Kathryn Strom Pathway Manager, Cumbria, Northumberland, Tyne & Wear NHS Foundation Trust, Newcastle, United Kingdom

Niki Sundström Clinical Psychologist, Psychotherapist, Director, The Programme for Personality Disorders, Karolinska University Hospital of Huddinge, Sweden

Elaine Swift Consultant Counselling Psychologist, Greater Manchester Mental Health NHS Foundation Trust (formerly North West Boroughs NHS Foundation Trust), Wigan, United Kingdom

Gordon Turkington Higher Research Assistant, Cumbria, Tyne & Wear NHS Foundation Trust, Newcastle, United Kingdom

Robert Watts Senior Clinical Psychologist, Cumbria, Northumberland, Tyne & Wear NHS Foundation Trust, Newcastle upon Tyne, United Kingdom

Lisa Weaving Systemic Psychotherapist, Mersey Care NHS Trust (formerly North West Boroughs NHS Foundation Trust), Halton, United Kingdom

PART 1
THEORY, RESEARCH, AND MODEL

1

Introduction and Rationale of Structured Clinical Management

Anthony Bateman

Introduction

Borderline personality disorder (BPD) is a serious mental health condition with a prevalence estimated to be between 0.7% and 2% in the general population (Torgersen, Kringlen, & Cramer, 2001). It is a disorder predominantly diagnosed in women (75%) although estimates vary and most studies have been in clinical populations, where women are more likely to seek treatment. The prevalence of BPD is particularly high in the psychiatric and prison population; in England and Wales it is estimated to be 23% among male remand prisoners, 14% among sentenced male prisoners, and 20% among female prisoners (Singleton, 1998). Given the costs to society and to the individual and the significant public health implications associated with the disorder—including extensive use of healthcare resources, high rates of suicide and self-harm, social and interpersonal dysfunction, and reduced life expectancy—the provision of accessible, effective treatment is a health emergency (Fok et al., 2012). Yet there is some complexity in how to provide treatment efficiently in public mental health services. The aim of this chapter is to outline SCM (Bateman & Krawitz, 2013) as the foundation for an effective treatment pathway for people diagnosed with personality disorder.

SCM follows the principles of consistency, coherence, and continuity of intervention whilst targeting the specific symptoms of an individual's diagnosed personality disorder. It has proven to be an effective psychological approach that can be implemented by generalist mental health professionals. SCM is not a specialist psychosocial treatment for a specific category of personality disorder but a psychological approach targeting the acute symptoms that make up personality disorder. Although it is an approach that meets the needs of people with a range of personality problems, it is organized primarily for the more emotionally expressive personality disorders diagnosed, such as borderline and antisocial, and histrionic disorders rather than those with avoidant personality functioning. SCM has been developed further for a range of other conditions and implemented in a variety of contexts and many of the chapters in this book attest to this adaptability of the model. Full details of the overall approach can be found in the original published manual (Bateman & Krawitz, 2013).

Rationale for Structured Clinical Management (SCM)

A number of factors need to be considered when organizing and implementing treatments for BPD in mental health services:

1. Identifying personality disorder accurately in mental health teams
2. Assessing effective treatments available and differentiating between treatments
3. Understanding mechanisms of change in treatment to maximize effectiveness
4. Training the workforce to deliver effective intervention

Identifying personality disorder

Mental health professionals have considerable difficulty in recognizing personality disorder. In part, this is related to the unsatisfactory definition. The categorical approach to personality disorders, as presented in Section II of the DSM-5 (American Psychiatric Association, 2013), provides ten discrete diagnostic categories of personality disorder. It is not fit for purpose. The attempt to categorize BPD, for instance, in this way is undermined by high comorbidity and within-diagnosis heterogeneity, marked temporal instability, the lack of a clear boundary between normal and pathological personality, and poor convergent and discriminant validity. The range of characteristics is so large that questions have been asked about whether BPD should be a category at all. All this suggests that the various available evidence-based treatments with seemingly equivalent outcomes may have been studied in different populations and may not in fact be equally applicable to all subtypes of BPD. For these reasons, the proposal for ICD-11 (World Health Organization, 2018) attempts to break away from categorization and uses the alternative concept of trait domains. This may be more appropriate. It allows a way of making sense of a service user's behaviour in terms of severity and typical styles of behaviour and their underlying cognitive processes. Treatment can then be organized not according to a categorical diagnosis but aligned to patterns of behaviour and personal experiences. SCM follows this dimensional approach and specifically targets the self-experience of the individual and their interactions with others, their behaviours that cause them and others distress, and managing their emotional states. The diagnostic status of the service user does not necessarily determine the offer of treatment.

Research has not yet caught up with this domain-based understanding of personality disorder and most available trials of treatment assume that people diagnosed with BPD are a homogeneous group when they are not. Even if they were, there is no clear agreement about the rating of levels of severity and so different treatments have been tested on different populations, even though all have a diagnosis of BPD. This makes comparing treatments across studies difficult.

Assessing treatments

Most of the evidence about effective treatment for personality disorder relates to BPD but there are indications that other personality disorders may also benefit from treatment. Recent meta-analyses for treatments of BPD report that several treatment approaches are effective (Cristea et al., 2017; Leichsenring, Leibing, Kruse, New, & Leweke, 2011; Stoffers et al., 2012). Cristea et al. included 33 studies of specialized psychotherapy either as a standalone treatment or as an add-on to non-specialized psychotherapies in adult service users diagnosed with BPD. Overall, specialized psychotherapy emerged as moderately more effective than non-specialized psychotherapy in reducing borderline-relevant and other outcomes, such as general psychopathology and service utilization, with no differences between specialized psychotherapy as a standalone or as an add-on to usual treatment. Importantly, the beneficial effects were typically maintained up to 2-year follow-up with very few adverse events being reported although this could be because most trials were not set up to measure harmful effects. With regard to the different specialist treatment approaches, both dialectical behaviour therapy (DBT) (Linehan, 1993) and mentalization based treatment (MBT) (Bateman & Fonagy, 2006, 2016) emerge as a little more effective than non-specialized psychotherapy or treatment as usual (TAU); no such differences were found for cognitive therapy and other interventions.

But the situation is more complicated. There is evidence of risk of bias in published studies and also publication bias, particularly with regard to studies reporting follow-up data which are few in number. Taking these problems into account, the differences in effectiveness between specialized and non-specialized treatments do not seem to be very substantial and any differences largely disappear at follow-up. More importantly, pre-2006 studies show more substantial differences between the specialist treatment and TAU and contribute mostly to the differences found in meta-analysis. In later studies where the control condition was strong (i.e. in manualized treatments such as general psychiatric management (GPM) (Gunderson & Links, 2014)) and SCM (Bateman & Krawitz, 2013) there were fewer significant differences in treatment effect. In fact, correcting for publication bias by adjusting effect sizes for missing studies leads to equivalence of effect.

Do these findings mean that specialized psychotherapies are actually no more effective than non-specialized psychotherapy and can we simply pick any treatment? Not quite! The case remains strong that specialist psychotherapies for personality disorder should be part of basic mental health service provision even though there is now evidence to suggest that many service users can do equally well with less specialist intervention. The most important question is which service users do *equally* well or perhaps better with non-specialist, well-structured intervention, and which service users *only* do well with more specialist intervention. There is limited evidence on which to base an answer to this question as we have incomplete understanding of how service users improve in treatment or who responds to what treatment. This lack of understanding is not solely related to treatment of personality disorder. There is only rudimentary knowledge about the moderators and mechanisms of change in psychotherapy itself, let alone in more complex psychosocial treatments. Since 1975, meta-analyses have found that no *bona fide* form of psychotherapy is superior to another, and that therapeutic change does not depend on specific, 'branded' techniques (American Psychological Association, 2012; Lutz, Leon, Martinovich, Lyons, & Stiles, 2007; Steinert, Munder, Rabung, Hoyer, & Leichsenring, 2017; Zuroff, Kelly, Leybman, Blatt, & Wampold, 2010).

Mechanisms of change

If we knew how service users changed for the better, we would bottle it! Certainly, it would allow treatment to be carefully targeted. Practitioners often assume that the techniques they use in the consulting room are the primary drivers of change. This seems unlikely and there is a danger of making assumptions about what constitutes the active ingredient(s) of treatments (Fonagy, Luyten, & Bateman, 2017). As an example, Neacsiu et al. (Neacsiu, Lungu, Harned, Rizvi, & Linehan, 2014) examined the role of DBT skills in improving treatment clinical outcomes in BPD. Unsurprisingly, participants treated with DBT reported using three times more behavioural skills by the end of treatment than participants assigned to a control treatment. Use of DBT skills was shown to mediate the decrease in suicide attempts and depression and the increase in control of anger, suggesting that skills acquisition and practice may be an important mechanism of change in DBT. However important this effort may be, though, it creates an illusion of an explanation, which fails to explain how service users treated with general psychiatric management in a randomized controlled trial (RCT) comparing this intervention with DBT changed equally without receiving any skills training (McMain, Guimond, Streiner, Cardish, & Links, 2012; McMain et al., 2009).

Cristea et al. suggest that the superior outcomes of specialized treatments and strong control conditions could be explained by the 'special attention' BPD service users received in such studies. This implies that the superiority of these outcomes is rooted in their highly structured and often carefully manualized design. In older studies, the control treatments were unstructured and poorly manualized. More recent studies have addressed this problem. The importance of structuring of subjective experience as part of treatment has influenced how therapists—including the therapists in the TAU arm of trials—work with service users diagnosed with BPD, so outcomes may have improved in TAU because iatrogenesis is likely to have decreased with the waning of unfocused exploratory and supportive interventions (Fonagy & Bateman, 2006). Control conditions, particularly those in more recent trials, thus were not truly 'non-specialized' treatments with smaller effects. They were in fact treatments which were better organized with structured intervention for the problems of people diagnosed with BPD. Consistent with this is an argument that the coherence, consistency, and continuity of all treatments for BPD are crucial because they provide cognitive structure for a patient group that lacks metacognitive organization (Fonagy, Luyten, & Allison, 2015). If this is true, it not only is evidently good news for service users and practitioners but it also offers pointers to how interventions can be made simpler without compromising their effectiveness. The finding that treatment intensity, in terms of duration and hours of therapy, is not related to outcomes also suggests further changes could be made to the current complex and long-term specialist treatments without losing effectiveness (Smits, Feenstra, Eeren, & Bales, 2020).

Training the workforce

Most people diagnosed with personality disorder are treated in general mental health community services. Skilful, effective intervention for the many in that context is more significant for population health outcomes than provision of highly skilled specialist intervention for a few people and it is not possible to train all mental health professionals in specialist treatments. This is time-consuming, costly, and some treatments may lie outside the skill level of many excellent practitioners. However, treating the many in community mental health services risks harmful effects from well-meaning but misguided intervention unless practitioners have an understanding of personality disorder and how people diagnosed with personality disorder experience themselves and the world. So, some level of additional training is necessary for SCM or general psychiatric management (Choi-Kain & Gunderson, 2019). Fortunately, it is possible to take the skills that generalist mental health professionals already have to generate consistency, coherence, and continuity in their application to people with personality disorder and to organize them as interventions relevant to people diagnosed with personality disorder. This increases the likelihood of good outcomes and reduces the risk of harmful intervention. It was these guiding principles that were used to develop SCM.

Cognitive Coherence and Three (or Four) 'Cs'

It seems that current effective interventions have aspects in common. These overlapping components between different treatments need more urgent attention from researchers who have been too inclined to promote comparative research into their cherished specialist treatments, hoping to demonstrate their superiority over other treatments and to promote their 'cause' using specious arguments about why their treatment is better than all others. Psychotherapeutic interventions that are able to create change in personality disorders share 'three Cs': *consistency*, *coherence*, and *continuity*. These qualities are particularly pertinent in the treatment of BPD, a disorder in which metacognitive organization is often substantially lacking (Fonagy et al., 2017). Indeed, metacognitive disorganization may be one of the key unifying features of the disorders currently categorized as personality disorders in the psychiatric classification systems. A fourth 'C' can be added to the list which is *communication*. Using an intervention style to bridge the communication gap between people diagnosed with BPD and others is necessary if a service user is to experience a practitioner as relating to them as a person rather than as someone who needs to desist from behaving in certain ways. A channel of understanding needs to open up between service user and practitioner for effective work to proceed (Fonagy & Allison, 2014).

There is some agreement about how the three 'Cs' are formulated in specialist treatments and how the fourth 'C' requires an attitude on the part of the clinician. First, all treatment manuals outline a structure for treatment and ask the practitioner to be clear about what can and what cannot be offered. This encourages proactivity and self-agency of the service user and requires commitment to the approach. Second, they make extensive effort to engage service users in treatment using a clear model of personality functioning that is explained to service users. This increases cognitive coherence for the individual and provides a joint lens through which service user and practitioner can view their problems. Third, a positive and validating active stance, generating a strong attachment relationship as a basis for a therapeutic alliance, is promoted. Fourth, there is a focus on emotion processing and connection between action and feeling to restore cognitive representation of emotion. Finally, to open up the communication channels there is detailed inquiry into service users' mental states (behavioural analysis, clarification, confrontation) to strengthen representations of those mental states. There can be no communication without the communicator having in mind the perspective of the receiver. In the first instance, this has to come from the practitioner understanding the mind of the service user from within.

The validation of the service user's sense of agency enables service users to make use of the techniques of the therapy to benefit from experiences in their day-to-day life. From this perspective, change is thought to be brought about by what happens beyond therapy, in the service user's social environment. Studies in which change has been monitored session by session have suggested that the service user–practitioner alliance in a given session predicts change in the next (Falkenstrom, Granstrom, & Holmqvist, 2013). This suggests that the change that occurs between sessions is a consequence of changed attitudes to learning from social experience engendered by therapy, which influences the service user's behaviour between sessions.

SCM

SCM was first developed as a non-specialist control condition in an RCT of MBT (Bateman & Fonagy, 2009). In most trials of specialist treatments for personality disorder the comparison intervention is commonly described as TAU; in practice this means no consistent treatment or poorly organized intervention by practitioners unskilled in treatments for people diagnosed with BPD. Even when skilled practitioners are used for a comparison treatment the variation in treatments in the control group and the context of treatments were substantially different. In effect, in most if not all RCTs for BPD, the odds are stacked against any comparator treatment. To address these problems, the protocol for an out-patient trial of MBT versus a comparator treatment required the control treatment, SCM, to meet the three 'Cs'. These were to be applied according to best practice, to be delivered by generalist mental health clinicians with the same level of training and experience as MBT therapists, and treatment was to be offered in the same frequency and format as MBT. Both MBT and SCM were to be learned with only limited additional training (3 days), building generic mental health skills so highly trained therapists were not essential for delivery. A manual for SCM was written and trial practitioners, who were nurses, graduate mental health workers, trainee psychologists and psychiatrists, were randomized to 3-day training in either MBT or SCM, thereby minimizing requirements for extensive training whilst reducing allegiance effects on treatment outcomes. All practitioners were given supervision in line with clinical service levels of support. This was a trial in the 'real world' of clinical services.

MBT was found to be superior to SCM in reducing self-harm, suicidality, and depression, and social and interpersonal function particularly in the long term. But comparing the average outcomes of service users between groups hides the fact that some service users do well in each group and some do badly. It is entirely likely that many service users who had MBT would have done just as well in SCM; the most important question is who needed MBT, that is who did badly in SCM but would have done well in MBT? A post-hoc analysis of moderators found that severity of condition as defined by the number of positive personality disorder

diagnoses in addition to BPD predicted the need for the MBT approach. SCM appeared to have less benefit on most outcome measures among these service users although SCM did well with service users who did not meet these severity criteria.
Given the evidence that SCM can

1. do well with service users diagnosed with BPD at a mild to moderately severe level, particularly in reducing suicide attempts and self-harm
2. be implemented by generalist mental health professionals
4. be delivered with flexibility in mental health teams rather than specialist services
5. minimize the likelihood of harmful intervention

and

6. the evidence of the superiority of any specialist treatment over well-constructed generalist treatment for most people diagnosed with BPD is limited
7. dropout rates from specialist treatments and SCM are equivalent at around 20%, indicating treatments are equally acceptable to service users although in general dropouts are higher when any treatment is implemented in general services outside research trials
8. our knowledge about mechanisms of change of complex psychosocial treatments indicates that the three Cs are important—consistency, coherence, and continuity
9. most people diagnosed with personality disorder are treated in general mental health services

It has been developed further as a psychological approach focusing on the three Cs and targeting the symptoms and behaviours specific to people diagnosed with BPD.

Principles of SCM—Consistency, Coherence, and Continuity

Stage 1

Practitioner
SCM requires practitioners to generate a therapeutic alliance right from the start using a compassionate and interested therapeutic stance. Practitioners should elect to work with people diagnosed with personality disorder rather than be forced to do so. Personal characteristics of the practitioner may affect treatment. Over-controlling, overprotective, reactive, anxious practitioners are unlikely to be

helpful to people diagnosed with BPD; those who are able to manage their anxiety around risk, are secure in their attitudes, and less reactive to excessive negative and overly positive emotional expression are likely to fare better and bring about superior outcomes. Level-headedness is the key.

SCM is implemented as a structured and sequential coherent programme so the service user knows what to expect and when to expect it. The programme is permissive in terms of number of sessions and the mode of treatment, which is group, individual, or both when necessary. Initially a series of preparatory sessions are offered as a framework for further treatment. These sessions are in fact treatment itself and may be considered as a stabilization phase. Expert consensus suggests that treatment for people diagnosed with BPD should be offered over the long term rather than the short term and so treatment length is commonly around 1 year. The initial sessions are task-orientated. The service user is given a series of dates agreed beforehand, each with an allocated task with the final session identified as a decision-making session focusing on a collaborative formulation for treatment or agreement about no treatment or referral to a more appropriate treatment. This process is commonly organized over six sessions but this is flexible, as is their frequency, which may be every 2 weeks rather than weekly, or even less frequent if this is agreed between the service user and practitioner. Although each session has a task, they join together to generate a shared perspective of the service user's problems.

Sessions 1 and 2
The first stage of any effective treatment involves the transmission of substantive content to the service user that helps them organize their problems into a coherent and credible frame that they can recognize and accept. The first session is a 'get to know you' session with history taking and identification of problem areas. To be accepted, it has to be personally relevant so the service user recognizes himself as an agentive self, that is, a person who has an active role in his experiences and as someone who has the potential to take control rather than be at the mercy of circumstances. SCM practitioners actively place the service user's problems into specific categories representing the main domains of problem found in people diagnosed with BPD. Therefore, the practitioner listens to the service user, identifying problems that relate to emotional regulation and mood control, impulsivity, and interpersonal sensitivities. In clinical practice, it is useful in the second session to organize these domains into column headings on a sheet of paper and populate each column with the problems and behaviours that the service user describes. This is the beginning of identifying and sharing the SCM framework with the service user and making the four problem areas the centre of the work. Service users need a framework within which to begin to consider their problems if they are to experience greater personal agency.

Sessions 3 and 4
Once the framework for thinking about problems is established, the next sessions require the practitioner to focus on establishing a diagnosis or agreed description of the problem, safety planning and developing a co-produced formulation. The final session is agreeing the treatment plan. Establishing a diagnosis is controversial and SCM leaves the decision about using a categorical diagnostic system in clinical practice and talking to the service user about this to the clinical team. Some teams discuss a categorical diagnosis with the service user prior to organizing a formulation around the five Ps—Predisposing, Precipitating, Presenting, Perpetuating, and Protective factors. Others avoid diagnostic categories and talk to the service user about their problem areas. The reasons for avoidance may be political for some, in terms of stigma and labelling people, whilst for others it is academic in terms of categorical diagnostic systems being an artefact not fit for purpose. In practical terms, many practitioners are not trained to make formal diagnoses and a professional with the skills to do this reliably may not be part of the team. In the end, it is for the clinical team to agree an approach to this dilemma and to take a decision one way or the other, which is then implemented by all. One advantage for the service user in discussing the diagnosis sensitively is that they have a reference point from which to access online information and peer group support systems, which are commonly organized around the term BPD.

Safety planning to maintain safety is a key element of SCM. The process follows normal safety planning in mental health services and has to be done systematically and collaboratively. The service user and practitioner develop a summary leaflet of their joint safety plan itemizing what the service user can do if risk and safety changes, what the practitioner can and cannot do, and what others can and cannot do. The main emphasis is on what the service user can do to increase their own responsibility for avoiding crisis or decreasing the level of risk when it escalates. The practitioner does not take over responsibility for the life of the service user but does take responsibility for generating a pathway to manage and reduce risk over time.

Sessions 5 and 6
The final task of the initial sessions is the development of a joint formulation that summarizes the key problem areas using the five 'Ps' and identifies goals related to the four clinical domains of SCM: emotional management, mood control, impulsivity, and interpersonal problems. This ushers in the second stage of treatment, which is for the service user to engage in a group to focus on their immediate goals related to the four clinical domains.

Prior to this transfer into the second stage of referral into a group SCM programme, the practitioner must address any factors that might interfere with service user attendance or ability to profit from the intervention. Practical factors such as housing, finance, and childcare might require the practitioner to become an advocate for the service user by jointly completing applications for support from other services and encouraging involvement in purposeful activity such as attending college or seeking voluntary work or employment. Crucially, the practitioner may have to decide to work for a few sessions on other problem areas before referring them into an SCM group. The most important of these is co-occurring severe anxiety and interpersonally triggered dissociative problems, which may indicate underlying complex trauma or a dissociative disorder. Unless dissociation and other trauma problems are reduced the service user will not be able to take advantage of the second stage.

The second stage

In the second stage, the service user is encouraged to attend groups in which the practitioner structures therapeutic work around the four SCM domains, namely groups on emotional management, mood control, impulsivity, and interpersonal problems, all of which are addressed using a problem-solving approach to difficulties. The number of groups allocated to each domain varies according to the needs of service users but as a rule of thumb, at least five consecutive groups on each domain in the first instance will be required. If a service user enters the group currently working on a domain that does not address their problems the practitioner encourages the service user's interest in others' and their ability to interact constructively to help others in the group whilst indicating that the focus will soon be on them and their difficulties. Alternatively, the practitioner organizes the service user to begin the group when a relevant module is starting.

Generic group skills are required by the practitioner to run SCM groups well. The practitioner needs to recognize the service users as an agent of their own futures and be able to validate and acknowledge their emotional states. The attitude is not solely educational but is facilitating of discovery and developing problem-solving skills. Problems are embraced, and if they cannot be solved they can be placed aside temporarily whilst other problems are examined. The domains of focus each have a series of treatment strategies associated with them, for example naming and describing emotions in the emotional management module, but the key factor is the ability of the practitioner to make the sessions personally relevant to each service user and demonstrate the social and interpersonal value of change. An open, trustworthy, and non-judgemental environment is fostered that is conducive to exploration and discovery.

SCM is timed (time-limited) and although there is discussion about length of treatment, most services limit treatment to 1 year. This is specified at the beginning of treatment. There is some merit to timed treatment. The overall evidence is that gains that people make in psychotherapy occur early rather than late and in research trials on treatment of people diagnosed with personality disorder measurable change tends to occur around 6 months. Indeed, in the trial of MBT versus SCM reduction in self-harm and suicide attempts started around 4–6 months.

Ending or termination in psychotherapy is an important and under-researched topic. SCM attempts to work overtly on ending and the emotion reactions and responses to it. There may have to be acceptance of what has been lost in the past, tolerance of the current level of adaptation to life, and regret about not achieving earlier life goals. On the other hand, there can be a review of positive changes and planning for the future. The practitioner finds a balance between exploring the failures and success of treatment. Decisions can be taken about follow-up and maintenance sessions. Again, SCM is permissive in this, leaving the decision to the service user and practitioner, only emphasizing the importance of ending treatment at the agreed time rather than continuing it and ensuring the service user rather than the practitioner takes responsibility for managing their life.

Other Features of SCM

1. Involving families of people diagnosed with personality disorder is often neglected by practitioners. SCM practitioners invite families to multi-family meetings. Relatives may live with and financially and emotionally support the person diagnosed with BPD and so are crucial in their recovery. Family members experience high levels of distress and burden and their involvement in treatment reduces their level of distress. In SCM, a two-session multi-family intervention is described in the original manual with a leaflet for families. It is important the practitioners provide accurate information about BPD as a diagnosis and about their treatment plans and ensure that families are validated in their attempts to support their family member. Multi-family interventions allow families to share their experiences and learn from each other and this in itself may enable them to respond more constructively to the person diagnosed with BPD.

2. The evidence for using medication to treat people with personality disorder is poor. Yet most people diagnosed with BPD are on one or more psychoactive medications and the number of different medications prescribed increases over time. Medication may be used for co-occurring disorders such as depression but medication may also be prescribed as a result of practitioner anxiety. Therefore, SCM requires a review of medication whenever possible and integration of prescribing within the SCM programme to address these issues. Concerns about risk and emotional and interpersonal reactivity for example are best addressed in the group treatment than suppressed with medication. Any medication prescribed should be monitored carefully in

terms of the target symptoms and if there is no improvement over an agreed period of time the medication is stopped.

3. Integration between the SCM programme and other services available to the service user such as in-patient facilities, drug addiction clinics, and eating disorder units is important to ensure treatment is coherent and coordinated.

Conclusions

SCM is a multifaceted approach to helping people diagnosed with personality disorder combining a range of interventions that are within the scope of generalist mental health practitioners. The approach is configured not only to deliver effective interventions but also to avoid harmful interactions between services, practitioners, and the person diagnosed with personality disorder. The majority of people diagnosed with personality disorder are treated within general mental health services rather than by specialist units and so skilful implementation of SCM by community mental health teams is efficient and ensures effective intervention is readily available.

References

American Psychiatric Association. (2013). *Diagnostic and statistical manual of mental disorders* (5th Ed.). Arlington, VA: American Psychiatric Publishing.

American Psychological Association. (2012). Recognition of psychotherapy effectiveness. Retrieved from http://www.apa.org/about/policy/resolution-psychotherapy.aspx.

Bateman, A., & Fonagy, P. (2006). *Mentalization based treatment: a practical guide.* Oxford: Oxford University Press.

Bateman, A., & Fonagy, P. (2009). Randomized controlled trial of out-patient mentalization based treatment versus structured clinical management for borderline personality disorder. *American Journal of Psychiatry, 1666*, 1355–1364.

Bateman, A., & Fonagy, P. (2016). *Mentalization based treatment for personality disorders: a practical guide.* Oxford: Oxford University Press.

Bateman, A., & Krawitz, R. (2013). *Borderline personality disorder: an evidence based guide for generalist mental health professionals.* Oxford: Oxford University Press.

Choi-Kain, L., & Gunderson, J. (2019). *Applications of good psychiatric management for borderline personality disorder: a practical guide.* Washington, DC: American Psychiatric Association Publishing.

Cristea, I. A., Gentili, C., Cotet, C. D., Palomba, D., Barbui, C., & Cuijpers, P. (2017). Efficacy of psychotherapies for borderline personality disorder: a systematic review and meta-analysis. *JAMA Psychiatry, 74*(4), 319–328. doi:10.1001/jamapsychiatry.2016.4287.

Falkenstrom, F., Granstrom, F., & Holmqvist, R. (2013). Therapeutic alliance predicts symptomatic improvement session by session. *Journal of Counseling Psychology, 60*(3), 317–328. doi:10.1037/a0032258

Fok, M., Hayes, R., Chang, C., Stewart, R., Callard, F., & Moran, P. (2012). Life expectancy at birth and all-cause mortality among people with personality disorder. *Journal of Psychosomatic Research, 73*, 104–107.

Fonagy, P., & Allison, E. (2014). The role of mentalizing and epistemic trust in the therapeutic relationship. *Psychotherapy, 51*, 372–380.

Fonagy, P., & Bateman, A. (2006). Progress in the treatment of borderline personality disorder. *British Journal of Psychiatry, 188*, 1–3. doi:10.1192/bjp.bp.105.012088

Fonagy, P., Luyten, P., & Allison, E. (2015). Epistemic petrification and the restoration of epistemic trust: a new conceptualization of borderline personality disorder and its psychosocial treatment. *Journal of Personality Disorders, 29*(5), 575–609. doi:10.1521/pedi.2015.29.5.575.

Fonagy, P., Luyten, P., & Bateman, A. (2017). Treating borderline personality disorder with psychotherapy: where do we go from here? *JAMA Psychiatry, 74*(4), 316–317. doi:10.1001/jamapsychiatry.2016.4302

Gunderson, J. G., & Links, P. L. (2014). *Handbook of good psychiatric management (GPM) for borderline patients.* Washington DC: American Psychiatric Press.

Leichsenring, F., Leibing, E., Kruse, J., New, A. S., & Leweke, F. (2011). Borderline personality disorder. *Lancet, 377*(9759), 74–84. doi:10.1016/S0140-6736(10)61422-5

Linehan, M. M. (1993). *Cognitive-behavioral treatment of borderline personality disorder.* New York, NY: Guilford.

Lutz, W., Leon, S. C., Martinovich, Z., Lyons, J. S., & Stiles, W. B. (2007). Therapist effects in outpatient psychotherapy: a three-level growth curve approach. *Journal of Counseling Psychology, 54*(1), 32–39. doi:10.1037/0022-0167.54.1.32

McMain, S. F., Guimond, T., Streiner, D. L., Cardish, R. J., & Links, P. S. (2012). Dialectical behavior therapy compared with general psychiatric management for borderline personality disorder: clinical outcomes and functioning over a 2-year follow-up. *American Journal of Psychiatry, 169*(6), 650–661. doi:10.1176/appi.ajp.2012.11091416

McMain, S. F., Links, P. S., Gnam, W. H., Guimond, T., Cardish, R. J., Korman, L., & Streiner, D. L. (2009). A randomized trial of dialectical behavior therapy versus general psychiatric management for borderline personality disorder. *American Journal of Psychiatry, 166*(12), 1365–1374. doi:10.1176/appi.ajp.2009.09010039

Neacsiu, A. D., Lungu, A., Harned, M. S., Rizvi, S. L., & Linehan, M. M. (2014). Impact of dialectical behavior therapy versus community treatment by experts on emotional experience, expression, and acceptance in borderline personality disorder. *Behaviour Research and Therapy, 53*, 47–54. doi:10.1016/j.brat.2013.12.004

Singleton, N. (1998). *Psychiatric morbidity among prisoners in England and Wales.* London: Office of National Statistics.

Smits, M., Feenstra, D., Eeren, H., & Bales, D. (2020). Day hospital versus intensive outpatient mentalization-based treatment for borderline personality disorder: multicentre randomised clinical trial. *British Journal of Psychiatry, 216*, 79–84.

Steinert, C., Munder, T., Rabung, S., Hoyer, J., & Leichsenring, F. (2017). Psychodynamic therapy: as efficacious as other empirically supported treatments? a meta-analysis testing equivalence of outcomes. *American Journal of Psychiatry*, 10.1176/appi.ajp.2017.17010057 [epub ahead of print].

Stoffers, J. M., Vollm, B. A., Rucker, G., Timmer, A., Huband, N., & Lieb, K. (2012). Psychological therapies for people with borderline personality disorder. *Cochrane Database of Systematic Reviews, 8*(8), CD005652. doi:10.1002/14651858.CD005652.pub2

Torgersen, S., Kringlen, E., & Cramer, V. (2001). The prevalence of personality disorders in a community sample. *Archives of General Psychiatry, 58,* 590–596.

World Health Organization. (2018). *International classification of diseases* (10 Ed.). Geneva: World Health Organization.

Zuroff, D. C., Kelly, A. C., Leybman, M. J., Blatt, S. J., & Wampold, B. E. (2010). Between-therapist and within-therapist differences in the quality of the therapeutic relationship: effects on maladjustment and self-critical perfectionism. *Journal of Clinical Psychology, 66*(7), 681–697. doi:10.1002/jclp.20683

2

Diagnosis, Formulation, and Assessment in SCM

Rachael Lester and Mark Sampson

Introduction

This chapter will review the history and epidemiology of the diagnosis of borderline personality disorder (BPD), including service users' experiences of receiving the diagnosis. It will then review how psychological formulation is used and applied to structured clinical management (SCM). Finally, the chapter will review how the assessment process is structured, organized, and delivered in the early sessions with the service user.

SCM and the Borderline Personality Disorder Diagnosis

The term 'borderline personality disorder' (BPD) was derived by practitioners in the 1930s to identify a group of individuals who did not fit into the usual categorization of 'neurotic', including what we now refer to as anxiety and depressive disorders, or 'psychotic', including what we now refer to as bipolar disorder and schizophrenia (Bateman & Krawitz, 2013). Practitioners found there was a group of individuals who, descriptively, in most ways fitted the 'neurotic' category except that they did not respond to the usual treatments at the time. The term 'borderline' referred to the belief during this time that this group of people were on the 'border' between 'neurotic' and 'psychotic'. Whilst some people diagnosed with BPD do have occasional psychotic or psychotic-like experiences, this definition of BPD, being on the 'border' no longer applies, but the term has become ingrained. There was a discussion in the 1970s of BPD as a variant of schizophrenia, in the 1980s as a variant of depression, in the 1990s as a variant of post-traumatic disorder, and since then as a variant of bipolar disorder. BPD was and is often described as a categorical disorder: you either have BPD or you don't. However, in reality many experts would acknowledge that there is a dimensional aspect to the disorder (Bateman & Krawitz, 2013).

There are two different mental health diagnostic manuals. There is the American-based system, the *Diagnostic and Statistical Manual of Mental Disorders*—now in its fifth edition (DSM-5; American Psychiatric Association, 2013). The term BPD originates from section II of this manual. The World Health Organization system is the International Classification of Diseases 11th Edition (ICD-11). Prior to this most recent edition, this diagnostic system used the term 'emotionally unstable borderline personality disorder—impulsive type or borderline type'. However, both DSM-5 and ICD-11 have moved towards trait dimensional approaches to personality disorder which have been replicated across different cultures and for which there is much research support (Bach & Presnall-Shvorin, 2020; McCabe & Widiger, 2019; Ofrat, Krueger, & Clark, 2018). Clinical assessment using this approach may now focus on assessing severity of functional impairment along with distress experienced, which may then be followed up by assessment of five to six trait-domain specifiers that illustrate how the person expresses their traits (Bach & First, 2018). New assessment tools have been developed with good psychometric properties which support trait-based clinical assessments of service users (Bach & Presnall-Shvorin, 2020; Clarkin et al., 2018; Oltmanns & Widiger, 2018).

For the purpose of this chapter and the book, section II of DSM-5 diagnosis will be the default system used. Most research evidence is for DSM diagnoses of BPD or antisocial personality disorder (ASPD). Research using the new personality levels of functioning and trait-based domains is new and developing. Using trait-based assessments will help reduce the stigma of personality disorder diagnosis in that functional impairment and trait expression become the issues of most concern for formulation and treatment planning rather than a binary approach to either 'having a personality disorder' or not. The National Institute for Health and Care Excellence (NICE) guidance was developed for BPD and supports the use of structured clinical assessments, such as SCID-II. NICE will need to catch up with newer assessment tools using the alternative trait-based models of personality disorder.

Epidemiological research estimates between 15–28% of service users in mental health services (including in-patients and out-patients) meet the BPD diagnostic threshold, with a prevalence of 1.7% in the general population (Gunderson et al., 2018).

Reviewing evidence for the diagnosis

Using psychiatric diagnoses in the care of people with mental health difficulties has generated great controversy in recent years, particularly amongst service users and health professionals regarding the diagnosis of BPD. The conceptual validity of BPD has provoked debate amongst health professionals—research has indicated that many service users have shared many different experiences of their difficulties to the clinical descriptions of BPD (Castillo, 1993; Ng et al., 2019; Rusch et al., 2006), with some preferring a diagnosis of bipolar disorder or anxiety and depression. In contrast, some individuals have been found to hold an internalized medical view of themselves and inadvertently defined themselves through their diagnosis (Dyson & Brown, 2016). For some people, this can protect their self-esteem by allowing them to distance themselves from their struggles. However, for others it can collude with avoidance and a feeling of 'defectiveness', whereby they see themselves as being 'sick' and needing to be 'fixed' by health professionals. Some people view the BPD diagnosis as one that is highly stigmatizing and leads to judgmental perceptions from some mental health professionals (Ng et al., 2019; Perseius et al., 2005).

That said, many experts in the field accept BPD as a valid recognizable condition, acknowledged because BPD exists as a DSM-5 diagnosis. This has led to much debate about the changes suggested in ICD-11 described earlier. The controversy about the diagnosis is set to continue for the near future.

BPD as a diagnosis is most often applied only to adults, referencing child and adolescence as a period when many BPD trait features begin to occur as part of normal adolescent development. Consequently, many practitioners tend not to make the diagnosis in adolescents. However, some experts emphasize the value of making an early diagnosis so as to be able to initiate effective treatments before the person and mental health system get locked into mutually reinforcing, ineffective behaviours. Chanen et al.'s (2008) randomized controlled trial demonstrated that it is possible to identify and effectively treat adolescents with full or sub-syndromal BPD, thereby also going some way to alleviate fears of iatrogenic dangers of diagnosis in adolescence (Chanen, Jovev, & Jackson, 2007).

Criteria for meeting the BPD diagnosis

What leads somebody to meet the diagnosis of BPD?

To meet the diagnosis of BPD, a person will experience problems which are persistent (usually starting in late adolescence or early adulthood), problematic (causing significant distress or impairment in functioning), and pervasive (affecting a number of different personal and social contexts). Box 2.1 below illustrates the diagnostic criteria for BPD.

To echo the above, individuals diagnosed with BPD show a pervasive pattern of instability of interpersonal relationships, self-image and affects, and marked impulsivity beginning by early adulthood and present in a variety of contexts. This is known as the 'ThreePs' and may be formally assessed in the Structured Clinical Interview for DSM IV Axis II Disorders (SCID-II). The assessing practitioner is looking for examples in the nine areas to see if a clinical threshold of the three Ps has been met. Any practitioner doing the diagnostic assessment for BPD should have training in undertaking a semi-structured interview around the diagnostic criterion around threshold to ensure validity and consistency. It is also important that this training ensures the diagnostic assessment is carried out in the correct way and that the information is shared effectively. Alternatively, the practitioner may use the user's guide to administer the Structured Clinical Interview for the DSM-5 Alternative Model for Personality Disorder (First et al., 2018), which is the trait-based equivalent alternative scheme.

Box 2.1 Diagnostic Criterion for Borderline Personality Disorder (DSM-5)

---

1. Frantic efforts to avoid real or imagined abandonment; this does not include suicidal or self-mutilating behaviour covered in criterion 5

2. Pattern of unstable and intense interpersonal relationships characterized by alternating between extremes of idealization and devaluation

3. Identity disturbance: markedly and persistently unstable self-image or sense of self

4. Impulsivity in at least two areas that are potentially self-damaging (e.g. spending, sex, substance abuse, reckless driving, binge eating); this does not include suicidal or self-mutilating behaviour covered in criterion 5

5. Recurrent suicidal behaviour, gestures or threats, or self-mutilating behaviour

6. Affective instability due to a marked reactivity of mood (e.g. intense episodic dysphoria, irritability or anxiety usually lasting a few hours and only rarely more than a few days)

7. Chronic feelings of emptiness

8. Inappropriate intense anger or difficulty controlling anger (e.g. frequent displays of temper, constant anger, recurrent physical fights)

9. Transient, stress-related paranoid ideation or severe dissociative symptoms

Note: It is important to look to ensure that the above difficulties are not caused by other acute symptoms e.g. depression/anxiety.

Service users' experiences of receiving the BPD diagnosis

As highlighted throughout this chapter, the concept of diagnosis, particularly BPD, has generated great controversy amongst both service users and healthcare professionals over many years. There is a plethora of existing research exploring the experiences of people living with the BPD diagnosis, though in more recent years, the focus of attention appears to have moved on to understanding more specifically peoples' subjective experiences of receiving the diagnosis.

Research exploring the effects of the diagnostic process more broadly has highlighted that service users are positively emotionally affected following diagnostic feedback provision (Holm-Denoma et al., 2008). This was no different for people receiving the diagnosis of BPD when the diagnosis was delivered in a particular way. A literature review of the current evidence base (Lester et al., 2020) captured a range of service user accounts offering different perspectives on receiving the

BPD diagnosis, with particular focus on their experiences of diagnosis delivery and their subsequent understanding and interpretation of the diagnosis. Negative experiences included a lack of information about the diagnosis, a reluctance of practitioners to communicate the diagnosis, and in some cases the diagnosis being withheld. It was found that this could adversely reinforce their perception of being stigmatized and rejected, particularly by practitioners and mental health services. Those who received less information and shared a more limited understanding about the diagnosis were found to view themselves in more undesirable ways, for example 'I am bad', and express negative emotional responses (shame, guilt, hopelessness). In contrast, experiences that are more positive were shared by service users surrounding the efficacy of the diagnosis in providing a clearer understanding of themselves and their difficulties, with many expressing a huge sense of relief and validation (Lester et al., 2020). Connecting with the person and 'seeing more' (beyond an individual's diagnosis and/or behaviour) epitomized helpful experiences. When practitioners in delivering the diagnosis took an empathic, careful, and non-judgemental approach, service users felt empowered and hopeful about their capacity for change. Clinical guidelines for best practice (Grenver et al., 2015) advocate this approach when communicating the diagnosis in that it helps to engage the service user in treatment and fosters a belief that a valuable and beneficial service is on offer. These findings emphasize that communication is key to distinguishing between a conversation that discusses diagnosis carefully and sensitively and one that does not.

Conclusion around diagnosis

In the United Kingdom, the NICE guideline for Borderline Personality Disorder (2009) covers the diagnosis and stigma associated with this, acknowledging that the 'label' has both positive and negative aspects. For some, it can provide clarity of their difficulties and a sense of control, whilst for others it feels labelling and stigmatizing. What is important however, is that any description or need for diagnosis should be a label of inclusion rather than one of rejection or exclusion. NICE's approach and recommendation is that knowledge about the service user's needs, including how the psychiatric system currently labels this, can empower them if delivered in the correct (sensitive) way. This includes open and honest discussions about diagnosis and the diagnostic label (NICE, 2009).

Using a diagnosis within an SCM pathway can also have the effect of service users being categorized by their diagnosis, for example 'she is on the BPD pathway/he has BPD'. If this is not managed effectively, practitioners and the organization can then forget to see the 'person' behind the diagnosis or reassess mental health need appropriately. Any assessment pathway/SCM pathway would need to address this if diagnosis is used. Labelling in this way is a form of a non-mentalizing communication style and is often unhelpful.

What any organized pathway needs to address however is organizational paralysis associated with the needs of people diagnosed with BPD which can mean that assessments are not completed properly, if at all.

It is important to look beyond the whole area of diagnosis and explore what the function should be, as described in this chapter. Service users want the assessment to provide them with clarity about their problems in daily life, a clearer understanding of why they behave as they do, hope regarding the future, and a pathway to be able to connect with others. These functions should be paramount in any assessment procedure around SCM for BPD.

Formulation and SCM

This section provides an overview for practitioners working with service users diagnosed with BPD, on the concepts, role, and value of the formulation process in SCM.

There is no universally agreed definition for formulation. Our view is that a case formulation is a theoretically based description of a person's mental states (thoughts, feelings, beliefs, and assumptions) and how they interact with their behaviour and the wider system, in a way that may be pertinent to the maintenance of their problems. It offers a hypothesis about the cause and maintenance of the presenting problems and provides a framework to developing the most suitable management or treatment approach (Eells, Kendjelic, & Lucas, 1998). In SCM, formulation looks to identify core psychological factors that could be contributing to the service user's difficulties, both most distressing and most amenable to change. It is a quasi-formulation in that the formulation tends to focus on the service user and their core difficulties. It is important to mention that SCM does in a sense place the 'problem' with the individual service user rather than the wider system. SCM acknowledges this; it is a pragmatic approach that focuses on controlling the 'controllables', acknowledging the fact that controlling the behaviour of others, world views, or in fact a less than perfect mental healthcare system is out of the remit of SCM. Consequently, service users who take up the programme accept the overarching goal is to help them to build competency in social problem-solving, the assumption being that a large part the service user's difficulties in problem-solving are due to psychological areas of relationships, impulsivity, and emotional regulation.

Consequently, a formulation in SCM focuses on the psychological factors that are underlying the service user's difficulties around their ability to solve problems. An SCM formulation provides explanations for behaviours related to BPD diagnosis. As many problems are also around relationships, it enables a collaborative discussion to open up between the practitioner and service user on what the service user views as the advantages and disadvantages of engaging in therapy. This allows the practitioner the opportunity to highlight the positive aspects associated with therapy as well as to identify any potential barriers that may hinder engagement.

Box 2.2 illustrates the Five Ps. These comprise a well-established generic framework in UK mental health NHS Trusts for organizing a formulation, and one that practitioners can grasp relatively easily.

To summarize, formulation is a collaborative, open, and ever-evolving process which offers a shared understanding of the relationship between target symptoms and problems, motivational factors, survival strategies, and interpersonal difficulties, in ways that diagnosis alone does not. It is individualized and tailored to the service user. Importantly, it can also provide a rationale and shared agenda for what areas to target and in what order, informing treatment approaches. Whilst there may be some risks involved in formulation, if approached sensitively and collaboratively, building on strengths, we suggest it can be a valuable clinical tool for answering the classic questions of 'why this person?', 'why this problem?', and 'why now?' As one SCM practitioner described, SCM sees problems like an 'onion'; throughout the programme you are working with the service user peeling the layers away and getting increasingly closer to the core problem.

The process of assessment, formulation, and treatment are synergistic and fluid, meaning that they continually respond to new insights as the service user develops and thus influence each other. As Persons (1989) noted, 'assessment and treatment are a continuous process of proposing, testing, re-evaluating, revising, rejecting, and creating new formulations'.

Assessment in Structured Clinical Management

SCM takes a pragmatic approach to care and the approach to diagnosis and formulation is no exception. As is repeatedly referenced throughout this book SCM has several core components and the assessment process is no different.

The key to a good assessment involves:

- The practitioner having the right approach.
- A clear 'structure' to the assessment.
- The assessment is delivered reliably and consistently.

What is the important function of an assessment in SCM?

What service users value from the assessment process is that it helps to provide them with a clearer understanding of their sense of self and identity, to make sense of their difficulties, and to connect with others (Lester et al., 2020).

Box 2.2 The Five Ps Formulation

1. Presenting problem. This goes deeper into the diagnostic categories to include what the service user and practitioner identify as difficulties underlying the traits (e.g. what could be underpinning the frantic efforts to avoid real or imagined abandonment?), how the service user's life is affected, and when a particular difficulty should be targeted for intervention. For example, while a service user may receive the borderline personality disorder diagnosis, presenting difficulties may include impulsivity, not being able to build and maintain relationships, and emotional dysregulation. In SCM, the practitioner aims to define the problems further using a process of curiosity and validation—the SCM clinical stance (SCM CV) to help the service user to identify areas they can work on e.g. being more aware of their emotional build-up and enhancing their self-soothing/tolerance. Specifying such difficulties can allow for a more focused intervention.

2. Predisposing factors. This incorporates possible genetic vulnerabilities (e.g. family history of mental health difficulties) and environmental factors (such as trauma and/or attachment history) which may put a person at risk of developing mental health difficulties. Here, it is important to take a trauma-informed approach by asking 'what has happened to you?' rather than 'what is wrong with you?'

3. Precipitating factors. This comprises significant events preceding the onset of the problem, such as interpersonal (over-giving due to insecurity and fear of abandonment) or financial stressors (in part caused by difficulties around impulsivity that could be also be related to relational difficulties fear of being on their own). This is usually about exploring triggers to emotional and behavioural vulnerability, both internal and external.

4. Perpetuating factors. This includes factors which maintain the current difficulties, such as repeating behavioural patterns (e.g. self-harm, aggression towards self or others, avoidance, re-enactments of trauma or abuse, or safety behaviours) or cognitive patterns (e.g. attentional biases, negative self-beliefs).

5. Protective factors. This involves identifying strengths, qualities, resources, or supports that may mitigate the impact of the problem. These can include social support, skills, interests, achievements, and some personal characteristics. Macneil et al. (2012) suggest that identification of protective factors also creates increased optimism in both the practitioner and service user and contributes to a positive therapeutic relationship. It can also help to reframe 'survival resources' into 'creative resources' that are focused on improving daily life functioning.

Organizations and care providers have similar aims in that for them, a good assessment should identify the core needs of the service users and provide guidance to effective treatments or care pathways.

From an SCM perspective, the function of the assessment is to help the organization and service users to understand the mental health needs effectively and then to navigate them through the correct care pathway to address these needs.

Discussing the diagnosis can be part of this process or alternatively the assessment process could be a 'needs' led assessment whereby diagnosis is not covered at all. Either way, the end point should be that the service user and organization has a clearer view on what care approach would be most helpful for the service user. The service user and their family/carers should also be given a clear message about how services work, what the care pathway is working on and aiming to do, along with clear expectations about what is expected from the service user and their family. All too often, care fails because treatment/therapy is started before the service user and family, and sometimes even the organization, is clear on what the service user's needs are and what are the tasks and goals they will be undertaking.

If diagnosis is used, the assessment should not stop with a diagnosis but rather focus on helping the service user, family/carer, and organization understand the key factors that contribute to the person meeting the diagnosis. With respect to BPD, you do not address or treat the diagnosis but rather the underlying psychological, behavioural, and social factors that contribute to behaviours/symptoms meeting the diagnostic profile. Sometimes this is referred to as the formulation (e.g. Five Ps), the key being it is a clear description of the service user's needs and an understanding of what areas need to be supported and enhanced.

Due to the importance of this assessment process for any care pathway/programme it is recommended that there is an organized, structured assessment procedure and that practitioners have additional training to be able to deliver the assessment correctly. There is no evidence that any one profession is better at conducting an assessment for service users with BPD than another. However, it is recommended that the assessing practitioner should be experienced in personality disorder, ideally having completed specialist training in personality disorder such as an awareness training or training in a therapy approach to working with personality (e.g. mentalization-based treatment (MBT), dialectical behaviour therapy (DBT), SCM, cognitive analytic therapy (CAT), Schema, etc.). They then have additional training in doing a semi-structured assessment of personality disorder. Box 2.3 illustrates what the training covers.

If diagnosis is used in your assessment it is extremely important that individuals whom services feel meet the diagnosis of BPD are accurately assessed. The NICE quality standards (2015) recommend that people should only be diagnosed if they have completed a semi-structured diagnostic assessment, due to the lack of

---

Box 2.3 Key Components for an Effective Assessment of Personality Disorder

---

- Having the right approach (clinical stance SCM CV)

- Interviewing skills

- Going through a structured clinical assessment of personality and personality disorder

- Feeding back the assessment results

- Having an ability to do a quasi-formulation, e.g. the Five Ps

- How to talk about the diagnosis and formulation

- Involving family and friends in the assessment process

- Discussions on therapies and treatment options

---

reliability if the diagnosis is made from a standard clinical assessment/interview. If practitioners are using the semi-structured clinical interview as part of the assessment, practitioners must complete additional training for the semi-structured interview process that focuses on having the right clinical approach along with covering reliably and validity particularly around threshold for meeting criterion for the diagnosis. The assessment process is seen as the beginning of the journey for the service user. It is crucial that the assessment is carried out in line with NICE recommendations with hope and optimism.

To summarize, the process of assessment involves several key components of which the diagnosis is only one. Other key functions are:

- To validate the service user's experiences
- Collaboratively to highlight the service user's strengths and goals as well as to define their needs
- To support the service user to develop an understanding of the diagnosis of BPD, including the limitations of diagnosis
- To develop a treatment plan that is deemed to build strength and resilience for living life well.

Through the identification of underlying difficulties and their potential mechanisms, the assessment process assists the practitioner to determine whether or not the SCM approach is likely to be effective for the service user.

Guidelines for considering SCM

- Does the service user have difficulties with emotional regulation?
- Does the service user have self-harming/risk behaviours associated that could be linked to problem solving?
- Is impulsivity associated with some of the service user's difficulties?
- Are they motivated and committed to learning different ways of solving their problems?
- Can they cope with a group intervention?

Note: acceptance for SCM should not be 'solely' based on meeting the diagnosis of BPD, it should be needs led.

Practical guide to an assessment

Below is a session-by-session illustration of what an assessment procedure can look like.

The assessment process generally takes around six sessions but may be fewer than this depending on what level of insight the service users possess when they attend the assessment. The next section provides session-by-session guidance to what an SCM informed assessment for BPD could look like. This is guidance; (see Chapter 1 for a slightly different structure) often the flow and what is covered will and can vary depending on what the service user brings/their needs. This is acceptable SCM is permissive in application as long as there is a frame and structure in the process.

Note: before the first session the service users should be given an information leaflet explaining the assessment procedure and what is expected of them. Figure 2.1 is an overview of the assessment sessions:

Session 1 (1 hour)

The initial session involves therapeutic rapport building—using the SCM CV as described in Chapter 3—and listening to the service user's experiences in a manner which is non-judgemental, supportive, and sensitive, validating their journey and needs, whilst exploring their current difficulties. The practitioner will support the service user to identify their strengths, aspirations, and interests, another key aspect to building positive, therapeutic relationships. The practitioner will also explain to the service user what they can expect from the assessment process, including the rationale for conducting the assessment.

The practitioner should also carry out a full and up-to-date risk assessment. The risk assessment should be made using the current risk assessment protocol

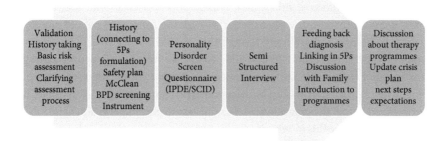

Figure 2.1 SCM Assessment Procedure Overview

of the mental health service with which the service user is currently comfortable. These commonly include information about past and present risks (both acute and chronic), indicators of increased risk, and factors that decrease risk. The practitioner should obtain a detailed history of previous suicide attempts and/or acts of self-harm and other areas of risk. Use of standardized clinical assessment tools such as the Columbia Suicide Severity Rating Scale (CSSRS) can also be helpful (Posner et al., 2008). Information from the risk assessment will inform the development of the crisis/safety plan. The practitioner should emphasize to the service user that the crisis/safety plan is a therapeutic tool that is ever-evolving and subject to change and/or enhancement through new experiences (see Chapter 4).

It is recommended that the assessing practitioner completes an assessment care plan in session 1 or 2 with the aim of further helping the service user to engage with the assessment process. Finally, the remaining sessions (usually 4–5) will be booked at this time. This will support the service user to feel safe and secure as well as to promote motivation and engagement.

Note: although it would be expected that previous mental health assessments would have looked at other mental health and coexisting needs, it is not unusual for these to have been missed or not evident at the time. The assessing practitioner should constantly be aware of other mental health-related problems such as an eating disorder, substance misuse, severe depression, anxiety, post-traumatic stress disorder (PTSD), bipolar, dissociative disorder, or psychosis. If these are identified then a further assessment of these may be required and decisions around primary treatment needs taken.

Session 2 (1 hour)

In this session, the practitioner will collate a life history from the service user, for example developmental milestones, childhood experiences and attachment history. Importantly here, the practitioner will ask the service user about any experiences of trauma and adversity though they should try not to explore this in emotional depth at this point, they should just get the 'headlines'; the overarching aim is to build the service user's resilience and support more adaptive ways of coping. If the service user wishes to discuss their trauma experiences in detail, it is recommended that the practitioner takes the case to peer supervision before deciding how to manage this in session.

The session will also seek to gain information about the service user's past and current coping patterns, problem-solving strategies, and triggers for self-harm, with focus on relationship stressors (linking to the Five Ps as mentioned earlier). Other problem areas associated with BPD will be explored, such as debt, impulsivity, anger/aggression, sleep and isolation, and social care concerns such as children. The practitioner will explore the service user's relationship patterns with services (care providers) and their expectations of care and treatment. Here the practitioner is particularly aiming to highlight any areas of interpersonal tension/sensitivity and service failures (note: 'taking it on the chin' and owning when services have let them down). Additionally, there will be an emphasis on assessing the service user's problem-solving abilities and their past and current coping styles, including internal (what can they do) versus external (what they want/need others to do) coping. Conversations surrounding medication, including any medication that the service user is currently taking, and their perceptions of this will be facilitated. The practitioner will discuss the expectations of services surrounding the prescription of medication, with rationale, at this point. It may be appropriate to initiate a review with a pharmacist or psychiatrist if there is evidence of over-reliance on medication or the service user expresses concerns surrounding aspects of their medication regime, such as withdrawal or side effects.

For some service users, it will be appropriate to begin discussions about personality disorder in this session and the practitioner may also complete a screening questionnaire, for example the McLean Screening Instrument for Borderline Personality Disorder (MSI-BPD) (Zanarini et al., 2003) which can be used for pre-assessment, though it can also be completed in sessions 2 and 3.

At the end of the session, practitioners should discuss the case in clinical supervision.

Sessions 3 and 4 (both 1 hour)

These sessions will provide the service user with an introduction to borderline personality disorder (if this categorical diagnostic approach is being taken by the organization). This will incorporate a discussion about what BPD is; the practitioner will highlight that it is a medical label which describes a person's difficulties, though it is subject to change and does not explain why a person may cope in a particular way or define them as a person. The practitioner will then complete the screening tool with the service user (or feedback scores if this was completed in an earlier session). There are two main semi-structured interview formats for DSM-5, the International Personality Disorder Examination (IPDE) and the Semi-Structured Clinical Interview (SCID-II), both of which have pre-screening questionnaires. Following this, the service user will engage in the IPDE semi- or SCID-II semi-structured interviews based on the criterion that scored highly on the screening tool. Here, the practitioner will look for criteria that meet the 3 Ps (i.e. is problematic, pervasive, and persistent). The practitioner will explore with the service user what the symptoms mean to them personally and if the service user meets the criteria for BPD, they will be provided with information about the diagnosis. *Note:* as long as this is an organizational-agreed approach, then a needs-based assessment is appropriate and diagnosis does not need to be addressed.

The practitioner is then looking to build on the diagnosis (if this is used) and start to develop a formulation using the Five Ps as described earlier.

Session 5 (1 hour)

If the service user has provided consent for their family/carer(s) to be involved in the assessment process, they will be invited into this session. This will enable the practitioner to facilitate a collaborative discussion around the BPD diagnosis and formulation of the 5 Ps and the service user's future care and treatment. Wherever possible, the practitioner will go through the SCID BPD questions and also the Five Ps with the service user and their family/carer(s) and explain what the findings of the assessment mean (even if the service user does not meet the diagnosis of BPD). Each outcome should be explored sensitively and compassionately, discussing what this means to the individual themselves. The family/carer(s) should be offered support which may take the form of a support group and/or a family/carer training programme if available. Again, the crisis/safety plan would be revisited and information from the assessment and particularly the formulation can be used to enhance this. As mentioned in Chapter 4, the safety plan covers what the service user wants services to do in a crisis, what others can do for them in a crisis, and, importantly, what they can do for themselves in a crisis (it is not uncommon for service users to struggle with this section).

Session 6 (1 hour)

In this session, the practitioner will begin by exploring the service user's individual goals for therapy, aiming to identify problem areas and areas to build strength, as well as to promote social inclusion. The safety and contingency plan will be collaboratively revisited again, building on what was covered in the previous session which will be reviewed and enhanced. As highlighted above, the safety plan should be reflected in the service user's care plan.

The practitioner will then discuss treatment options with the service user, using a stepped care approach (i.e. the level and intensity of treatment that they require). Generally, service users should be offered the least intrusive treatment possible. If there is an evident risk of suicide and/or engagement in self-harming behaviours, then a full multimodal minimum 12-month treatment programme such as SCM will be recommended to the service user. *Note:* organizations are recommended to give service users a choice of therapies/treatment approaches, for example SCM or DBT/MBT, etc.

If the service user agrees to engage with the full programme, they will be given clear, in-depth information about the pathway and their treatment programme. It is useful to discuss commitment and highlight that the programmes require active participation at this point. It can also be useful to discuss the group component of the therapy, acknowledging and validating the service user's difficulties and potential anxieties about engaging in a group. For service users who really feel that they are unable to engage in the group in SCM there can be the option for them to complete the 12-week SCM socialization phase to support their future participation in this part of the treatment programme.

Conclusion

As implied throughout this chapter, the primary aims of the assessment and formulation process for service users and practitioners are to capture a clear understanding of the service user's difficulties and decide on and navigate the most recovery-focused treatment/therapy pathway aligned to their needs. It is clear that the concept of the BPD diagnosis continues to elicit mixed views amongst service users, though the assessment process appears fundamental to shaping such perceptions. When a collaborative, sensitive, and validating communication process is used, which is conversational rather than solely educational, service users tend to gain a greater understanding of their diagnosis and interpret it much more positively (Lester et al., 2020). This highlights the importance of the 'how' rather than the 'what' for service users during the assessment and diagnostic process and this can shape their views about hope for recovery and engagement with services. For any SCM programme there are dilemmas around whether to use the diagnosis. It is crucial that the diagnosis question does not loom too large and therefore becomes a reason to avoid establishing a pathway for people diagnosed with BPD or complex relational and emotional needs. Service users value and deserve having a clear explanation of their problems and one that provides them with an explanation of their behaviours and difficulties, along with offering a clear pathway/direction for recovery (Lester et al., 2020). This can be achieved with or without giving the diagnosis. We would strongly recommend that irrespective of whether or not the diagnosis is used, the function of the assessment is not lost.

References

American Psychiatric Association. (2013). *Diagnostic and statistical manual of mental disorders* (5th Ed.) *DSM-*. Washington, DC: American Psychiatric Association.

Bach, B., & Presnall-Shvorin, J. (2020). Using DSM-5 and ICD-11 personality traits in clinical treatment. In C. W. Lejuez & K. L. Gratz (Eds.), *The Cambridge handbook of personality disorders*. Cambridge: Cambridge University Press.

Bach, B., & First, M. B. (2018). Application of the ICD-11 classification of personality disorders. *BMC Psychiatry, 18*, 351. https://doi.org/10.1186/s12888-018-1908-3.

Bateman, A. W., & Krawitz, R. (2013). *Borderline personality disorder: an evidence-based guide for generalist mental health professionals*. Oxford: Oxford University Press

Castillo, H. (2003). *Personality disorder: temperament or trauma? an account of an emancipatory research study carried out by service users diagnosed with personality disorder* (Vol. 23). Jessica Kingsley Publishers.

Chanen, A. M., Jackson, H. J., McCutcheon, L. K., Jovev, M., Dudgeon, P., Yuen, H. P., ... McGorry, P. D. (2008). Early intervention for adolescents with borderline personality disorder using cognitive analytic therapy: randomised controlled trial. *British Journal of Psychiatry, 193*(6), 477–484.

Chanen, A. M., Jovev, M., & Jackson, H. J. (2007). Adaptive functioning and psychiatric symptoms in adolescents with borderline personality disorder. *Journal of Clinical Psychiatry, 68*(2), 297.

Clarkin, J. F., Livesley, W. J., & Meehan, K. B. (2018). Clinical assessment. In W. J. Livesley & R. Larstone (Eds.), *Handbook of personality disorders: theory, research and treatment* (2nd Ed.). London: Guilford Press.

Dyson, H., & Brown, D. (2016). The experience of mentalization-based treatment: an interpretative phenomenological study. *Issues in mental health nursing, 37*(8), 586–595.

Eells, T. D., Kendjelic, E. M., & Lucas, C. P. (1998). What's in a case formulation? development and use of a content coding manual. *The Journal of Psychotherapy Practice and Research, 7*(2), 144.

First, M. B., Skodol, A. E., Bender, D. S., & Oldham, J. M. (2018). *User's guide for the structured clinical interview for the DSM-5 alternative model for personality disorders*. Washington, DC: American Psychiatric Association Publishing.

Gunderson, J. G., Herpertz, S. C., Skodol, A. E., Torgersen, S., & Zanarini, M. C. (2018). Borderline personality disorder. *Nature Reviews Disease Primers, 4*, 18029.

Holm-Denoma, J. M., Gordon, K. H., Donohue, K. F., Waesche, M. C., Castro, Y., Brown, J. S., ... Joiner Jr, T. E. (2008). Patients' affective reactions to receiving diagnostic feedback. *Journal of Social and Clinical Psychology, 27*(6), 555–575.

Lester, R., Prescott, L., McCormack, M., & Sampson, M. (2020). Service users' experiences of receiving a diagnosis of borderline personality disorder: a systematic review. *Personality & Mental Health, 14*(3), 263–283.

Macneil, C. A., Hasty, M. K., Conus, P., & Berk, M. (2012). Is diagnosis enough to guide interventions in mental health? using case formulation in clinical practice. *BMC Medicine, 10*(1), 111.

McCabe, G. A., & Widiger, T. A. (2020). A comprehensive comparison of the ICD-11 and DSM-5 section III personality disorder models. *Psychological Assessment,* Jan *32*(1):72–84. doi: 10.1037/pas0000772.

MIND. (2019). *The Consensus Statement for People with Complex Mental Health Difficulties who are diagnosed with a Personality Disorder—'Shining lights in dark corners of people's lives'.* Retrieved from https://www.mind.org.uk/media/21163353/consensus-statement-final.pdf.

NICE. (2009). *Borderline personality disorder: recognition and management.* London: NICE.

Ng, F. Y., Townsend, M. L., Miller, C. E., Jewell, M., & Grenyer, B. F. (2019). The lived experience of recovery in borderline personality disorder: a qualitative study. *Borderline Personality Disorder and Emotion Dysregulation, 6*(1), 10.

Ofrat, S., Krueger, F., & Clark, L. A. (2018). Dimensional approaches to personality disorder classification. In W. J. Livesley & R. Larstone. (Eds.), *Handbook of personality disorders: theory, research and treatment* (2nd Ed.). London: Guilford Press.

Oltmanns, J. R., & Widiger. T. A. (2018). A self-report measure for the ICD-11 dimensional trait model proposal: the personality inventory for ICD-11. *Psychological Assessment, 30*(2), 154–169. doi:10.1037/pas0000459.

Perseius, K. I., Ekdahl, S., Asberg, M., & Samuelsson, M. (2005). To tame a volcano: patients with borderline personality disorder and their perceptions of suffering. *Archives of Psychiatric Nursing, 19*(4), 160–168.

Persons, J. B. (1989). *Cognitive therapy in practice: a case formulation approach.* New York, NY: Norton.

Posner, K., Brent, D., Lucas, C., Gould, M., Stanley, B., Brown, G. & Mann, J. (2008). *Columbia-Suicide Severity Rating Scale (C-SSRS).* New York, NY: Columbia University Medical Center.

Rüsch, N., Hölzer, A., Hermann, C., Schramm, E., Jacob, G. A., Bohus, M., ... & Corrigan, P. W. (2006). Self-stigma in women with borderline personality disorder and women with social phobia. *The Journal of Nervous and Mental Disease, 194*(10), 766–773.

Zanarini, M. C., Vujanovic, A. A., Parachini, E. A., Boulanger, J. L., Frankenburg, F. R., & Hennen, J. (2003). A screening measure for BPD: the McLean screening instrument for borderline personality disorder (MSI-BPD). *Journal of Personality Disorders, 17*(6), 568–573.

3

The Clinical Stance and Individual SCM Sessions

Mark Sampson and Sharron Kayes

Introduction

Structured clinical management (SCM) is an attachment-focused, coordinated, and organized programme of care for service users diagnosed with borderline personality disorder (BPD). Although, SCM in name can sound clinical, fundamentally it is a programme of care that is wholeheartedly focused around developing a therapeutic relationship with service users who find relationships difficult. In SCM the relationship between the service user and practitioner is central to an effective SCM care programme.

It is hoped that this therapeutic relationship with the service user and their bond with their peers (if in a group) who are on the recovery programme leads to improvements in mental health that lasts between appointments and facilitates recovery beyond the end of the programme. SCM achieves this by embodying well-established core components evident in most effective therapy programmes for BPD. As described in Chapter 1, SCM, is a coherent, consistent, well-organized programme with high levels of continuity.

This chapter provides guidance on communication and 'how to be' when working with somebody who diagnosed with BPD. These core qualities can be applied to all clinical interactions including assessment, socialization, care coordination, in-patient work, and crisis management. Although 'how to interact' or what is often referred as the clinical stance in SCM focuses in this chapter on working with people diagnosed with BPD, these core competencies for effective communication will be invaluable for all service users. At the end of the chapter we will describe how SCM problem-solving clinical sessions can be structured.

Clinical Stance for SCM Interactions—The SCM-CV (Curiosity and Validation)

In SCM, the clinical stance is the anchor for all interactions. It is embedded in SCM training and constantly revisited in supervision or reflective practice. The clinical stance gives a practitioner a compassionate therapeutic base to hold on to when systemic, relational, or personal stressors are pulling at them to act in a less therapeutic way.

In SCM, curiosity and validation can be seen as the core components of the clinical stance in SCM and central to individual sessions or interactions. They are the spine of SCM interactions. In training, this is often referred to as the SCM-CV (curiosity and validation). Curiosity and validation are at the heart of the SCM practitioner's communication style. Practitioners use these in all interactions, whether assessment, socialization, crisis management, in-patient work, or problem-solving.

Curiosity and the 'not knowing stance'

Curiosity in SCM has been largely borrowed from mentalization-based treatment (MBT). In SCM, the practitioner intentionally takes a 'non-expert' stance of curious interest and an open, 'not knowing' position with regard to what the service user is thinking or what would be the most effective solutions. This therapeutic position helps the practitioner maintain a non-judgemental attitude. It also provides an environment that encourages and enables the service user to become more active in the interaction or session, as they have to work (with respect to reflective thinking) to answer the curious questions. This process of enabling the service user to reflect on their thoughts, feelings, and assumptions can eventually help the service user to become more aware of their own mental states (thoughts, feelings, and urges) that could be influencing their problem-solving, particularly around the choices they can or can't make. It can also help prevent practitioners and teams jumping to the wrong assumptions or hypotheses as to what the service user is wanting, thinking, or needing.

Curiosity in SCM individual interactions or sessions is best delivered in a natural, conversational way. It is important to highlight here the danger of slipping into interrogation mode or the 'why, why, why' trap. One service user describing this as the Woody Woodpecker approach: 'you are always pecking at my head'. This should be avoided. The practitioner should use reflective statements, questions, and normalizing, all within an authentic interaction. Supervision is a safe place to practice delivering curiosity in a way that is not too interrogatory.

Validation

Validation is the V in the SCM-CV. Validation comes in many forms; on a basic level it is about being human, active, responding, listening, and being interested in the service user. This is essential in SCM and comes under the umbrella of good customer care. It is vital that the SCM practitioner accepts the service users' internal experiences without judgement.

In SCM, validation is seen as an intervention in its own right and has been broken down into three components (Bateman & Krawitz, 2013):

- It involves working hard to see the situation from the service user's perspective with an emphasis on how they are feeling or what they are trying to communicate or do.
- Once the practitioner has identified the feelings, efforts, and intentions from the service user's perspective the skill is to feed this back effectively and authentically, in a way that allows the service user to connect with the practitioner (*Note:* whilst the practitioner must try to avoid sounding like a 'therapist').
- The final component is that the service user believes the practitioner is being genuine in their feedback and they feel listened to and heard.

In SCM, validation focuses on the mind, thoughts, and feelings of the service user. The practitioner is validating how the service user is feeling, their efforts and intentions rather than their behaviour and coping responses (e.g. focusing on the anger not the aggression).

Validation can be difficult, particularly when working in an acute mental health setting and requires practice and refinement.

It is important to stress that validation is a very effective intervention in its own right and the very act of validation can lead to significant reduction in emotional distress as well as being a crucial first step before problem-solving. This helps the service user feel heard and that someone is 'sitting alongside' them whilst they experience emotional distress. When done carefully, with close attention to the felt sense of connection and safety, it can often produce co-regulation of affect through safe and secure attachment. Validation is a very useful counterbalance to curiosity.

The Clinical Stance—Skills for Enabling Effective Interactions

In reality, clinical interactions with service users with who are in high emotional distress can be challenging. Below are some key strategies/approaches that can help facilitate effective sessions.

Holding on to the bigger picture

Belief in a model (in this case SCM) is vital for enabling effective coherent care. Having a clear therapeutic direction helps keep the practitioner focused on the long-term therapeutic goal, particularly at times of heightened emotional tension. In SCM, in all their interactions the practitioner is trying to enable the service user to build self-agency and autonomy through the medium of problem-solving. This in turn aims to build the service user's confidence in their ability to manage their mind more effectively. It is important for continuity and coherency to have a model to 'hold on to' at times of emotional tension (sometimes referred to as emotional storms), otherwise short-term solutions become tempting and it is easy for both service user and practitioner to lose sight of the longer-term goals. The SCM model can be the anchor to manage these emotional storms.

Being able to 'hold the bigger picture' helps the practitioner keep on track in their interactions and stay in the 'middle ground'. Holding the 'middle ground' is another useful anchor point for maintaining this therapeutic direction. In SCM, the practitioner seeks to manage the external and internal pulls of a polarizing approach to care which can often mirror extreme attachment positions. Commonly, this involves the SCM practitioner aiming to avoid becoming too rigid, restrictive, and withholding (a position that can expect too much from the service user), or the opposite position which can be described as too accommodating, placating, and one that expects too little from the service user. Hamilton (2010) refers to this as the boundary seesaw.

Therapeutic activeness

'Therapeutic activeness' is how much responsibility the SCM practitioner takes in session, particularly around problem-solving. Being aware of how active you are managing the situation or solving problems is really important. In SCM, the practitioner does not want to be too active as this can hinder building self-agency. Likewise, the practitioner does not want to be too inactive as this may lead service users to become frustrated, confused, or even terrified (Bateman & Krawitz, 2013).

Managing the emotional intensity of the session

A component of therapeutic activeness is managing the emotional intensity of the session. It is important that the SCM practitioner is active in doing this. This skill is crucial to both individual and group facilitation. If the session is emotionally void and emotions are absent the practitioner may probe and focus more on feelings. If the interaction or session is too intense to a level whereby the service user is too caught up in their emotions then the practitioner needs to be more active in reducing the emotional intensity. Reducing intensity may involve a gentle subject distraction (subtle change away from the emotional content), validation, or a behavioural intervention such as deep breathing.

Reduce advice giving

In SCM, it is recommended that advice is used sparingly for several reasons.

- Advice can reduce self-agency as the practitioner is generating solutions rather than the service user.
- Advice can easily be invalidating particularly when it comes from the practitioners; clues to this are when you hear yourself say 'you need to' or 'you should do'.
- Advice is often delivered too early, before the problems are fully defined.
- Advice often reduces exploration curiosity around mental states.

Despite there being very few benefits to giving advice, there are times when practitioners feel compelled to offer advice (and the service user may also expect this), particularly when the service user is in a place of solution paralysis and passivity. At these times the practitioner should consider reframing the advice in a way that facilitates discussion. For example, 'in this situation other people have tried XXX and found it helpful? Is this a solution you have tried?'

Language

For services users with trauma and/or BPD, language (words and statements, etc.) is very important. Even slight assumptions or errors can cause intense emotional reactions. Although misunderstandings and language errors will occur, it is helpful if the practitioner is thoughtful around the language they use, particularly with regard to how it could be viewed by a service user.

Typical examples of language triggers can be obvious:

- Practitioner: 'what brought this on all of a *sudden*'—practitioner assuming the service users has poor tolerance;
- Practitioner: 'you *need* to go for a walk'—the practitioner is telling the person what they should do; although this can work as a challenge if delivered slightly differently (occasionally encouraging the service user to flip from passivity), more often than not it is unhelpful and more about the practitioner needing to 'fix' the situation;

or more subtle:

- Practitioner: 'I can see you have *genuine* emotions about that.' To the service user, this can be interpreted as implying that at other times, their feelings are not genuine. The practitioner might consider using the word 'intense' which may be more appropriate;

- Practitioner: 'I am interested to hear your *story*.' A story can infer that a situation has been made up or invented. 'I am really interested to hear about your life' is often a better way to phrase this.

Another important area related to language is ambiguity. Service users diagnosed with BPD can struggle with ambiguity as it can activate their threat-based mind-reading. Therefore, practitioners should avoid ambiguity and, where possible, explain their own thinking and actions; for example, 'I need to cancel this appointment because ...' or 'I was late because ...'.

Clinical stance of 'taking it on the chin'

In SCM, the aim is to reduce misunderstandings. However, misunderstandings are still inevitable. When these occur, the approach the practitioner should adopt is to 'take it on the chin' and 'own' their part in any misunderstanding.

The process of 'taking it on the chin' and owning your role in the process can also have several useful functions

- It validates the service user's perspective and often reduces the emotion;
- It can model fallibility;
- It can open discussions around the service user's interpersonal difficulties because what occurred in the session is likely to occur in other settings.

Guidance for the Practical Structure, Consistency, and Continuity of SCM Individual Sessions

During the sections above we covered the generic clinical stance or approach in SCM that can be used in most interactions. Now we focus on the structure and content of SCM 'clinical' sessions as part of the formalized SCM programme (see Figure 3.1).

Structure, reliability, consistency, and continuity of the individual sessions are essential for setting the foundations for developing a secure therapeutic attachment required for effective one-to-one sessions in SCM. Although at a glance there are obvious systemic pressures within an organization which can make this difficult, if you are offering SCM it cannot be stressed enough how crucial these are for the programme. Many service users diagnosed with BPD can struggle with disorganized thinking about themselves and others. The order and structure of a

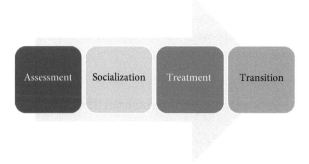

Figure 3.1 SCM Programme Structure

SCM programme helps organize the care system for a service user, helping them become more aware of what to expect from the practitioner and what is expected from themselves. Get this right and there will be significant reductions in crisis presentations.

Reliability

Consistency and continuity are vital in SCM. Where possible, keep the sessions to the same time on the same day each week. Try to avoid cancelling too many sessions. If you have to cancel, always explain the reasons for this (reducing ambiguity). In trials, SCM was delivered weekly. However, if weekly sessions are not possible, then whatever is agreed should be reliably delivered. Reliability also extends to the way the practitioner works and includes the stance (way of being), model, and therapeutic strategies employed. This means that the practitioner reliably does what they said they would do within the agreed therapeutic contract with the service user. There are many pressures on practitioners that can make it difficult to be reliable, however reliability is central to enabling the foundations of recovery. Consequently, SCM practitioners pride themselves for being reliable and on time for appointments.

Consistency of the session length

How long should formal SCM sessions be? In the randomized trial where SCM emerged as an effective approach the sessions were 40 minutes in length (Bateman & Fonagy, 2009). Therefore, 40 minutes is a good reference point for session length. However, the length is probably less crucial than the consistency. Whatever is agreed in your SCM this should be adhered for 'all' service users. If you go with 40 minutes sessions, try and keep to 40 minutes for all service users on the SCM programmes. If you want sessions to be 50 minutes or an hour, then that is your time frame and try and keep to this throughout the programme. Consistency also refers to the practitioner's approach and the application of the SCM model/programme (see later sections in this chapter).

Risk adaptability—structured flexibility

There will be times, particularly when the service user is presenting in acute distress, when the practitioner may, on occasion, need to extend the session length. An example may be that the service user has declared just before leaving that they intend to commit suicide and may not see the practitioner for the subsequent session. During these times, the practitioner would negotiate an extension with the service user, acknowledging that the session needs to be extended and explaining the reasons for this. They would then rapidly assess the degree of intent and communicative function behind the service user's comments and agree any further safety measures as part of an interim enhanced plan. Although the session has been extended, there is still a new negotiated structure, which would remain a temporary measure until the service user's risk returned to the low (or chronic) level. If this is repeated on other occasions, then this would be addressed as a (attachment) problem to be solved, as with any problem. It is also OK within SCM to offer an additional crisis session (generally 30 minutes) when needed, in between the agreed sessions (for more on this see Safety Planning in Chapter 4). As with extending sessions, if this becomes a frequent pattern, this would be explored with the service user and factors contributing to the repeated nature of the behaviour defined. An agreed revised plan to address this can then be introduced.

Managing cancellations and 'did not attends' (DNAs)

In research trials, cancellations and missed appointments (not attending) are often managed very differently from how mental health services routinely operate. In SCM, the aim is to bring some of the procedures from research trials into normal care. Consequently, in SCM, as in research trials, there is a strong emphasis on trying to retain people in the programme. If a service user does not attend their appointment, the practitioner or group facilitator is expected to telephone the service user. The practitioner would curiously enquire about the reasons for the service user not attending. Crucially, whilst doing this there is still a consistent message of self-agency and building autonomy. The way of addressing cancellations follows a similar process. The practitioner would validate the barriers for attending and then curiously explore ways of overcoming these barriers.

Attendance

Like most therapy programmes, SCM monitors attendance. It is important for the success of the programme that people attend regularly. We recommend SCM follows a similar model to that used in MBT, expecting a 75% attendance. Drop in attendance is discussed with the service user and barriers to attendance explored. It is important to address poor attendance early. Sometimes it may be necessary to transition the service user out of the programme if attendance does not improve. SCM follows an 'easy back in' approach for service users who were not able to commit to the programme previously (this process can be repeated several times).

Where to hold the SCM sessions?

Whenever possible, SCM tries to facilitate active participation from the service user. Consequently, where possible the session should be delivered outside the service user's home, preferably in an out-patient or a community clinic (e.g. general practice surgery). Encouraging the service user to leave their home and travel to a place for the session potentially has several therapeutic benefits beyond the session itself. For instance, by leaving their home and travelling somewhere, you are helping them break out of isolation and negative rumination whilst also providing structure. Having the sessions take place in a 'safe', neutral venue can help them keep focused on the therapeutic 'work' (intervention versus befriending). It can also be protective of boundaries for the service user and practitioner.

Sometimes it is not possible for the service user to come to clinic/appointments, for example due to problems with travel or the 2020 pandemic. We would suggest video sessions are preferable to telephone, and in some cases home visits. If the sessions are delivered virtually via video link, then the practitioner would encourage the service user to be as active as possible during these sessions.

Implementing the SCM Programme—Individual Problem-Solving Sessions

Attitudes, expectations, and belief in the model

Believing in the programme of care (model) and believing in the possibility that a service user can change is fundamental to SCM. For effective delivery of a SCM programme the practitioner authentically believes in the service user and their ability to change along with a belief that SCM is an effective approach and model to do this (by enhancing the service user's problem-solving abilities). Practitioners who do not believe in the approach or service users diagnosed with BPD should not be delivering SCM.

The SCM Problem-Solving Session

In SCM the practitioner does not exist to solve problems but rather to help the service user be able to define the problem as effectively as possible whilst also enhancing their confidence to solve their own problems.

Being less active as a practitioner in problem-solving can be a challenge for some mental health practitioners whose previous roles and internal desire to help can lead them to be 'active' problem-solvers. Note, it is important at the start of treatment to discuss this with the service user, explaining that in SCM the practitioner will be less active at solving their problems.

Problem-solving structure

Problem-solving in SCM follows a standard problem-solving format:

- Defining the problem.
- Exploring solutions.
- Implementation.
- Evaluation.

Defining the problem

At the beginning of SCM a problem hierarchy is collaboratively developed. Generally high-risk problem behaviours are prioritized. Once problems are identified the SCM practitioner uses the SCM-CV (described earlier) as an approach when helping the service user to define the problem.

A crucial first part of SCM problem-solving is to define the problem effectively. In SCM the practitioner is looking (via gentle questioning and curiosity) to define problems in terms of service users' mental states (their thoughts, feelings, and assumptions) in the problem domains relevant to a diagnosis of BPD (e.g. the SCM focus for recurrent debt could be addressing the causes of their impulsive spending on top of ensuring the person is on appropriate benefits if they are unemployed). Validation is crucial here as many service users initially see the problem as the world and/or other people (partly because for many, the world and other people have let them down or hurt them in some way).

Below is a problem-solving example taken from SCM training:

A service user feels that their mental health practitioner has let them down, adding they are not professional and should always be available for them. The fact they were not means the practitioner was not professional.

In the SCM session, the aim would be to define this problem. However, first it requires some foundation work using effective communication and the SCM-CV. The practitioner owns the issue of when they weren't available ('takes it on the chin', as discussed earlier), authentically validates the service user's position, listens, and then has a conversation about why it is so important to the service user that the practitioner is always available when the service user calls. The aim is to broaden the problem area away from 'the problem is the practitioner' to at least also acknowledging that there is also problem of emotional regulation in this context (e.g. the service user feels they can't manage unless somebody is always there and available to them). The practitioner would spend sufficient time validating the service user's struggle managing their feelings, what they were hoping for and struggling with, in wanting an immediate response from the practitioner. The aim is to help the service user feel safe to see that at least part of the problem is their difficulty in managing attachment insecurity and their emotions (e.g. 'I need others there all the time because I feel overwhelmed, can't think straight and my feelings getting too much to handle').

Note: a key aspect of SCM is effective defining of the problem. It cannot be stressed enough how important this is. All too often solutions are implemented before the problems are fully defined.

The Problem Areas in SCM

To help structure the sessions in SCM the problems are defined in core areas or domains. In the full programme, these areas are covered in the SCM groups (see Chapter 5 on Groups for more information). As in many multi-modal therapies (group and individual together), a strength of is how the information from the group and individual sessions complement each other.

SCM's problem domain categories are related to the areas below.

- Impulsivity (including self-harm, risky behaviours, and suicidality)
- Emotional understanding, tolerance, and regulation (including managing mood states)
- Getting on with others, including interpersonal sensitivity, mentalizing attachment, and fostering safe and secure relationships

The SCM practitioner uses these categories as reference points when working with the service user, exploring how these areas relate to their problems.

Box 3.1 Components of Impulsivity

- Not attending and decreased attention
- Not planning and lack of preparation
- Action without reflection—acting rashly
- Difficulties or an inability to tolerate boredom and a need for stimulation
- Difficulty tolerating urges and a need for immediate gratification

---

Impulsivity

Impulsivity is a diagnostic criterion for BPD and thus prevalent in many service users who meet this diagnosis. Impulsivity is often related to difficulties with effective problem-solving. Box 3.1 illustrates the components that make up impulsivity.

In SCM, the practitioner together with the service user explores thoughts, urges, feelings, and behaviours related to their specific type of impulsivity. Initially, the practitioner is looking to increase conscious awareness around how impulsivity affects the service user, slow down their thinking around this, and 'extend the fuse', so that the impulse or urge can begin to subside. Once impulsivity is understood, solutions can be explored. For example, for one service user, their 'impulsive' stealing was related to a heightened sense of entitlement stemming from childhood neglect and repeated patterns of self to self neglect reinforced by a high level of care for others, which made sense to the service user. They felt validated and heard and the solution, weekly self-care (time in a coffee shop with a cake), seemed to correlate with a reduction of the self-reported stealing behaviour (practising assertiveness could have been another solution).

In summary, managing impulsivity is often about helping the service user to learn to pause on the urge, helping them to reflect on and name the impulse and associated urges, strong emotion (including boredom), and emptiness. They can then, together with the practitioner, explore helpful coping responses.

Emotional understanding

With respect to emotional understanding, the practitioner uses the SCM-CV approach to explore and then validate the service user's emotions. This approach enables the service user to reflect on their mind and emotions, and clarify what emotions they are feeling, along with what thoughts, feelings, and fears they have about these emotions. Emotional understanding can include education about what types of emotions there are and what is the different between a thought and feeling. Labelling and naming emotions are really important.

Emotional tolerance

Here, the practitioner is trying to work with the service user to help them to stay with, tolerate, describe, and self-validate their emotions. Modelling a calm approach, curiosity, and validation are vital components for emotional tolerance. The practitioner is modelling it is OK to feel these emotions. With reference to emotion tolerance, the SCM practitioner does not assume that a service user's emotional tolerance is reduced (this can be a common practitioner assumption and can be invalidating). Rather, the practitioner works with the service user to explore their emotional experience and define the complex interplay between emotions and thoughts.

Emotional regulation

Emotional regulation is the service user's ability to be able to stay with and then turn up or down their emotional intensity, using various emotion regulation strategies and skills. There are many excellent books and articles available on emotional regulation. It is often helpful exploring books/strategies together whilst also bringing in the examples covered in the group sessions. In SCM, the practitioner and service user would collaboratively explore emotional regulation strategies. It is important to look at different emotional regulation skills, linking these to different emotions, and work out what works and what doesn't work for the service user.

Case Example

One service user repeatedly ligatured at home. The practitioner worked with the service user to define the problem as management of the feelings around helplessness and despair. Further defining linked this to a sense of feeling powerless in his life. The ligaturing appeared to have several functions; it was related to distraction from the emotion as it provided an alternative emotional state via adrenaline. It also gave him a sense of control and power. Once the problem was defined solutions could be explored. The solutions are often very simple but tend to be more effective as they are more accurately targeted to the problem and thus personalized and owned by the service user. In this case, the solution was around doing press ups and exercise in this state as an alternative coping option. It is also important to highlight that the very process of talking about his emotional states was equally as therapeutic as the coping action.

When looking for coping strategies it can be useful to break coping and emotional regulation into different domains/areas/types (see Folkman & Lazarus, 1984; Porr, 2010). Box 3.2 provides some examples.

Box 3.2 Examples of Coping Approaches

- Releasing pent-up emotions—e.g. cathartic expression sharing/talking
- Distracting oneself—e.g. reading/jigsaw/computer game/work
- Managing hostile feelings—e.g. reappraisal of negatively viewed emotions e.g. anger
- Mindfulness/meditation strategies
- Using relaxation procedures—e.g. deep breathing, applied relaxation
- Behavioural management—e.g. acting opposite to the emotion
- Acceptance (owning/accepting the problem event or emotion)
- Self-validation (allowing oneself to feel emotionally heard)
- Self-soothing/calming via self-talk, smells, touch, taste, hearing, and vision

---

A strength of SCM is its ability to link coping strategies more accurately to coping with specific problems.

Getting on with others and mentalizing attachment

Relationships are highly complex behaviours and inherently difficult for most of us. However, in general they are even more difficult for those diagnosed with BPD. Relationships are a complex balance of being aware of your own needs and being able to assert them whilst simultaneously acknowledging the other person's needs, and then determining your actions based on this understanding. For clients diagnosed with BPD this can be particularly difficult and a key problem area as they become too fixed in one state so are either too focused on the self ('it's all about me') or too focused on the other ('it's all about them') in their interactions.

Problems in this area can be around:

- Helping the service user identify what they want or exactly what their needs and urges are.
- How to manage their wants/needs/urges, for example impulsivity/emotional regulation.
- Work with them to help them get/ask for want they want effectively (this can involve exploring emotions and barriers such as fear/embarrassment to being able to do this). If there is a skills deficit, this can be addressed with training such as assertiveness training.

- Working on assumptions about other people's mental states—building curiosity.
- Mentalizing self and others—how do we understand ourselves and others, and what helps us develop safe and secure relationships? How do we resolve misunderstandings?

Note: in the individual session the practitioner breaks down interpersonal problems into these domains and then collaboratively works with the service user on these. Often the problems around getting on with others will also involve emotional regulation/tolerance and impulsivity.

Problem-solving suicidality and self-harm

Problem-solving suicidality and/or self-harm follows a similar process in SCM.

- The practitioner will use the approach as per clinical stance/SCM-CV
- The practitioner will look to identify thoughts/feelings/urges associated with self-harm or suicidal intent. The practitioner will also look to explore internal and external triggers.
- The practitioner will validate the service user's emotional state and then look to explore alternative solutions to the current state as opposed to suicide/self-harm. Any risk would be explored as per the safety management plans.

Box 3.3 provides an overview of a SCM session format.

Box 3.3 Session Structure

- Review the questionnaire scores.
- Curiously explore any variation in these.
- Curiously review the previous events/week.
- Validation of mental state and difficulties.
- Curiously look to find any particular problem areas.
- Choose an area/s on which to work.
- Look to define the problem.
- Look to define mental states related to problem.
- Explore possible solutions and service user's thoughts/beliefs about these.
- Explore with the service user what solutions are available to them.
- Implementation of solution if appropriate (e.g. problem is defined).

It is important to be aware that sessions do not follow a linear trajectory but rather they are a journey between the two points that often zig-zags significantly along the way.

Conclusion

Individual sessions in SCM are about fostering a therapeutic relationship that will facilitate recovery and build autonomy for people diagnosed with BPD. The sessions are about having the right approach (clinical stance or the SCM-CV). They involve having a clear and coherent approach and organized structure that is delivered reliably and consistently. The sessions always look to build the services user's understanding of their own mind and seek to help them through the language of problem-solving and build on their ability to manage their own thoughts, feelings, and urges.

Continuity, coherency, and consistency provide the structure of SCM individual sessions that help build the therapeutic bond and protect both practitioner and service user. One key function of structure is its containing function for both service user and practitioner. As described by one SCM practitioner who has over 20 years of experience working as a psychiatric nurse: 'SCM has fundamentally changed how I work for many reasons but crucially, for me the structure within SCM helps me organize my mind and this allows me to deliver more effective care.' A key therapeutic component of SCM or any structured programme is that it allows practitioners and service users to obtain a clear and coherent understanding of their relationship and the programme of care. This can help them to understand how to work with each other and together embark on a recovery journey. The clinical stance or SCM-CV helps provide the practitioner with an anchor point to help them navigate through emotional storms and it further ensures continuity and consistency in care during what can be difficult moments.

Although this chapter describes the key characteristics that make up an individual session it is important to remember that many mental health practitioners already possess these qualities and practice this way. In fact, they are abundant. SCM is about ensuring these qualities are valued by the system (organization) and that practitioners are sufficiently supported to be able to be clinically effective.

References

Bateman, A., & Fonagy, P. (2009). Randomized controlled trial of outpatient mentalization-based treatment versus structured clinical management for borderline personality disorder. *American Journal of Psychiatry*, *166*(12), 1355–1364.

Bateman, A. W., & Krawitz, R. (2013). *Borderline personality disorder: an evidence-based guide for generalist mental health professionals.* Oxford: Oxford University Press.

Hamilton, L. (2010). Boundary seesaw model: good fences make for good neighbours. In A. Tennant, & K. Howells (Eds.), *Using time, not doing time: practitioner perspectives on personality disorder & risk* (pp. 181–194). Chichester: Wiley-Blackwell.

Lazarus, R. S., & Folkman, S. (1984). *Stress, appraisal, and coping.* New York, NY: Springer.

Porr, V. (2010). *Overcoming borderline personality disorder: a family guide for healing and change.* Oxford: Oxford University Press.

4

Crisis Work and Safety Planning

Rebecca Bevington, Ashleigh McGuinness, and Mark Sampson

Introduction

A general dictionary definition of crisis is a 'time of intense difficulty or danger'. In states of mental health, a crisis is described as a 'state of mind that can lead to imminent danger for themselves or others'. Mental health services generally respond to a mental health crisis with a crisis intervention and crisis planning. A crisis intervention described by Borschmann et al. (2012) in their systematic review as 'an immediate response by one or more individuals to the acute distress experienced by another individual, which is designed to ensure safety and recovery and lasts no longer than one month'.

A safety plan is a collaboratively pre-agreed set of actions and support systems that aim to help service users when they *are* in a state of mental health crisis or impending crisis. Safety planning is ideally delivered prior to a 'crisis' emerging; however, in reality, crisis planning and crisis interventions are often linked and occur simultaneously. For the purpose of this chapter, safety planning will include an element of crisis intervention.

Safety planning is as important for service users diagnosed with borderline personality disorder (BPD) as with any other mental health presentation. In fact, it could be argued even more so due to the often recurrent nature of crises that can occur in service users diagnosed with BPD. This chapter outlines the core features of an SCM safety plan and the processes involved in its development and how to conduct safety assessments and manage current crises during sessions.

SCM and Safety Planning

In SCM, safety planning is a dynamic activity that goes beyond giving out telephone contact numbers for support (whilst acknowledging that these are important). Safety planning focuses on how to undertake safety planning with service users with recurrent 'crises' and elevated levels of risk. Obviously, safety plans are best done prior to a crisis when the service user is in a state of mind to be able to reflect on their mental states (thoughts and feelings) and coping options. It is important to note that even when service users with recurrent crises are not in 'crisis' the process of reflecting on crisis situations can be very difficult. Often, service users do not want to reflect on situations and events that have previously caused them distress, harm, or shame. This can lead to resistance and is sometimes one reason why safety planning is not fully implemented.

The SCM safety plan (Bateman & Krawitz, 2013) aims to help the service user:

- Increase awareness of what they can do to help themselves when they are in a mental health crisis.
- Increase clarity and review expectations around what they want others to do in a crisis.
- Increase clarity and review expectations around what they want services to do.

SCM safety plans look to address these points by reviewing three previous crises with the service user. In summary, an SCM safety plan not only focuses on how the service user can keep themselves or others safe, for example by giving them crisis numbers and support, but also aims to increase self-awareness, start the process of building self-agency, and also explore relational aspects of help seeking and expectations from others.

Developing a SCM Safety Plan

As described in previous chapters, SCM is more than a structured approach to care. A key fundamental of any SCM approach is actually about the practitioner's approach and relationship with the service user. Safety planning is no different.

The process of developing a safety plan collaboratively with a service user can be a reassuring and soothing process particularly if they have attempted to access support previously and their needs were not sufficiently met or their problems were exacerbated due to their interaction with services (Bateman & Krawitz, 2013). Henderson et al. (2009) found that through completing safety planning with service users they felt more in control of their mental health states of mind and empowered to obtain their chosen treatment and care outcomes in crisis.

Safety plans are completed collaboratively with the service user during a period of relative stability in order to plan ahead for managing potential future crises. The purpose of a safety plan is to develop with the service user a set of options to consider when experiencing a crisis and for the plan to clearly state what support could be accessed during this period, if self-management is insufficient. The plan acts as a conscious prompt or cue for action during moments or periods of instability. Bateman and Fonagy (2009) reported that the process of development of the plan itself can be as important as the content.

Therapeutic approach and stance

In SCM, prior to any safety planning intervention taking place, training to help guide the practitioner's clinical stance and therapeutic approach to the sessions and their content is helpful. As with a SCM clinical session, this clinical stance lays the foundations for future sessions and sets a structure and expectation for the service provided as it progresses. Communication comes in various forms and often an impression has already been made prior to any verbal interactions. Developing a positive and trusting therapeutic alliance with the service user is a priority as it has been found that effective therapeutic relationships will maximize and enhance the model of treatment, which in turn enhances and maximizes the effectiveness of the model (Bateman & Krawitz, 2013).

An active, authentic, interested, and responsive practitioner (as illustrated in Chapter 3) will portray to the service user that they are being listened to, taken seriously, and that what they have to say is valuable. The service user is then more likely to participate actively in safety planning because a trusting and safe therapeutic alliance is being developed. Additionally, empathy and hopefulness in the practitioner is thought to be an essential characteristic as research shows that hopelessness in both practitioner and service user can increase suicide risk (Wright, Basco, & Thase, 2006). Practitioners should also ensure they avoid presenting as distant or rigid with the service user. It is important for the service user to feel able to express any concerns or worries regarding the therapeutic relationship otherwise this could potentially cause problems later in the relationship.

In the early stages of building rapport and mutual respect, appropriate boundaries (frame and function of the sessions) need to be agreed between the service user and the practitioner. A particularly important boundary in the implementation of safety planning sessions is regarding the handling of trauma disclosures. When a service user feels listened to and heard, it is often the case that they feel safe to share traumatic experiences and attempt to use the sessions to disclose their difficult experiences. However, this is not the function of safety planning sessions and rather than interrupt a distressed service user who is sharing personal details of such traumatic life events, it is more appropriate and helpful for them to be informed of the purpose of the sessions before commencing the intervention. Safety planning sessions are structured sessions aimed at developing robust collaborative plans to aid the client when in crisis, when it is often more difficult to think clearly. In contrast, service users may present as passive and avoidant within sessions and this is equally important to address and requires complete transparency.

Talking about the person's thoughts, feelings, and crisis/suicidal behaviour

Despite widely held beliefs to the contrary, research suggests that talking about suicide may in fact reduce suicidal ideation and behaviour rather than increase it

(Dazzi, Gribble, Wessely & Fear, 2014). This is equally valid for people with recurrent suicidal behaviour. It can be all too easy to become avoidant when undertaking effective safety planning for people with recurrent crisis or suicidal behaviour through unconscious assumptions and fears about life and death from both the service user and practitioner.

In SCM safety planning, there is an emphasis on validating and talking with the service users about their thoughts and feelings associated with crisis/suicidal behaviour. There is a focus on the service user's mental states and their ability to reflect and seek solutions to these. This is sometimes referred to as mentalizing. Mentalizing, as described in previous chapters, is the ability to focus on and try to understand your own and others inner mental states, often simultaneously. SCM safety planning is not a 'pure' mentalization therapy strategy as per mentalization-based treatment (MBT), but there is a strong emphasis on focusing on the subjective experience of the service user, encouraging them to share their thoughts and feelings and their beliefs about the thoughts and feelings of others. By doing this, the practitioner is attempting to understand the world from the service user's point of view, helping to clarify the service user's understanding of their mind, and also the assumptions that they have about other people's minds, including services.

Many crises occur because of a service user's distressing experience of their own thoughts and feelings that can be felt more intensely due to interpretations of what they think other people may think and feel about them. A person in crisis may think that their loved ones would be better off without them in their life, or that they are a burden, or that services don't care and are not taking them seriously. When a service user is not aware of their own thoughts or emotional state, it makes it very difficult for them to interpret the thoughts and emotional states of others accurately. By encouraging and exploring their own mental states and their thoughts around the mental states of others, it may enable the service user to understand the thoughts and feelings of others and regulate their own problematic emotional states.

Curiosity

As mentioned in previous chapters, curiosity is a core component throughout SCM and safety planning is no different. It is a powerful approach to engaging service users and is extremely effective in crisis planning, especially for service users who are not forthcoming about their own risk behaviours. An approach taken with a high degree of curiosity can be used to discuss all areas of safety planning and can be used to encourage a service user to become more aware of their thinking around crises and beyond. By displaying curiosity, practitioners can ask service users what it must have been like for them to experience crises and what it must be like for others also. The inclusion of such information will inevitably produce a more personal and robust safety plan. Motivating questions and reflective statements can also be used to build a conversational scaffold and help to validate a person's experiences. Reflective statements can be powerful in safety planning sessions as often people do not accept their own thoughts or feelings as real until they are reflected back to them.

Validation

Another essential and often overlooked skill in crisis work is validation. Validation involves active observing, reflection, and direct validation. It is the recognition, acknowledgment, and acceptance of a person's subjective experience. It is important to highlight that you do not have to agree with the person's opinions, thoughts, and/or feelings related to a situation to validate them. Validation is more about acknowledgment and acceptance of one's right to experience them. Additionally, in SCM it is generally the service user's inner experience, effort, or intentions rather than their behaviour that is validated. Effective validation can make a substantial difference to the service user feeling listened to and heard, which is why it is important to include this on a crisis plan either as a preventative or reactive approach to crisis. SCM training, particularly the clinical stance or SCM-CV, provides a great foundation for effective safety planning.

Structure and Safety Planning Guidance

In SCM safety planning, emphasis is placed on having a clear structure with a clear therapeutic aim. It is helpful if practitioners are clear and provide the structure. For example, if the safety planning is an intervention in its own right, then clarifying the focus of the sessions, number of sessions, and booking in the sessions with the person in advance can be very helpful. Bateman and Krawitz (2013) reported that providing regular structured sessions can ameliorate some abandonment anxieties held by the service user.

As mentioned earlier, safety planning for people with recurrent crises explores previous ones in order to identify any patterns in behaviour. Identifying triggers and points of vulnerability is a vital step in supporting the service user to act preventatively rather than reactively and again should be explored in relation to previous crises. It is also encouraged at this stage to explore potential helpful or unhelpful coping strategies that the person has adopted that could be maintaining or worsening their problems. Furthermore, the expectation that the service user may have of services and their support system may need to be addressed, particularly if they have identified accessing services and support as unhelpful in the past. This process in itself often leads to eliciting areas to work on in SCM or any other therapy programme.

Boxes 4.1 and 4.2 present a guide for implementing an SCM informed safety planning programme.

Box 4.1 Stabilization and Crisis Containment

Session 1
- Exploration of presenting problems
- Talking about the person's thoughts and feelings related to the crisis/suicidal behaviour
- Validation
- Complete safety assessments, i.e. Columbia Suicide Severity Rating Scale (C-SSRS; Posner et al., 2008)
- Complete outcomes measures, i.e. Patient Health Questionnaire-9 (PHQ-9)
- Crisis contact numbers

Session 2
- Explore brief timeline of crisis events
- Discuss signs of a crisis and need for safety
- Who do they get support from and how are they supported?

Session 3
- Build on who can be contacted in a crisis
- Goals for future treatment
- Previous experience with services
- Advanced decisions
- Complete safety assessments, i.e. Columbia Suicide Severity Rating Scale (C-SSRS)
- Complete outcomes measures, i.e. Patient Health Questionnaire-9 (PHQ-9)

Box 4.2 Personal Resilience Component of Crisis Planning

Sessions 4–6
- Identify psychological vulnerabilities for their crises
- Helping explore their own resilience profile with a focus on helping them to build on their own coping strengths
- If therapy input/help is required there will be a focus on developing goals and motivation for change
- Completing a Keeping Safe Recovery Action Plan
- Complete necessary measures
- Update safety screenings

The Safety Plan

Once a secure therapeutic alliance has been established and rapport is being built, the safety plan structure needs to be developed. As previously mentioned, the structure is a vital component and supports the service user until they feel better equipped to take some responsibility in their own care. An example of an SCM approach in safety planning is the SCM-informed personal resilience programme (PRP; McGuinness, Bevington, Sampson, Bass, & Fisher, in preparation), which provided 3 sessions for safety planning and then 3 sessions focusing on personal resilience and effective help seeking for service users who presented with self-harm and suicidality.

In the PRP programme, the safety planning sessions were delivered over a one- to 2-week period following a suicide attempt or acute crisis presentation to a service. The time period was adapted in order to facilitate a rapid access, brief intervention; however, all safety planning sessions do not need to have the same structure. Safety planning can be adapted to the needs of the service user with an appropriate rationale; if a person has recently made a suicide attempt and is struggling to keep themselves safe in the community, it may be more appropriate to provide intervention/stabilization sessions first as it may take longer to develop the safety plan collaboratively. Alternatively, if a service user is admitted into hospital and needs a safety plan to be discharged into the community, it may be more appropriate to complete the safety plan on the ward prior to discharge, in collaboration with the clinical treatment (community) team.

The PRP (McGuinness et al., in preparation) sessions were 40 minutes long, occurred in an out-patient setting, and were arranged with the service user over a 2-week period. This programme was offered to service users presenting with/in a crisis (feel they can't manage without input from mental health services), recent self-harm, or suicide attempt.

Managing a 'Crisis' in Safety Planning

Service users who will engage with safety planning in SCM are likely to have experienced a crisis, are in a crisis, or their presentation is escalating towards a crisis. There are a number of requirements in the risk assessment of service users that practitioners need to keep in mind, one of which is ascertaining whether the person is able to keep themselves safe prior to the next meeting and access support appropriately if it is believed they cannot. This can be a sticking point in completing risk assessments when engaging with safety planning as it is likely that the service user has presented with some suicidality recently. Additionally, some service users can feel that their mental healthcare is dependent (probably quite correctly) on risk and suicidality. Without this, they fear they may not be helped by services. In effect, suicidality becomes the 'currency' that 'buys' the treatment. Therefore, it is vital that practitioners and services explore expectations of care and talk openly and honestly about this.

There is no one factor to look for when trying to separate out acute and chronic risk. Key factors in understanding a service user's ability to keep them safe are presented in Box 4.3.

If a person is reporting plans for the future, for example attending a return-to-work interview, they are demonstrating that they see themselves engaging with these plans and subsequently are most likely able to keep themselves safe. If a person reports that they have suicidal thoughts but would not act on them due to their children, the risk is likely to reduce. Factors that may increase the risk are access to means. Many people receive monthly prescriptions of their medication in the community, which leaves the person with large quantities of medication in their possession, easy access to the means to self-harm or commit suicide.

Managing access to means can be complicated with service users with recurrent long-standing self-harming. Although for acute crises it is often important to remove access to lethal means, for recurrent risk, this requires more analysis because 'other' people (including services) can then become drawn into taking responsibility for the service user's 'coping' and these actions can have detrimental effects for building self-agency. Additionally, if a service user presents with increased risk when engaging with safety planning sessions, their ability to engage fully with the intervention needs to be reassessed regularly. If the service user has experienced deterioration in mental state and/or is experiencing a great deal of distress, it may not be possible to continue with the safety plan as they may not be able to focus on the content of the plan.

Box 4.3 Factors to Consider When Determining Risk

Lack of future planning

Currently engaged in abusive relationship, acute relationship breakdown

Acute plans

Access to means

Increase in or high use alcohol and/or drug taking

Previous self-harming behaviours

Evidence of acute depression, psychosis, or extreme anxiety agitation

Lack of protective factors

An indication that they are not seeking help and support

The practitioner may need to be more active when the service user is in an acute distress/crisis in session. The practitioner needs to take the lead in managing the intensity of the distress in the session, whilst assessing risk. Where possible, try to bring the intensity down via validation, distraction, or behavioural intervention (e.g. deep breathing).

Sometimes it may be the case that the service user may require stepped-up care such as enhanced home treatment or a hospital admission to manage escalating acute risk temporarily. If stepped-up care is required, (if possible) it is useful to work with the service user on what their expectations and goals are for this. If the service user is seeking an admission (which is their solution to their problem), it can be useful to have a conversation about what it is about hospital that makes this the right solution for them. Here, striking the right balance between validating the severity of their current difficulty and distress versus the gentle, curious probing around their solution can be helpful if the service user is in a position to engage in this exploration. This can lead into discussions about goals and what they want from a hospital admission: is it about helping them keep themselves safe from their own mind, getting them out of their current situation, a need for something to change, an assessment or a need for compassionate care and for other people to recognize just how difficult things are? These can all be reasons for seeking an admission but are often not explicitly raised. Goals and how they might be monitored, expectations of care and estimated length of admission can all be equally helpful conversations if the situation enables these.

The Safety Assessment

In SCM, safety assessments are a vital component because the information collected helps to inform the safety plan. When completing a safety assessment, the practitioner needs to document a thorough history of the service user's risk and loss of safety history including suicide attempts, preparations and intent, self-harm, and suicidal thoughts and actions. A formal risk assessment can be helpful as this can help structure the risk assessment, for example Columbia Suicide Severity Rating Scale (Posner et al., 2008). *Note:* practitioners need appropriate training to ensure any risk assessment is carried out correctly. This training should be completed as per their service protocol.

With high-risk situations a practitioner should never make care decisions without the support of a multidisciplinary team. This can both help them to support the service user's own safety plan but also the practitioner managing the associated risk. If, which is often the case, the situation requires a quick clinical decision, then getting an immediate 'second opinion' from a senior colleague in the team can help provide the 'observing eye' for what are at times very difficult risk-taking decisions.

How can people spot the signs of a crisis?

One early task in SCM safety planning is for the practitioner to establish if the service user is aware of the early 'signs' of a crisis emerging. Even if a service user feels unable to identify such signs, their engagement and active participation in this process is in itself therapeutic, and discussions should be encouraged to explore this further. Furthermore, it is important that the practitioner empathizes with a service user who is unable to make sense of their thoughts, feelings, and behaviours in crisis, and acknowledge how difficult this could be for them. Nevertheless, identifying the early signs of a service user's crisis, and what makes them feel vulnerable, is an important component of SCM and, therefore, the practitioner will need to use their curiosity, non-judgemental manner, and reflective statements to draw out these early warning signs.

If service users particularly struggle to highlight any signs, the following change areas could be suggested as prompts for further discussion: communication with others, routine, behaviours, self-care, risk, and internal signs. Most service users completing safety plans will notice changes in behaviour, for example lack of motivation, but many do not consider them as signs until these curious and validating conversations take place. Additionally, it is often the case that people say that their loved ones can quickly recognize changes in their presentation, but further exploration reveals that they have not discussed what it is that has changed that has been recognizable with their friends and family. Practitioners should encourage such discussions with family and friends in order to enhance their safety plan. Ideally, effective safety planning would also include a member of their support network to engage with one of the sessions to build on the crisis plan. *Note:* most SCM care programmes should have a carer/family programme that sits within the pathway; it can be useful to consider referring the family member, friend, partner to this service.

What might help me in a crisis? How would I like people to help me in a crisis?

If the service user has a positive support network in place, each member should be identified with the level and type of support they receive documented. Many people will describe different types of support being offered by different individuals and this is essential to document in the safety plan. It may be the case that a person's mother provides practical support, for example she takes responsibility for distributing their medication when they need it. If this is mentioned, the practitioner can curiously explore the pros and cons of this behaviour for the service user. A conversation about this and the reasons why other people are taking responsibility for managing their risk can be helpful.

This section of the plan should identify the range of support (whilst also defining what the service user means by support) offered to them to ensure they do not utilize one source in crisis and that one source alone. It is also essential to identify what the service user finds unhelpful in each of the relationships; for example, being shouted at/criticized for self-harming rather than validated for the difficult feelings leading to the self-harm.

Most importantly, when completing this section of the plan there should be a discussion around what ways the service user can support themselves in a crisis and what they can do to keep themselves safe. If a person is unable to self-soothe (talking or acting in a validating, calming way) or distract themselves and relies on external support or sources, they will struggle to develop coping strategies in managing their own crisis. This can also result in an escalation in risk if all external sources are not available when the service user is experiencing a crisis.

One aspect of an effective safety plan is to promote development of skills in self-management. When the service user feels that they are struggling to manage, how do they tolerate their emotions? As well as highlighting coping strategies, it is important to explore and document when these strategies are effective and when they are ineffective. Regularly, service users may state that a particular strategy is helpful until they reach a certain level of distress, therefore the crisis plan should highlight when this strategy should be implemented and when alternative strategies should be tried. Each service user has endless knowledge of their crises and what has or hasn't helped previously. It is worth revisiting this throughout the safety planning sessions and building upon the knowledge as the sessions progress. If the service user is in SCM then the safety plan should be intermittently revisited and enhanced as understanding develops.

Who should they contact?

If in crisis, what support would be utilized and who would be contacted? Sometimes, service users will highlight their immediate support network for first contact when experiencing a crisis and report that their support network would contact additional services, such as their GP, on their behalf if required. At other times, service users state that they don't trust others to help or don't want to burden other people so they contact services as a first option.

It is important to explore all this further and work on barriers around appropriate help-seeking in this stage of the plan as there could be an over or under reliance on services. The General Help Seeking Questionnaire (Wilson et al., 2005) can be a useful questionnaire to go through with the service user. It can be useful to explore their responses and discuss the reasons for the responses around their help-seeking behaviour.

In SCM, it is not appropriate to highlight attending Accident and Emergency departments or admission to hospital as the sole response to crisis, even if this is the only option that the service user suggests on their crisis plan. If a service user does this, the practitioner will gently need to explore what the function of this is (as described earlier regarding if they feel they need an admission to hospitalization) and explore alternative (less active/restrictive) options, such as using the crisis team or Home Treatment Team (HTT). Whenever possible, the practitioner is trying to support the provision of the least 'active' or intensive external support to manage the crisis. At this time, it is vital that the service user's emotional state of mind feels heard and taken seriously by the practitioner (thus authentic validation is the key).

In SCM safety planning, an important intervention is exploring the service user's perceptions of support services, discussing what they want from services and any barriers to why they don't want to engage in them. Sometimes service users have negative perceptions of crisis services and/or the HTT for various reasons. It is recommended that the practitioner works with the crisis service and/or HTT to address any concerns or issues about accessing appropriate support in the safety plan. Inviting them into a safety planning session and/or doing the plan collaboratively with them if appropriate can be helpful. It can be equally important to facilitate discussions around psychiatric admissions and defining the purpose and goals of admission before they are in a crisis. If the service user is in or about to start the SCM programme or another therapy programme designed to build autonomy, this can be a good opportunity to revisit the programmes and goals around building autonomy and self-agency. Having conversations about crisis responses and admissions prior to a crisis can be especially useful if frequent in-patient admissions are proving counter-therapeutic.

Safety planning can also cover what services should not do as well as what they should. This part of the safety plan can be as important to the assisting practitioner as for the service user. All too often, the crisis practitioner feels under extreme pressure to 'fix' the current crisis. The intense internal pressure on the crisis practitioner to alleviate the service user's distress quickly and the systemic pressure (so they can go onto the next service user in crisis) can lead them to problem-solve quickly, tell the service user what to do, or suggest a coping strategy (hence the 'you need to ...' statement). Thus, the responses to 'fix' the situation quickly, that often invalidate service users, are often due to systemic pressure and their own anxieties. Having a safety plan that also states what 'not to do' can help protect against this reaction.

What treatment/care would I like?

Treatment options can cover medical input, psychological intervention, and social care needs. This part of the safety plan gives the service users the opportunity to discuss any previous treatment and/or care that they have received and what their experience of this was. Additionally, the service user can identify and share potential goals they may have for the future regarding engaging with treatment. Some service users may not know what they want with regard to their care, in which case open discussions can be facilitated around what they think could or could not be beneficial for them. Other service users are clear and sometimes request interventions and treatments that can help in the short term (e.g. a short course of diazepam) but may cause more problems by building external dependency and loss of self-agency in the long term. Medication is not the only challenge; practitioner input, for example reassurance or advice giving, can also have a detrimental long-term impact on building self-agency. Having open discussions exploring the pros and cons of all medical interventions, psychological or social input can be helpful.

Do I have any advanced statements or decisions?

Service user involvement is a vital part of safety planning in SCM as the plan allows them to take some control over potential future crises and decision-making. Advanced statements and decisions allow service users to communicate through the safety plan what should be done in a crisis that will act in line with their thoughts, feelings, and emotions. Essentially, what would a service user want to happen in their best interests if they were in crisis? As previously mentioned, it is important to be realistic regarding expectations of a service user's support network and services. It is also important to note that sometimes the service user can say one thing in one state of mind and contradict it in another; that is, a non-emotional reasonable state may present as 'I don't ever want to be admitted', whereas an emotional irrational state may present as 'I can't cope, please admit me'.

Practitioners may want to have open conversations about risk and what the service user feels is best for their care. If in crisis, would an admission be helpful? Has it been helpful in the past? Would input from a Home Treatment/Crisis Team be more effective? When would their support network know when community support was no longer effective? Who would make those decisions if the person was unwell and/or did not have capacity? These are all very important questions to be raising as well as documenting outcomes in the crisis plan. It may not be the case that the person is aware of the answers but the conversations can be facilitated with their support network to provide a more robust plan. Alternatively, if someone does not have a support network, what would need to happen in their best interests and how would services know when to offer that support? It can be useful when doing this to try and ask the person to check whether or not different states of mind would have different expectations.

See Box 4.4 for an example of a safety plan.

Box 4.4 Example of a Completed Safety Plan

Case example of a brief safety plan

How can people spot the signs of a crisis?

Spending more time alone in my bedroom, not eating regular meals or looking after myself (washing and getting dressed), not wanting to speak to my family and friends. When things get worse I sometimes self-harm by cutting myself and I have suicidal thoughts. When I am at a crisis point, I will sometimes go missing as I don't want to burden everyone.

How would you like people to help you?

I don't want people to tell me to 'cheer up' as this makes me feel worse. I want my family just to listen to me rather than try and keep me busy. I don't want them to shout at me if they see I have self-harmed as that makes me not want to speak to them and I'm less likely to ask them for help. I do not want to be judged if I need to get checked out when I have self-harmed.

Who should they contact?

I would want my boyfriend to be contacted first as he understands what I am going through. If I don't feel I can keep myself safe I can call Samaritans to talk to someone or speak to the mental health team about getting some help.

What treatment would you like?

I would like to be asked what I want rather than people assuming they know best. I would like to understand how to manage my emotions better and to be taken seriously. I have tried different medication and that can make me feel worse.

Have you made an advanced statement or decision?

I do not want to go into hospital again as I struggle to manage being alone afterwards. I seem to manage better if getting extra help from home. I do not want my work to find out about my mental health.

After completing the initial safety plan, you can go on to develop an enhanced safety plan. This includes coping responses for the service user. *Note:* how much you are able to put in the plan will vary from service user to service user. Less is often more in that you should only put in what has been collaboratively agreed. When completed, the plan would ideally be written up and given to the service user. Figure 4.1 is a template example of what 'could' go into a safety plan. It was developed by one of our colleagues, Elaine Swift. Our experience has been that time spent developing a collaborative safety plan is well worth it. Many service users keep their plan close by and repeatedly refer to it during times of crisis. It does appear for some to provide a 'go-to place' that can help them to regain their thinking/mentalizing at times of acute distress or detachment.

(a)

Goals

It may be helpful to include my positive future goals to help me to feel more hopeful in times of crisis.

People I can ask for support

It might be helpful to think about people who you can approach for support. This might include members of your family or friends; it may also include NHS mental health services, or any other services that are available to you.

A Guide to Working on My Safety Plan

Developing skills to prevent and cope with crisis

(b)

My Triggers
These may include

- Being told no
- Feeling rejected
- Social media
- Not being listened to
- Lack of privacy
- Certain smells/tastes
- Darkness
- Hunger/pain
- Hormonal imbalances
- Arguments
- Room checks
- Loud noises
- People yelling
- Not having control
- Important anniversaries
- Feeling overwhelmed
- Feeling disrespected
- Feeling lonely/empty

My Early Warning Signs
These may include

- Feeling very excited
- Being quiet and withdrawn
- The urge to be violent
- The urge to injure self
- Feeling tired
- Sleeping a lot
- Pacing
- Eating more
- Swearing
- Shaking
- Difficulty concentrating
- Not feeling like eating
- Having aches and pains
- Struggling to relax
- Being snappy with others
- Crying
- Clenching teeth

Skills I can work on and develop

In order to help me to work on My Safety Plan with my team, I will be offered information and guidance on:

- Distraction skills
- Self-soothing skills
- Grounding skills
- Problem-solving
- Surfing the urge
- Groups available to me

What others can do to support me

- Staff will help me to develop my skills and will support me to use them
- There will be opportunities to practice any new skills that I learn and revisit any skills I have previously used
- Support to develop my skills will be provided during my named-nurse sessions
- I will also be offered support to us my safety plan at times when I am struggling

Figure 4.1 A Guide to Working on My Safety Plan

Conclusion

Safety planning is a key strategic process in supporting service users to manage their mental health crises particularly when presenting with a diagnosis of BPD. The safety plan enables service users to have greater insight into how to manage their crises as well as their expectations of how they want their support network and services to respond.

In order to facilitate effective safety planning, practitioners should attempt to build a positive and trusting therapeutic alliance through open communication as well as presenting as active, interested, and responsive to the service user. In SCM safety planning, a greater emphasis is placed on the importance of discussions with service users about their thoughts and feelings related to their crisis. A curious approach will demonstrate interest in the client whilst observing, reflecting, and directly validating their state will display that they are being listened to and heard.

Safety planning in SCM requires an initial period of stabilization and crisis containment through a structured approach. The SCM safety plan focuses on the service user's previous crises and triggers in order to provide a robust plan to work preventatively rather than reactively to potential future crises. By establishing a service user's advanced decisions in how they access support, they are able to have more control when crisis situations occur and potentially seek support in more productive ways. Following stabilization, service users find it is useful to develop their resilience profile and build on their strengths, which can provide the necessary motivation to work towards their goals. They can build their own safety management plan that can be their go-to place at times of crisis.

Safety planning enables service users to have greater control over their care whilst also providing their support network and relevant services with the guidance needed to support them more effectively. The safety plan is part of an ongoing process for the service user to be actively involved in and build on whilst ultimately becoming an expert in their own experience.

References

Bateman, A., & Fonagy, P. (2009). Randomized controlled trial of outpatient mentalization-based treatment versus structured clinical management for borderline personality disorder. *American Journal of Psychiatry*, 166(12), 1355–1364.

Bateman, A. W., & Krawitz, R. (2013). *Borderline personality disorder: an evidence-based guide for generalist mental health professionals*. Oxford: Oxford University Press.

Borschmann, R., Barrett, B., Hellier, J. M., Byford, S., Henderson, C., Rose, D., … Hogg, J. (2013). Joint crisis plans for people with borderline personality disorder: feasibility and outcomes in a randomised controlled trial. *British Journal of Psychiatry*, 202(5), 357–364.

Borschmann, R., Henderson, C., Hogg, J., Phillips, R., & Moran, P. (2012). Crisis interventions for people with borderline personality disorder. *Cochrane Database of Systematic Reviews*, (6).

Dazzi, T., Gribble, R., Wessely, S., & Fear, N. T. (2014). Does asking about suicide and related behaviours induce suicidal ideation? what is the evidence? *Psychological Medicine*, 44(16), 3361–3363.

Department of Health. (1999). *A national service framework for mental health.* London: Department of Health.

Department of Health. (2008). *Refocusing the care programme approach: policy and positive practice guidance.* London: Department of Health.

Henderson, C., Flood, C., Leese, M., Thornicroft, G., Sutherby, K., & Szmukler, G. (2009). Views of service users and providers on joint crisis plans. *Social Psychiatry and Psychiatric Epidemiology*, 44(5), 369.

McGuinness, A., Bevington, R., Sampson, M., Bass, E. & Fisher, D. (in prep). *An evaluation of the personal resilience programme: the impact of a brief rapid-access intervention for suicidality on resilience and help seeking behaviours.* Manuscript submitted for publication.

Posner, K., Brent, D., Lucas, C., Gould, M., Stanley, B., Brown, G. & Mann, J. (2008). *Columbia-Suicide Severity Rating Scale (C-SSRS).* New York, NY: Columbia University Medical Center.

Wilson, C. J., Deane, F. P., Ciarrochi, J. V., & Rickwood, D. (2005). Measuring help seeking intentions: properties of the general help seeking questionnaire. *Canadian Journal of Counselling*, 39(1), 15–28.

Wright, J. H., Basco, M. R., & Thase, M. E. (2006). *Learning cognitive-behavior therapy: an illustrated guide.* Washington, DC: American Psychiatric Association Publishing.

5

Group SCM Sessions

Stuart Mitchell

Introduction

The group component of structured clinical management (SCM) is a key 'socializing' element of the model along with fostering a sense of social connectivity. It is here where service users feel connected to other people with similar difficulties along with learning to put into practice the social element of skills in problem-solving, managing emotions, urges, and impulsive behaviour, and developing relational trust and safety. This is not easy to do, and many service users may initially prefer individual therapy only or may find themselves re-enacting some of their problems within the group therapy context. Here the practitioner needs skills to manage these re-enactments in a compassionate but firm way so that the practical elements of the therapy can continue. In SCM group sessions, there is a large element of learning in a social situation from others, sharing with fellow service users, and developing a shared felt sense (Gendlin, 1981; Steele, Boon, & Van Der Hart, 2017) of normalizing and universality, which may help mitigate feelings of shame or unworthiness. Group work is both challenging and highly rewarding for the practitioner. It is satisfying to see how many service users benefit from being in a group and in SCM gain much also from the practical problem-solving style of therapy.

The group facilitator does not take an 'expert' delivery style but more of an informed practitioner who is able to hold the SCM-CV stance (curiosity and validation as described in Chapter 3), being able to keep an awareness of their own mind and a curiosity of the service user's mind simultaneously (mentalize) when they are under pressure, and remain focused on the task in hand. This is at a level of intensity that most service users can tolerate, provided they are not experiencing too many or too severe additional problems of complex trauma, dissociation, or avoidance. This chapter outlines the content of group sessions, the processes of delivery, and offers some guidance on how practitioners may overcome frequently seen problems that occur.

Why SCM Group Work?

SCM group therapy complements the individual SCM sessions. Since the service user's problems may involve a strong pattern of attachment, motivational, and relationship difficulties that can be activated in the group, the individual sessions provide a great place to review and problem-solve these. Here, the service user can feel more fully understood as an individual and attached to the therapist in the joint endeavour of working on their problems. Motivational work, alliance formation, understanding group issues, exploring crises, and agreeing progress monitoring (general therapeutic strategies) can all be employed here. The group therapy component is more a 'socializing' component where the service user can learn skills and strategies to solve problems in the presence of others with similar problems. This could be regarded as a sort of 'training ground' for working both on skill and insight into increasing awareness of their own and other peoples mind by their interactions with others in the group and in relationships outside the group. Learning from others may also help to foster greater capacity to understand (mentalize) oneself 'from the outside' and others 'from the inside' (Allen, Fonagy, & Bateman, 2008; Bateman & Fonagy, 2016). By focusing on both the individual and group session, the service user is able to have a greater sense of feeling contained in two sessions per week whilst learning new skills in a relationship context. This helps promote a faster recovery process without overstimulating the (insecure) attachment system (Bateman & Fonagy, 2016).

The evidence-based model for SCM for the full programme involves weekly group and weekly individual sessions. However, SCM can be delivered flexibly but be mindful there is less research on whether this produces good outcomes. For people with high-risk behaviours, it is not recommended to deliver SCM group sessions only however, as this may lead to less containment for the service user without the security of regular individual sessions. Although group-only interventions can be offered for people with less severe symptoms.

What Happens in SCM Group Therapy?

The skills components of the group can vary depending on needs of the service users but generally they should cover the four main modules, where group members can learn and practice skills which relate to the problems they find themselves coming up against in their lives. These include problem-solving, managing emotions, increasing awareness of their own and other people's mind (mindfulness, mentalizing), managing impulsivity and alternatives to self-harm, and fostering safe and secure relationships skilfully. Two practitioners facilitate each session. They each have a practitioner guidance manual, whilst service users have a corresponding workbook which contains all the handouts, worksheets, and exercises which will be discussed in the group sessions. We recommend that the manual is used as a guide or template to follow as practitioners teach and implement problem-solving within each session. There is a generic session plan template that is included at the start of each module which outlines a rough three-phase structure to follow. It is important that this is followed, so that equal time is given over to both teaching skills and problem-solving within the session. The session plan looks like:

1. **Homework review** (implementing problem-solving plans; practising skills—up to ten minutes).
2. **Skills teaching**—problem-solving and other skills as part of four modules (30–40 minutes).
3. **Application of problem-solving** to the problems identified by service users whilst in the group (40 minutes).

There is a risk if this structure isn't followed that there is too much teaching, and this leaves little time left for actual problem-solving in the group. The essence of SCM group therapy is to practise problem-solving in the group and not solely as a homework task. In this way, it is different from some other skills groups, which tend to focus more on skills acquisition (Linehan, 1993, 2015). We suggest discussion and teaching of a skill focuses on one to two handouts and one to two exercise worksheets that are the focus of the group discussion, problem-solving, then application of problem-solving, including new skills learned, as homework or 'application in daily life'. We think workbooks, flipcharts, pens and paper work best; PowerPoint presentations do not as they tend to limit the 'group' interaction for group members and lead to greater service user passivity.

The group and individual SCM programme combined should last about between 12 and 18 months, in line with the research evidence (Bateman & Fonagy, 2009). The four modules may be completed in 6 months, or 24 weeks. Although different group formats can be used, we find a structure similar to dialectical behaviour therapy (DBT) in terms of length of modules, structure, and repetition of them (Linehan, 1993, 2015) is appropriate but with some differences. Modules may be flexibly repeated as requested by the group, and the group therapy is not skills teaching only but a mixture of skills teaching and *in vivo* problem-solving. Programmes can vary on whether they are open or closed; most SCM groups are either closed or semi-open, meaning they have set start times. The start times, modules, and timing/sequencing of them are shown in Figure 5.1.

Each of the four specific modules are 'taught' for 6–7 weeks, but the practitioner should return to these within the problem-solving steps discussed in the first module when indicated to be of relevance to the problem identified during the solution analysis step of problem-solving. For example, a self-harm problem indicates material and skills covered in the self-harm module, or if there is an

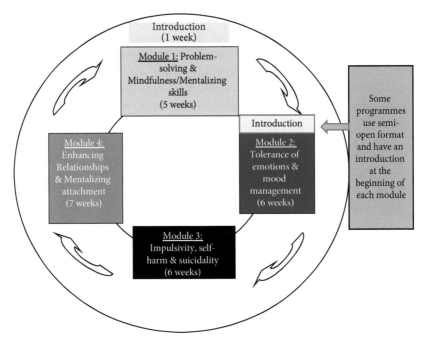

Figure 5.1 Sequencing and Timing of Modules in SCM Group Therapy

interpersonal sensitivity issue, the enhancing relationships module can be applied (Bateman & Krawitz, 2013). Steps in this specific group process for the practitioner are shown in Table 5.1.

SCM group size

There is no exact set criterion for how big SCM groups should be. SCM groups ideally group should be between six and 12 service users for face-to-face groups. This number needs to be lower for virtual (online) group sessions with four to eight being more the optimum number.

Content of SCM Group Sessions

In SCM group therapy, there is a Practitioner's Manual and a Service User Workbook, so the two can be used together to ensure practitioners and service users are working on the same areas, including handouts, worksheets, and exercises. It is based on research evidence and expert practice guidance about what helps people with personality and trauma-related problems recover

Table 5.1 Group Practitioners' Strategic Steps in SCM Group Therapy

	Strategic step	Rationale
1.	Identify clients' problems in one-to-one and/or group sessions Generate a hierarchy or problem checklist	Step 1 of problem-solving Strategy
2.	Agree first problem to be tackled from the list	Step 1 of problem-solving Strategy
*3.	Brainstorm solutions to the problem—within the group setting	Step 2 of problem-solving strategy
*4.	Share own possible solutions alongside group-generated solutions but remain neutral about choices	Step 2 of problem-solving strategy
5.	Discuss pros and cons of each solution suggested	Step 3 of problem-solving strategy
6.	Develop action plan with the group	Step 4 of problem-solving strategy
7.	Ask client to report back next week on results	Step 4 of problem-solving strategy
8.	Evaluate progress on the action plan and see if solutions can be improved	Step 5 of problem-solving strategy
9.	Apply module specific skills for solutions when generating action plans	Link modules on specific skills taught to problem-solving strategy

* These steps may include step 9 whenever possible and these additional skills are known and/or have been taught previously

(McMurran, 2008; D'Zurilla & Nezu, 2007). It can be used to help practitioners and group members focus on the tasks necessary, so that all are doing more or less the things that the group members specifically need to help them recover quickly and safely.

The first SCM group session is usually about discussing the goals (e.g. reduce misunderstandings and impulsivity and increase skills in mentalizing, managing urges and emotions, and problem-solving), establishing the format (e.g. how each session is structured and how to limit discussion of problems), and agreeing some guidelines or agreements for how the group sessions will run (group agreements/ values). Guidelines might cover things such as how to handle an event when someone becomes distressed or leaves the room, aggression or violence, substance use, confidentiality, social contact between members outside the group, and absences or communications from practitioners or service users. This can be tricky, especially if some people object to the authority of the practitioners in facilitating the group, or prefer to have no rules, or take over the running of the group themselves. Consequently, enabling everyone in the group to be active participants in developing the group rules addresses some of the resistance (see later below). It is better to do this at the start so that if problems with the boundaries or frame of the group sessions are tested, the guidelines can be returned to as a benchmark for how the group as a whole may handle them.

Module 1 (problem-solving, mindfulness, and mentalizing—SCM foundations)

This module provides the underpinning framework and skills which run through the whole of SCM group therapy. These are problem-solving, mindfulness, and mentalizing (PSMM). These skills help with everything that is discussed or taught in the four modules. The session titles and the numbers of handouts and worksheets are shown in Table 5.2

Table 5.2 Module 1 Problem-solving, Mindfulness, and Mentalizing (PSMM): Session Content

Session number	Session title
1	Problem-solving skills
2	What is mindfulness and states of mind?
3	Mindfulness 'what' and 'how' skills
4	What is mentalizing, why do it, and different (non-mentalizing) states of mind
5	Mentalizing and core skills: being balanced, doing it well and not so well
6	More mentalizing skills: what gets in the way, how to 'press pause' and become 'more flexible'

Module 2 (enhancing emotional regulation and mood management skills)

This module provides skills which help service users learn to identify, name, and regulate their emotions in a mindful and reflective way so that they don't get too caught up in them, or find they interfere with them being able to achieve their goals. It is about enhancing their ability to tolerate emotions and manage moods. The module will also cover how service users can monitor, identify, and manage mood states so they are less of a problem. The session titles and the numbers of handouts and worksheets are shown in Table 5.3.

Table 5.3 Module 2 Tolerance of Emotions and Managing Moods (TEMM): Session Content

Session number	Session title
1	Recognizing and naming emotions
2	Learning to reflect, not react
3	Opposite action
4	Relaxation, distraction, and self-monitoring
5	Recognizing and naming moods and triggers
6	Managing moods

Module 3 (impulsivity, self-harm, and suicidality)

This module provides skills which help service users learn to take a step back from their urges to act, slow things down, and become more mindful and reflective. It is about managing impulsivity, self-harm, and suicidal urges and behaviour. These issues are difficult to talk about and learn to manage as service users may experience strong feelings and urges to act, but they can be very helpful to developing overall safety and well-being, so it is important to encourage service users to stick with it. The session titles and the numbers of handouts and worksheets are shown in Table 5.4.

Table 5.4 Module 3 Impulsivity, Self-harm, and Suicidal Behaviour (ISS): Session Content

Session number	Session title
1	Recognizing aspects of impulsivity and 'risky' behaviours
2	Recognizing triggers for actions
3	Understanding self-harm
4	Strategies for reducing self-harm
5	Recognizing and managing suicidal behaviour
6	Recognizing and managing suicidal behaviour

Module 4 (enhancing relationship skills and mentalizing attachment)

This module provides skills which help service users learn to manage their relationships more effectively, so they can feel more safe and secure. It is about enhancing relationships and mentalizing attachment. In the module, they will learn to recognize areas of sensitivity and ways of managing this, skills which might help them develop positive relationships, recognize their own attachment pattern, and how to foster greater security in current relationships. This module can be quite difficult, so it is recommended to encourage service users to take their time with it and go at their own pace, so they can really learn from it and apply it to their outside daily life. The take-home strapline to this module is 'be wise and mentalize'. The session titles and the numbers of handouts and worksheets are shown in Table 5.5.

Process of SCM Group Sessions

It is important to recognize that SCM group therapy is not a 'process' type of group therapy, nor is it MBT or DBT. It does however include some aspects of teaching skills, such as problem-solving, mindfulness, emotional regulation, interpersonal skills, and chain analysis. The SCM group also aims to facilitate an enhanced self-awareness for the service users around their own emotions, thoughts, and feelings and also those of other people (awareness of themselves from the inside, others from the outside); this is often referred to as mentalizing. This mentalizing ability is a seen as a central and common therapeutic factor in accounting for mechanisms

Table 5.5 Module 4 Enhancing Relationships and Mentalizing
Attachment (ERMA): Session Content

Session number	Session title
1	Goals and barriers
2	Mentalizing attachment: recognizing attachment styles and current safety
3	Handling interpersonal sensitivity
4	Getting needs met effectively
5	Building relationships and maintaining self-respect
6	Resolving conflict and moving on
7	Mentalizing attachment: resolving insecure attachment problems

of therapeutic change for service users diagnosed with borderline personality disorder (BPD) (Bateman & Krawitz, 2013). The process generally just happens in SCM group therapy as service users form some kind of alliance or bond with each other and the practitioners, and this should be carefully managed through the structure, format, and clinical stance of the practitioners. We suggest there should be two practitioners per SCM therapy group. This reduces the demands on the sole group practitioner and also assists with managing difficult issues such as a distressed service user leaving the session and in managing the group during the problem-solving application phase. There are key tasks for the group practitioners to undertake, which we divide into 'therapy' and 'management' or 'dynamic administrator' tasks (Behr & Hearst, 2005).

Therapy tasks are about one SCM group practitioner adhering to the model of therapy, undertaking problem-solving using an agreed number of stages, teaching service users skills in problem-solving and other areas, integrating the individual and group components of therapy, monitoring their own reactions to service users within supervision, and monitoring service users progress on stuck points and problem-solving these. Management tasks are about the various 'tests' the SCM group practitioners encounter on maintaining the structure, frame, purpose, and integrity of the group (Behr & Hearst, 2005). It may be helpful to develop with the group some group 'guidance' in the first session on what has been found through experience to help therapy groups run well (Bateman & Krawitz, 2013). It is best not to do this in an authoritarian way with the implicit message 'you must do this', but more with a suggested guidance that 'this will help the group work best and if we can't do this then lets problem solve why not'.

It is helpful for group SCM practitioners to agree what their respective roles will be in the group sessions, and who will undertake what task. A suggested simple division of this labour is to divide the 'management' from the 'therapy' tasks. However, on occasions, such as when one practitioner becomes stuck or lost in their task, the other practitioner may step in to support them (Linehan, 1993, 2015). A summary of these various tasks for the SCM group practitioners is shown in Table 5.6.

Challenges and Solutions to Problems in SCM Group Sessions

There are many problems which might arise in the running of any therapy group for service users diagnosed with personality disorder (Bateman & Krawitz, 2013; Gunderson, 2008; Linehan, 1993, 2015). Some of these have been described within the 'management tasks' discussed previously. Common blocks to service users progressing in group therapy may include their preference for individual therapy, a wish to talk about problems excessively, acting out urges within groups, objecting to other group members comments or behaviour (including practitioners), hyper- or hypo-arousal, significant stressful life events, suicidal intentions and behaviour, dominating aggressive or narcissistic group members, and not attending sessions or encouraging others to do the same (Bateman & Krawitz, 2013; Linehan, 1993, 2015). Service users themselves may also temporarily lose their self-awareness and thus mentalizing capacity due to a current stressful trigger which leads them to resort to non-mentalizing modes, such as being stuck in a highly aroused state accompanied by rigidity in thinking, detached from any current felt reality, or feeling that the only way to obtain relief is through acting on their urges or encouraging others to do so (Bateman & Fonagy, 2016). A further complication may occur when a service user's own insecure attachment to the practitioner, room, building, or other staff is overstimulated. This may result in the service user becoming regressed, clingy, anxious, or demanding requests for more and more contact with the practitioner. When the attachment system is activated, as is all too commonly seen in service users diagnosed with personality disorder (Bateman & Fonagy, 2016), service users may seek excessive contact with their attachment figures or service/building, detach and avoid, or show a chaotic mixture of both (Bateman & Krawitz, 2013' Gonzalez & Mosquera, 2012).

Group SCM practitioners need to monitor closely their own emotional and behavioural reactions to service users, reflect on the nature of these, and manage them in a professional manner, with support from a senior colleague or supervisor (Bateman & Krawitz, 2013; Sedlak, 2003). We have found that generalist practitioners may initially struggle with this, but with supportive and reflective supervision, they learn how to contain their own feelings and impulses and make good

Table 5.6 SCM Group Clinician Tasks

Management tasks	Therapy tasks
1. Attending to the frame, setting, and boundaries of the group so it is secure.	1. Adhering to the SCM model of therapy with fidelity to each individual service user.
2. Finding and keeping a suitable venue that is free from noise, interruptions, and is comfortable.	2. Undertaking problem-solving using generic and specific skills on problems identified and agreed with service user at assessment (or later).
3. Dealing with communications (letters, phone messages) from group members.	3. Teaching the service users skills and strategies in problem-solving and within the four modules (as detailed in the manual).
4. Dealing with requests for travel expenses etc. (via admin.).	4. Integrating the individual and group SCM components of therapy carefully.
5. Managing challenges to the frame, etc. as they arise.	5. Monitoring own reactions to service users, reflecting on these, and discussing solutions to manage these professionally in clinical supervision and team discussions.
6. Maintaining consistency in the time, setting, staffing, etc.	6. Monitoring and evaluating service users individual progress in liaison with the SCM individual practitioner.
7. Developing 'group guidance' with the group on how to manage distress, absences, equity, relationships outside the group setting, and confidentiality.	7. Problem-solving with service users who appear 'stuck' in the group and progress is difficult and linking this to the modules for potential solutions.
8. 'Group problems' (e.g. no single person bringing problems) to problem-solve these.	8. Managing the structure and timing of the phases of each group session—review, skills teaching, problem-solving.
9. Group clinician issues—experience, anxiety, confidence, defensiveness, conflicting roles, etc.	
10. Looking after the group process: parking, siding, and triangulation.	

use of them in service of the therapeutic process. Supervision of the SCM group practitioners' may be a helpful place to discuss and reflect on the different group dynamics so they do not become behaviourally communicated and harmful or iatrogenic. Should the group practitioner find it difficult to contain or manage their own feelings despite good supportive clinical supervision which are engendered by the clinical work, then it may be that further support or therapy should be recommended for them by the supervisor. A summary of these multiple problems and suggested initial solutions is shown in Table 5.7.

Table 5.7 SCM Group Therapy Troubleshooting

Problem/Issue	Solution(s)
1. Service user prefers individual therapy.	1. Discuss with SCM individual practitioner; pros and cons of group vs individual; build motivation/commitment to goals whilst acknowledging how hard the 'tasks' are; target this in group as 'a problem to be solved'.
2. Service user wants to talk about problems excessively.	2. Validate both sides of the problem; remind them of timing/structure of each session; anticipate effect of this (e.g. lack of time to generate solutions, make progress, etc.); seek group views on potential solutions.
3. Acting out urges in groups	3. Recognize and validate the feeling behind the urge and the pressure to act; refer to the module and skills which might help (e.g. impulsivity, self-harm); encourage reflection on solutions as a group (i.e. a thinking/planning phase in the strategies of solving problems and preventing further problems later on).
4. Objection to other group members or practitioners	4. Validate service users feelings; 'side' with service user if they feel victimized; encourage reflection on the problem and link to the modules as appropriate; recognize and validate awareness of different perspectives and respect for each other; acknowledge own contribution and problem-solve this if appropriate.
5. Service user appears severely regressed, has recent experience of stressful life events, or strong suicidal intentions or behaviour	5. Outside of the group ask service user if they are having a problem being in the group right now; ask if something has happened to make them feel like this and validate this struggle and related feelings or urges; ask if they feel able to stay today or prefer to leave; one practitioner may leave with them and undertake brief risk assessment and safety plan as appropriate; liaise with individual SCM practitioner at earliest opportunity.

Table 5.7 *Continued*

Problem/Issue	Solution(s)
6. Dominating, aggressive, or narcissistic group members	6. Recognize and validate their need to have time, etc. to work on their problems vs the need for equity and balance in the group; stress the importance of this in a non-authoritarian way; maintain structure and timing of phases of each session; intervene to stop aggressive behaviour immediately and ask the member to think of better ways to speak to the service user/others; liaise with individual SCM practitioner as required.
7. Not attending sessions or encouraging others to be absent.	7. Identify this as a service user issue or problem to be solved in the group; briefly acknowledge the effect of absences in the group (e.g. other members miss them, wonder why they are not attending, etc.) or making progress on solving problems and maintaining this outside the group; revisiting group guidance on relationships outside and what modules to invoke (e.g. enhancing relationships) to address this. However, ultimately in order for them to continue the programme, they have to address attendance issues.

Managing the group process

Group facilitation is a skill in itself. SCM group facilitation covers three components:

- The education and group content as described above.
- The approach of the facilitator—clinical stance or SCM-CV
- Managing the group process

The approach of the group facilitators

The structure and content of the groups has been covered earlier in the chapter. This section focuses more on the dynamic process of running the group. SCM group practitioners essentially model the SCM clinical stance and SCM-CV. In summary, this involves the practitioner in their interactions taking a curious stance on all areas discussed, being open to people's views, and then exploring the thoughts, feelings, and beliefs that underpin group participants' problem-solving or opinions. The group facilitators should work hard to take a non-judgemental approach. They should also focus on the validation in the SCM-CV with effective listening and communication along with an emphasis on looking to understand and then validate group participants' opinions. This is key to SCM as the practitioner is modelling curiosity and validation whilst also trying to encourage participants to reflect and describe their own thoughts feelings and beliefs.

The facilitator would also focus on managing the intensity of the group as per individual sessions. For example, if the group becomes too emotive then the facilitator seeks to calm the intensity down. Alternately, if the group is too cut off or detached the facilitator seeks to ask more probing emotive questions.

Other general communication competencies for SCM group facilitation are consistent with the clinical stance taken in the individual session and should be around:

- Language—the practitioner being mindful about language used and how this could be judgemental.
- Taking it on the chin—owning their own mistakes and modelling fallibility.
- Reducing advice giving—as this can often prevent active participation in group participants.

SCM core group facilitation skills

SCM core group facilitation for clarity is put into three core areas: parking, triangulation and siding. It is essential for an effective SCM group that practitioners are active in all three areas, which are taken from MBT. At the end of the randomized controlled trial comparing MBT with SCM, the effective processes of each treatment were studied. Some effective elements of specialist group intervention in MBT, of which these three are the most important, were incorporated into SCM as they could be implemented skilfully by generic mental health practitioners.

Parking

Parking is when the facilitator is active at asking one of the group members just to pause what they are saying to allow other group members to contribute to the topic. It is normal group dynamics that some participants will speak more than others. What is also common in SCM groups is that some participants struggle to regulate their actions and can overtalk. The long-term aim is for group participants to become aware of these tendencies and to self-regulate. However, initially for some individuals this is really difficult and facilitators often need to help them by encouraging the parking/pause. At first, some SCM group facilitators can struggle with this as they are essentially asking a group member to defer to others and keep quiet just when they are in mid-flow and this can create tension. However, it can't be stressed enough how important this is in creating an effective group and also for the service user who is struggling to self-regulate with respect to their participation as the group may well turn on them.

Triangulation

Triangulation is about trying to encourage group discussions rather than one-to-one discussions. The facilitator is trying to encourage group discussion and avoid one-to-one therapy with the facilitators.

Siding

The final core competency is siding. This can be misunderstood as it is not about the practitioner taking a 'side' of the participant but rather encouraging diversity in thinking and allowing all points of view to be explored. This means being open to the reasons for the service user to hold a particular point of view.

As illustrated, there is a lot the SCM group practitioners must do. This is why it is recommended where possible that there are two practitioners, with one delivering the material whilst the other facilitates the group with the competencies described.

Conclusion

Group sessions in SCM comprise an important 'socializing' element to implementing the SCM model. Here, service users learn to develop mentalizing, problem-solving, and other skills in a safe social context in order to practise skills with their fellow service users. This is akin to an 'SCM training ground'. Since most service users have significant interpersonal and social functioning difficulties, if they can tolerate and attend group SCM regularly, this will provide a greater opportunity to consolidate social learning in a way that is less dependent on attachment to an individual SCM practitioner.

In group SCM, service users are taught skills and then practise them in a series of sessions covering four key areas, which are delivered sequentially:

1. Problem-solving, mindfulness, and mentalizing.
2. Tolerance of emotions and managing moods.
3. Impulsivity, self-harm, and suicidality.
4. Enhancing relationships and mentalizing attachment.

Group SCM practitioners' adopt a practical problem-solving style as the fundamental platform in all group sessions which are then structured around a particular topic, as part of one of four modules. It is important to have a balance within each session between reviewing homework and implementation of action plans, skills teaching, and application of *in vivo* problem-solving in the session. It is not recommend to use PowerPoint presentations of the skills for face-to-face groups being taught as this all too easily leads to an excess of didactic teaching, a reduction in active participation from group members, and omission of *in vivo* problem-solving. However, for group work conducted by video, PowerPoint clearly has a place. It is also recommended SCM group practitioners agree roles and responsibilities so that 'managing the group' and SCM therapy tasks are distinguished, as shown in Table 5.6.

References

Allen, J. G., Fonagy, P., & Bateman, A. W. (2008). *Mentalizing in clinical practice*. Washington, DC: American Psychiatric Publishing, Inc.

Bateman, A., & Fonagy, P. (2009). Randomized controlled trial of outpatient mentalization-based treatment versus structured clinical management for borderline personality disorder. *American Journal of Psychiatry, 166*, 1355–1364.

Bateman, A. W., & Krawitz, R. (2013). *Borderline personality disorder: an evidence-based guide for generalist mental health professionals*. Oxford: Oxford University Press.

Bateman, A., & Fonagy, P. (2016). *Mentalization-based treatment for personality disorders*. Oxford: Oxford University Press.

Behr, H., & Hearst, L. (2005). *Group-analytic psychotherapy: a meeting of minds*. Philadelphia, PA: Whurr Publishers.

D'Zurilla, T. J. D., & Nezu, A. M. (2007). *Problem-solving therapy: a positive approach to clinical intervention* (3rd Ed.). New York, NY: Springer Publishing Company.

Gonzalez, A. & Mosquera, D. (2012). *EMDR and dissociation: the progressive approach* (1st Ed., rev.). Available via Info@itradis.com.

Gendlin, E. (1981) Focusing and the development of creativity. *The Folio, 1*(1), 13–16.

Gunderson, J. G. (2008). *Borderline personality disorder: a clinical guide* (2nd Ed.). Washington, DC: American Psychiatric Publishing.

Linehan, M. M. (1993). *Cognitive-behavioural therapy of borderline personality disorder*. New York, NY: Guilford Press.

Linehan, M. M. (2015). *DBT skills training: handouts and worksheets* (2nd Ed.). New York, NY: Guilford Press.

McMurran, M. (2008). *Stop & think! problem-solving therapy for people with personality difficulties*. University of Nottingham, July 2008.

Sedlak, V. (2003). The patient's material as an aid to the disciplined working through of the countertransference and supervision. *International Journal of Psychoanalysis, 84*(6), 1487–1500.

Steele, K., Boon, S., & Van Der Hart, O. (2017). *Treating trauma-related dissociation: a practical integrative approach*. New York, NY: Norton & Co.

PART 2

IMPLEMENTATION MODELS

6

Models of SCM Implementation—
United Kingdom

Mark Sampson, Christopher Berry, Allyson Jerry, and Catriona Gray

Introduction

Since the publication of the National Institute for Health and Care Excellence (NICE) guideline for the treatment of borderline personality disorder (BPD) in 2009, there have been substantial improvements in the care and treatment for people so diagnosed. In the 2017 National Personality Disorder Survey, 84% of specialist mental health Trusts in England reported that they had a dedicated service for personality disorder and 77% reported that they offered some form of care/therapy within generic mental healthcare (Dale et al., 2017). Although encouraged in their review, Dale et al. (2017) concluded that 'despite this progress, data presented here provides evidence that there remains continued exclusion, variability of practice and inconsistencies in the availability of services'.

Structured clinical management (SCM) and structured care pathways are one way to enable services to address exclusion, variability, and inconsistency. The SCM approach enables generalist (non-specialist) mental health practitioners to deliver care for people diagnosed with BPD in a way that is structured, organized, and focused on recovery. It enables organizations to increase their capacity to provide effective care for people diagnosed with BPD with relatively limited additional investment. This chapter describes three structured care pathways from different UK organizations, all of which have been strongly influenced by SCM. Their pathways are presented as case examples. Their services are contextualized and their implementation process described before going on to illustrate their pathway. The chapter concludes by identifying commonalities in these pathways along with the shared 'key enablers' that are considered to have helped in the successful implementation.

The Pathways

We will now consider three different Trusts and their implementation of the pathways.

North West Boroughs Healthcare Foundation Trust

North West Boroughs Healthcare (NWBH) Foundation Trust is situated between Manchester and Liverpool in the United Kingdom. It covers a wide demographic of approximately 1 million people. Note: in 2021 NWBH Foundation Trust disbanded/split—Wigan joined Manchester Mental Health and Social Care Trust—with the Boroughs of Halton, Knowsley, St Helen's and Warrington joining Mersey Care foundation Trust.

Journey to pathway implementation

In 2009, funding was obtained to establish a Personality Disorder Hub Service. This was a small team of practitioners (four psychologists and one specialist practitioner for multi-agency work). Their role was to provide specialist assessment and training for personality disorder for the whole Trust and the wider system (for one area).

To address the training component, the Personality Disorder Hub service worked with the Institute of Mental Health with the aim of training as many staff as possible from their organization in the Knowledge and Understanding Framework (KUF; see Davies et al., 2014 for review of this). In order to do this at such 'scale', a team of experts by experience (service users with experience of personality disorder diagnosis and care) and experts by occupation were trained as trainers in the KUF. This team of practitioners and experts by experience not knowingly at the time were to become the foundation of a 'working together approach' that would lead to co-production in service development and governance for the personality disorder pathway.

In 2013, external training in SCM for general mental health professionals was commissioned. This led to a cultural change in services for people with personality disorder because non-psychological therapists now had a model and clear framework to treat people diagnosed with BPD. This laid the groundwork for a more structured clinical approach and was a key enabler for the development of a pathway. The pathway was collaboratively developed (in a set of workshops) between a multidisciplinary group of experts by experience, carers, nurse practitioners, psychologists, psychiatrists, and occupational therapists.

Whether or not to use the BPD diagnosis?

The first hurdle to overcome in developing the pathway was whether or not to use the categorical diagnosis of BPD. It was decided via a Multi-Disciplinary Team (MDT; including carers and service users) working group to use the diagnosis initially with the aim of moving away from this as soon as possible. The pathway was to be diagnostically informed but not diagnostically driven or led. The pathway would be needs-led and service users did not require a diagnosis to go on the pathway.

Principles underpinning the pathway

The underlying principles of the pathway were drawn directly from NICE guidelines 77 and 78 (the guidelines on Antisocial and Borderline, 2009), the Personality Disorder Consensus Document (2018), and Safer Care for Personality Disorder (2018).

Stepping away from care coordination

The first operational and organizational decision around the pathway was to re-focus and reframe, stepping outside and away from care coordination and the Care Programme Approach (CPA) towards a care pathway approach or recovery journey to service delivery. Service users who met criterion for the pathway based on clinical need would be aligned to a care pathway rather than care coordination. This had two important enablers; it freed up staff who would ordinarily be coord-inating care in order to use this time to work differently and provide care in a more structured, evidenced-based approach following SCM principles. It also provided more clarity for services users, enabling them to be able to navigate the care system more effectively. The NWBH pathway is illustrated in Figure 6.1.

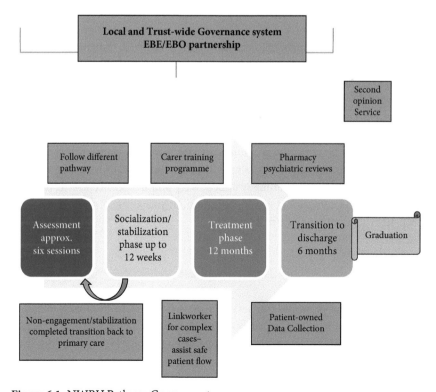

Figure 6.1 NWBH Pathway Components

Assessment phase

NWBH's pathway emphasizes the importance of the assessment process. The assessment process is seen as the start of the journey for the service user. The assessment (up to six sessions) involves several key components of which the diagnosis (semi structured assessment) is only one. Other key functions include: validating the service user's experiences, safety planning, identifying strengths and goals, formulation of needs, and involvement of family/carers.

The final part of the assessment process involves socialization to the pathway and models of treatment. The aim here is to promote understanding of the treatments offered, including what is expected of the service user and what to expect from services. Sometimes service users may not feel ready at the end of the assessment process to engage in the active treatment part of the pathway; in these cases the service user is referred to the socialization phase. All assessors have completed a generalist (SCM) and specialist training in personality disorder (dialectical behaviour therapy (DBT) or mentalization-based treatment (MBT)) and also a 2-day in house assessment training (covers therapeutic stance, SCID including threshold reliability).

Socialization phase

The socialization phase (up to 12 weeks) is the bridge between the assessment and starting therapy/treatment. In line with NICE guidance, the treatments offered for 'severe' BPD are multimodal, meaning group plus individual treatment. For many service users the prospect of group treatment provokes anxiety. The socialization phase addresses their concerns and fears about group work. Another important part of the socialization phase is developing safety plans, care plans and short- and long-term goals. *Note:* the pathway is linked to a stepped care approach; sometimes at the end of the assessment or socialization phase the service user and assessor concluded that the full programme is unnecessary and the service user is transitioned back to the community or offered group only therapy or offered a more appropriate therapy/treatment/pathway.

Treatment phase

All the treatment programmes (for service users who need the multimodal treatment) are the same length. The programmes on offer include a choice of at least two from SCM, MBT, or DBT. Although preparation for the programmes vary, the active treatment is 12 months. Service users then know how long they will be in active treatment. This gives them time to prepare for the ending as well as helping to keep them and their practitioner focused on the short- and long-term goals.

Transition phase

Endings and transitions can be difficult for service users, as discussed in Chapter 11 in this book. Consequently, all treatment programmes offer a 6-month transition phase. Within this phase, service users have continued access to the team and practitioner. They also have the option of taking three 'banked' (these can be planned or safety-driven appointments) sessions. These aim to support transition. For a service user who does not complete the assessment process or is unable to commit to the treatment programme, a safety plan is put in place. Ideally, this is completed with the service user. They will also be made aware that no judgement is made for not being able to participate in the programme at this time and they will be able to re-refer at any point in the future.

Graduation

At the end of treatment all service users are presented with a graduation certificate. This is an important acknowledgement of their effort and diligence in completing their intensive programme.

Linkworker

The Linkworker is a Personality Disorder-Trained Practitioner who specializes in working with people who have complex relational and emotional needs. This role provides the counterbalance to the very recovery-focused aspect of the pathway as well as supporting the system (in-Trust and wider system). The role includes:

- provision of an extended socialization phase for people who cannot engage in the programme and cannot be safely discharged back to their General Practitioner (GP).
- coordination of wider system working to help the system work more effectively with people diagnosed with BPD.

This roles is described in more detail in Chapter 14.

Carer training programme

The pathway acknowledges the needs of carers of people who meet the diagnostic criteria of BPD. The programme focuses on carers. It is co-delivered by a carer and a practitioner. The programme aims to educate carers about what a personality disorder is, how services work, and what treatments are available. The programme also offers a second phase of skills training which helps carers develop skills that will enable them to support the person in their care more effectively. The programme is delivered in a multi-carers group format. It involves education and peer support.

Patient-owned database

Evaluation of the treatment programmes involves using the Patient-Owned Database (POD) system. This is an electronic outcome monitoring system (via questionnaires). The difference with this system is that service users take responsibility themselves for completing the questionnaires. They can do this on their own tablet, computer, or phone. The key aspect of the database is that service users are able to see and monitor their own progress by looking at their graphs/scores, which promotes self-agency and motivation to work towards goal achievement.

Psychiatric and pharmacy reviews

The pathway offers the option of psychiatric and pharmacy reviews (including educational sessions about medication) to assess and treat any comorbid disorders as well as providing advice and guidance on medication. In particular, the aim is to support service users and the organization to use medication appropriately. This is covered in greater depth in Chapter 9.

Limitations of the pathway

Having a separate specialist pathway for borderline personality disorder has strengths and limitations. A major strength of having specialist practitioners is that service users on the pathway tend to get high-quality, consistent, and reliable care from a motivated workforce which believes in the model of care and is respectful of the service user. However, the limitations are that staff outside the pathway can feel deskilled at working with people diagnosed with BPD. The pathway can also have points of failure; for example, when staff are off sick or on maternity leave, limited cover is available and this significantly affects the care offered through the specialist pathway. Finally, use of the personality disorder diagnosis can lead some staff to see service users on the pathway as embodying a label such as 'BPD', and this prevents the organization and staff seeing the person behind the diagnosis.

Northamptonshire Healthcare NHS Foundation Trust

Northamptonshire Healthcare NHS Foundation Trust's (NHFT) pathway provides a structured and system-wide approach to providing high-quality and compassionate care to people diagnosed with personality disorder. Their ambition is to achieve a NICE standards-driven pathway that excels at delivering what service users and carers value, and actively seeks to enhance the capabilities and resilience of professionals across the pathway.

The pathway strives to enable practitioners to know 'what to do next', irrespective of service setting, and be guided by shared underlying principles of care that enable them and service users to evaluate the potential benefits and costs of particular treatment decisions and interventions critically.

NHFT's pathway has been informed by:

- A range of research and practice developments;
- Consultation with a range of stakeholders regarding important shared challenges and priorities;
- Building relationships with other NHS Trusts that clearly articulate the principles underpinning their pathways, actively support practitioners to engage in reflective practice, and strongly promote the needs of carers and supporters within the system;
- Valuing genuine co-production (between experts by experience and experts by occupation; EBE and EBO) as an essential component in improving services.

Local context

Since 2005, the Trust has had a countywide specialist personality disorder service (i.e. the Northants Personality Disorder Hub) that provides DBT, supervision and training to practitioners across general services, and coordinates and leads a range of pathway developments. The service also co-facilitates SCM in partnership with a range of colleagues within general mental health services and adopts a 'hub and spoke' model, placing linkworkers in all community mental health team (CMHT) localities.

Implementation: shared challenges and priorities

NHFT staff attended SCM training in 2015. At this time, there was a clear need for service development. For example, community mental health teams at the time tended to apply the Care Programme Approach (CPA) and coordinate care for individuals diagnosed with personality disorder. There were no limits set on duration of treatment, and interactions tended to be unstructured, crisis-driven, and were strongly influenced by the orientation of the practitioner offering individual sessions. In some in-patient areas there were also lengthy hospital admissions, with escalating levels of risk becoming a barrier to discharge. The specialist service provided 'awareness' and 'practitioner' level training, but this was not supported or maintained by ongoing supervision nor was it related to a broader strategy that was adopted across the services that staff returned to after training.

The process of change

In 2014, the Personality Disorder Hub adopted the strategy of continuing to provide DBT centrally whilst increasing the capabilities of other services within the system. This involved collaboratively offering an additional treatment programme within community mental health services, and delivering training backed up by ongoing supervision. The service adopted a hub and spoke model in which specialist practitioners were allocated a community locality and fulfilled a linkworker role. The initial aim was to make the service more accessible to a range of practitioners and to increase access to treatment (e.g. linkworkers assertively sought out referrals and identified service users whom teams felt presented them with challenges). This involved continuing to offer team formulation/consultation sessions locally, providing assessment in cases of team uncertainty/difficulty, and providing localized training. Via consultation with other Trusts, SCM was identified as a helpful unifying model and way of establishing a core set of principles and skills.

Early SCM practitioners and programmes benefited from operational managers who were proactive in attending training and peer supervision themselves, and planning and protecting SCM activities in the context of flexible patterns of activity and competing team demands. Alongside this, the Personality Disorder Hub endeavoured to model the principles of the approach with teams (e.g. validating needs whilst challenging passivity, expecting change whilst providing consistent and accessible sources of support, identifying core difficulties/barriers to implementation, and promoting problem-solving). The Hub also produced guidelines on structuring treatment intervention and a framework for facilitating reflective practice in peer supervision. Early implementation was also reinforced by countywide SCM strategy meetings/CPD sessions that brought localities together. Practitioner's motivation and development within SCM was also enhanced by taking up group facilitation roles and being informed of the shared outcomes and benefits of their practice (e.g. summaries of programme outcomes, POD (outcome) graphs demonstrating significant change).

The pathway has continued to receive support from senior managers and it has been helpful to link explicitly how changes in the pathway and the principles of the approach can help with a range of organizational issues/priorities (e.g. SCM training and further implementation was supported to decrease serious incidents, and avoidable and/or prolonged hospital admissions). This led to the Trust hosting a completely co-produced and co-attended Personality Disorder Strategy Day.

As outlined above by NWBH, increasing co-production with EBE and investing in this group has been important in promoting change in the pathway. The development of a Governance Group enabled 'high influence and high interest' stakeholders to have a direct impact on services. This has been facilitated by involvement from senior managers and actively approaching individuals identified in a 'stakeholder influence' mapping exercise.

NHFT pathway structure

NHFT's community treatment pathway takes the form of a stepped care model and access to interventions is largely determined by assessment of need, risk, and/ or complexity (see Figure 6.2).

4. Dialectical Behaviour Therapy

- Delivered by the Personality Disorder Hub and offering trauma-focused interventions during DBT
- A DBT-Adolescent programme is also provided to young people in CAMHS and mid-transition to adult services

3. Structured Clinical Management

- Co-delivered within each locality by the specialist service and CMHT practitioners (including psychologists)

2. Psychological Therapies

- Accessed within CMHT and offering a range of 1:1 approaches including CAT, Schema- and trauma-focused approaches

1. 18-Week DBT skills group

- Accessed via our Urgent Care and Assessment Team and available to people who have traditionally fallen through the gap between primary and secondary care services due to not meeting inclusion criteria

Figure 6.2 NHFT Pathway Structure: Interventions Available within Each Community Locality

The aim of the pathway is to enable service users to access and engage with a range of structured, evidence-based interventions. Whilst service user choice is a factor, and the pros and cons of particular approaches are discussed, SCM and DBT are particularly considered when we identify persistent, problematic, and pervasive difficulties associated with the diagnosis of BPD. In the pathway, DBT is considered when the individual is engaging in more frequent and severe forms of self-harm or risk behaviour, and/or reporting high levels of post-traumatic stress disorder (PTSD) symptoms or other strong interpersonal patterns (e.g. avoidance, dependence) that may inhibit their progress, or which have led to repeated break-downs in treatment with other therapeutic approaches.

Principles of the pathway

NHFTs overarching pathway is organized using the principles of SCM. Whilst these are common to a range of effective personality disorder therapies, having an approach that is accessible to all practitioners has led to a more rapid rate of system-wide change and embedded these principles more extensively in general mental health services. The large number of staff trained in the SCM approach are supported in their use of the principles to aid reflection and evaluate clinical decisions, allowing the majority to develop competencies in their own right and instigate further pathway innovations. System changes and skill development have benefited all interventions provided within the pathway and are not exclusive to the community SCM programme.

The primary principle that is emphasized is one where there is increasing access to evidence-based approaches with clear aims and principles of care. The approaches selected regard regular staff supervision as an integral component of what makes treatment effective. Traditional care coordination roles under the CPA are minimized and/or time-limited and focus on 'coordination' of agencies and interventions (if required) or decreasing barriers to engagement in the agreed evidence-based approach. In addition, the treatment approach sets a tone of high behavioural expectation and requires a high level of collaboration between practitioner and service user. This requires service users to be active contributors in developing meaningful short- and long-term goals, analysing events leading to unhelpful coping strategies and crisis-driven behaviour, applying new strategies, and working towards building relationships and opportunities outside services. Service users are also supported to leave secondary services at the end of an evidence-based intervention by discussing this early in the assessment and engagement phase of SCM.

Other principles focus on a 6-month ending/transition phase after the individual and group treatments have been completed, detailed safety planning, and

---

Box 6.1 Principles of NHFT SCM Pathway

- A primary emphasis on increasing access to evidence-based approaches with clear aims and principles of care.
- Our treatment approaches set a tone of high behavioural expectation and require a high level of collaboration between practitioner and service user.
- Our programmes also include a 6-month ending/transition phase.
- Service specific interventions (e.g. pharmacotherapy, acute risk management strategies) are evaluated in the context of the attachment model that informs SCM, and the pathway's overarching aim of enabling individuals diagnosed with EUPD to develop greater autonomy.
- The pathway promotes and values detailed safety planning and reflection on the causes of crises.
- Co-production of training and further pathway developments with service users and carers.
- Provision of a 12-week co-produced and co-delivered carers' skills group.
- Ensuring interventions provided within the crisis management component of the pathway adhere to the principles of SCM and NICE guidance.
- The pathway includes an in-patient linkworker whose role is to train other in-patient practitioners and model the use of particular SCM skills.

---

reflection on the causes of crises, establishing measures (e.g. SCID) to aid assessment, and work with carers and service users on how best to understand a person beyond the use of diagnosis. The principles on which the pathway is based are summarized in Box 6.1. These have contributed to increasing the effectiveness of the pathway and promoting change across the whole system.

Cumbria, Northumberland, Tyne & Wear (CNTW)

When Cumbria, Northumberland, Tyne & Wear (CNTW) Trust began the SCM Implementation Project in Community Treatment Teams (CTTs) there was already a proposed pathway for people with emotionally unstable personality disorder (EUPD) and a newly commissioned specialist Personality Disorder Hub team working throughout the Trust. The proposed pathway was based on the generic framework developed by Livesley (2003). Livesley's model is based on the following four principles:

- Knowledge of the structure/origins of personality disorder and evidence about what interventions work (*treatment efficacy*).

- The assumptions that the main features of personality disorder form a hierarchy of stability and change and treatment progresses through a *series of phases*.
- Those features *most susceptible to change* should be targeted first.
- Those features that are *most stable and difficult to change* should be targeted later (i.e. core self-identity and entrenched relational problems).

Based on these principles, Livesley outlined five phases of change through which a service user's journey may move, which are targeted by treatment interventions appropriate to that phase. The five phases are shown in Table 6.1.

Various treatment models were mapped against these five phases according to when the treatment model is likely to be most effective and at which point within the service user's care pathway it is best delivered, as shown in Figure 6.3.

Within the first three phases, SCM, DBT, and MBT are recommended since these evidence-based approaches are most suited to service users who present with high levels of instability, risk, and emotional dysregulation. It is only when sufficient stability and emotion regulation has been achieved that therapies such as cognitive behaviour therapy (CBT), eye-movement desensitization and reprocessing (EMDR), crisis assessment and treatment (CAT), and treatment-focused psychotherapy (TFP) are best offered. Similarly, service users are only referred to specialist individual therapies, such as psychodynamic psychotherapy, or structured therapies such as CBT, when their reflective ability or emotional stability have been improved and maintained in daily life. Clinical experience and research have shown that service users may deteriorate in these specialist therapies if they do not have sufficient emotion regulation or mentalizing skills and capacities to use the therapy to change (Bateman & Fonagy, 2004; Fonagy, 1989).

Table 6.1. Livesley's Phases of Change Model (Livesley, 2003, 2019)

Phases	Focus
1. Safety and crisis management	1. Unstable affects, crisis behaviour
	2. Unstable affects, crisis behaviour
2. Containment	3. Intense distress, self-harming behaviour and
3. Control and regulation	other symptoms, impulsivity
4. Exploration and change	4. Maladaptive schemas, interpersonal problems,
5. Synthesis	and effects of trauma.
	5. Identity problems, fragmented sense of self

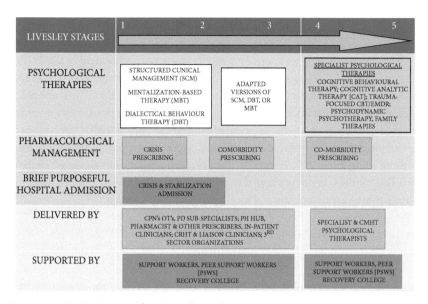

Figure 6.3 CNTW Personality Disorder Pathway

Psychological treatments offered in the pathway are delivered by practitioners who are specialist or partly specialist trained or who have generic mental health skills and are based within community mental health settings. These practitioners work closely, often jointly, with service users in allocating them to the most appropriate treatment model based on clinical assessment and resource availability. DBT and MBT are offered to a small number of people presenting with the most complex and high-risk difficulties by specialist practitioners, working within the hub but attached to each locality CTT offering 'scaffolding' to GPs. Scaffolding in this context refers to any activity which indirectly supports other practitioners in their work with the service user, and includes advice, support, and reformulation. This was generally well received but tended to be on an *ad hoc* basis with no consistent service model across different community teams.

Inevitably, access to appropriate services from experienced and trained practitioners for most people with a personality disorder diagnosis, or similar difficulties undiagnosed, was very limited. For service users in CTTs, treatments were often directed to managing comorbidities associated with personality disorder rather than addressing the problems associated with the primary diagnosis. CTT practitioners were doing the best they could using a generic care coordination approach. This often led to ineffective treatment over many years, continued high-risk behaviours, or discharge due to 'non-engagement' and 'inappropriate' use of services followed by rapid re-referral and reassessment due to ongoing crises.

Subspecialist practitioners

As a first step to offering an alternative model and a key component of the EUPD pathway, 'subspecialist practitioners', one community psychiatric nurse (CPN) and one occupational therapist (OT), were identified in each locality CTT. These practitioners had a specific interest in working with people with a personality disorder diagnosis and caseloads were capped at around 20. Subspecialist practitioners therefore had capacity to build their clinical expertise supported by strong links and scaffolding from the personality disorder hub practitioner allocated to their team. This model was not replicated in other localities in the Trust due to different commissioning arrangements and local operational differences.

Training

To address the lack of coordination between specialist services and general mental health services and the unskilled delivery of generalist treatment for people diagnosed with personality disorder, a programme of externally commissioned SCM training was offered to a number of senior psychological therapists who could act as supervisors in the new pathway. This was later developed through in-house training by a group of senior professionals highly skilled in treatment of people with personality disorder. Participants included psychologists, psychological therapists, Hub practitioners, CTT subspecialist CPNs and OTs, CTT clinical leads, and pathway managers, all of whom worked in the adult non-psychosis, older adults, or learning disabilities pathways.

Development of the pilot SCM service

Practitioners identified positively with the principles and practices of SCM following completion of the training programme and this became the first-line CTT intervention for people with a personality disorder presenting to adult generic mental health services. To determine whether it was feasible to implement both the individual and group components within current CTT resources, a pilot implementation site identified and a multi-professional steering group was formed including pathway managers and clinical leads from nursing, occupational therapy, and psychology professions as well as some 'subspecialist' practitioners. The Steering Group met monthly. Its core tasks are shown in Box 6.2.

Box 6.2 SCM Steering Group Tasks

- Identifying staff with job plans that included one day a week dedicated to SCM implementation. For the pilot, staff were the CTT subspecialists, a CTT psychologist, and a hub clinician.
- Development of referral criteria—this was to help practitioners identify people on their caseloads who might benefit best from the full service including individual and group components. It also allowed the service to move towards a needs-led rather than diagnosis-driven service.
- Development of an SCM information leaflet for referring practitioners and potential service users.
- Contributing to the development and revision of SCM individual and group workbooks for both service users and practitioners.
- Planning the pilot evaluation by identifying psychometrics, evaluation points, data gathering processes, storage, and analysis.
- Trouble shooting

The SCM pilot

Assessment and psychiatric review

Service users referred to the pilot first completed a thorough core assessment with the CTT. This often but not always included a psychiatric review. It was agreed with CTT psychiatrists that each service user accepted on to the SCM programme would receive at least one psychiatric review in accordance with NICE guidelines. As a result, some service users were seen for further sessions to review medication prescribed for co-occurring conditions whilst over time others reduced or stopped taking medication.

The socialization phase

This phase is undertaken in individual sessions and completed regardless of whether the person is then offered group work. In the pilot, this was offered by either a subspecialist or Hub practitioner but it became apparent over time that the work is within the skill set of anyone who had completed SCM training. The socialization phase lasts about 3 months, although there is some flexibility for service users who may require further work before beginning a group. The tasks of this phase are shown in box 6.3.

Sometimes the prospect of group work is daunting for a service user, an issue which is also addressed during the socialization phase.

Box 6.3 SCM Socialization Phase—Key Tasks

- Assess the person's willingness to engage in treatment
- Develop a co-produced formulation using the 5P + Plan model
- Develop co-produced intervention goals
- Develop co-produced safety and crisis management plans
- Share information and understanding around the diagnosis
- Introduce grounding skills

Treatment phase

The treatment phase lasts between 6 and 18 months depending on service user clinical need and comprises several components, as shown in Box 6.4.

Although the SCM group is essentially a problem-solving, skills-based group, important relationships are formed between participants over the treatment phase. The supportive nature of these relationships has been a key aspect in the positive therapeutic experience for service users, but at times there have been complex

---

Box 6.4 SCM Treatment Components

- An individual session for up to 60 mins per week which attends to both SCM and care coordination tasks.
- Group therapy for 90 mins once per week. Group cycles last for 6 months and service users are encouraged to attend for a minimum of two group cycles (12 months). Service users occasionally ask to attend a third cycle and this can be accommodated.
- Psychiatric review.
- Peer supervision/preparation for group facilitators for 2 hours per week. This includes preparation and debrief for the SCM group. In the pilot this was led by a clinical psychologist. In the roll-out this was led by any of the group facilitators.
- Psychodynamic supervision—monthly group supervision from a psychodynamic psychotherapist for SCM practitioners offering group work, exploring dynamics in the service user group and clinical team. This was not part of the agreed overall EUPD pathway or SCM model, but a locally agreed support structure.

dynamics to negotiate between group members and between service users and clinical staff. Monthly psychodynamic supervision is an additional optional element of the SCM programme assisting the SCM team to understand the relational dynamics and seek resolution to problematic aspects with service users empathically. This occurred in one locality only, based on local interest and capacity.

Achievement certificates

Certificates of completion are given out at the last session of every group cycle (6 months) and acknowledge the work that the service user has achieved through regularly attending and working in the group programme.

Work in individual sessions

Throughout the group programme, service users meet with their care coordinator who is usually also one of their SCM group facilitators. Tasks for individual sessions are shown in box 6.5.

Transition and ending stage
This stage is for consolidation of skills and consideration of options following the end of treatment such as vocational work, referral for specific therapies not addressed through standard SCM (e.g. trauma-focused interventions), Recovery College, or discharge from services. The ending phase typically lasts between 3 and 6 months and requires careful handling. There are sometimes limited vocational

---

Box 6.5 SCM Individual Sessions—Key Tasks

- Care coordination
- Review individualized group homework and group participation
- Problem-solve any group issues
- Problem-solve any additional problems
- Revise/update formulation
- Other work, as per individual SCM—update safety/crisis plans, family involvement, advocacy, pharmacy, etc.
- Review progress

options and the transition to other provider organizations will be carefully negotiated. Recently, the options have been enhanced by employment support practitioners recruited to and based in CTTs. 'Endings' need to be addressed including the bitter/sweet nature of reflecting on what has been achieved whilst acknowledging the sadness involved in saying 'goodbye'.

Occasionally during the group a service user is unable to maintain 75% attendance of the individual and group sessions combined, due to events outside of their control. This can be addressed, often successfully, in an individual session taking a problem-solving approach to resolve any obstacles preventing their attendance at the programme. Service users are given a number of sessions to achieve appropriate resolution. On occasion, if it is not possible to resolve the difficulties and following discussion with the person, a decision is made about whether they leave the programme, be referred for alternative treatment options, or be discharged from services. The person is encouraged to return to the programme when they are more able to commit to the requirements. For the few people who do defer, most return at a later date.

Roll out and maintaining fidelity to the model

Evaluation

Evaluation of the pilot programme and first group cycle in one locality was very positive. Psychometric measures indicated that service users were making progress. Focus group evaluations were even more positive from both service users and participating practitioners. All service users commented that they had found the group valuable, that they had made positive life changes as a result, and that they would recommend the group to others. Particularly valued topics were mentalizing and understanding attachment. Group facilitators commented on enjoying and valuing this part of their working week. There were no hospital admissions of service users during the programme and gains made during treatment were maintained over time.

Training

Since their initial training, CTT practitioners and Hub workers have continued to deliver the 3-day basic training within their own localities. This occurs usually twice a year and all new staff are encouraged to attend. More recently, the training is being co-delivered by SCM programme graduates who are either registered as trust volunteers or employed as peer support workers.

All practitioners offering group work complete a 2-day training course offered by the Trust's personality disorders lead and experienced SCM group facilitators.

They also complete one 6-month cycle as an apprentice before co-facilitating further groups themselves. More recently, the training has been converted to 3 days, covering both basic and advanced skills in running groups, based on the SCM UK National Curriculum (HEE, 2020).

Supervision

In addition to the supervision provided for the group programme, clinical leads are trained in SCM and provide clinical supervision to all staff delivering individual work. The Hub team have developed a SCM competencies checklist to aid self-reflection and supervision discussions. Hub practitioners continue to provide scaffolding to CTT practitioners through monthly 'Share, Learn, and Do' (peer supervision) groups.

Steering groups

The pilot steering group meets bi-monthly to ensure the local group programme is maintained by trouble-shooting difficulties such as staffing reductions, and supervision and training requests, and the group contributes to Trust-wide SCM developments, including developing service user co-produced resources. Local implementation groups are replicated in other localities and there is now also a Trust-wide SCM implementation group so that learning from all localities is shared and standard principles followed in implementation of the pathway as a whole.

Carer and family work

Families of service users open to the Hub have access to a carers' group. However, there is no routine access to carer and family support from CTTs. This work is currently being developed within the Trust and in partnership with local carer forums. See Figure 6.4 for CNTW SCM pathway.

Three SCM-UK Models Compared

The three SCM-UK pathways outlined in this chapter have been compared (see Table 6.2). The basic components in terms of structure, focus, phases, and links to other services are mostly similar with minor variations. All three pathways have a clear structure, with careful phasing of the treatment pathway. All pathways provide group SCM and some family- and carer-structured skills-based interventions. Service users and carers are involved in co-producing and delivering the pathways. Medication management is an area of development of all three pathways, even though prescribing guidelines had been produced in one pathway, but integration and adherence to guidelines requires further work. A final area in need

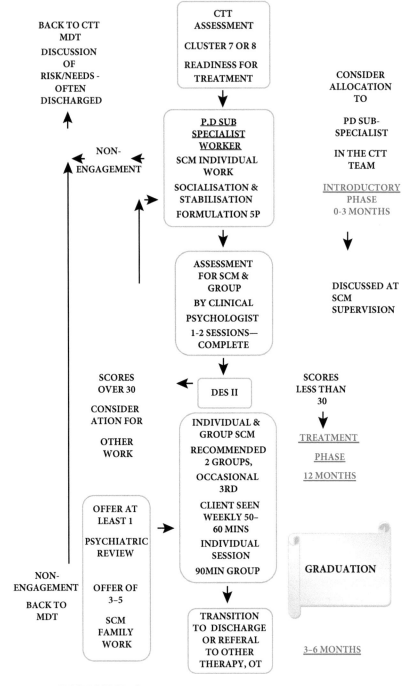

Figure 6.4 CNTW SCM Pathway

of development in all three pathways is occupational and vocational functioning. This was an area of impairment of many service users, and some pathways made some developments with third sector partner and employment specialists but further work is needed to ensure gains are developed in functioning in daily life.

Crucial to the successful development and operation of the SCM pathway is the strategic and operational support provided by the host organization. There are many factors that are required for any organizational change. These 'enablers' are essential for the SCM programmes and pathways to succeed. They require continual support and organizational commitment in order to sustain them. All three pathways had some committed degree of organizational support, including operational management. This was not clear at the start in two pathways, but gained momentum as they became more established, and demonstrated efficacy. There was strong leadership in all three pathways, including a specialist personality disorder lead clinician or specialist service lead. Service user groups were well engaged in all three pathways, and all received external SCM training in the early stages of development of their pathways. Staff identified to implement the pathways all had clear roles and some protected time that was dedicated to their pathway work, but this needed further protection as staff leave and services came under pressure. These enablers have been summarized in Table 6.3.

The operational aspects of these pathways require clear governance structures, systems, and procedures. All three pathways had developed a governance group for monitoring the effectiveness of the pathway, which includes service users. There was regular in-house training, which is refreshed with updates and training for managers and pathway leads. Clinical supervision was established in all three pathways on a weekly basis, including team and peer supervision in one pathway. Outcome measures were used in all three pathways, but these were different in each and require further refinement and greater consistency in use, including the use of the health service utilization data. Finally, there was standard operating and pathway procedure guidance in all three pathways in place. These governance enablers are summarized in Table 6.4.

Table 6.2 Three SCM-UK Pathways Compared

Model	NWBH	NHFT	CNTW
Structured programme with clear model and philosophy	Yes	Yes	Yes
Informed by NICE guidelines	Yes	Yes	Yes
Timed care	Yes	Yes	Yes
Diagnostically informed	Yes, but not diagnostically driven	Yes, but not a requirement to access the pathway	Yes, but diagnosis not required, based on needs and formulation
Formulation-driven care	Partial as there is an option for formulation-driven care	Partial—more so available within psychological therapies and DBT	Yes, everyone has a CTT 5ps and plan formulation in the first instance
Stepped care	Partial	Yes	Only between CTT and hub for a small number of SUs with more complex needs.
Socialization stage	Yes	Yes	Yes
Assessment stage	Yes	Yes	Yes
Group involvement	Yes	Yes	Yes
Multi-modal option	Yes	Yes	SCM only in CTTs.
Structured Ending/ Transition	Yes	Yes	Yes
Family programme	Yes	Yes	Partial Carer's programme for service users open to the hub. Family sessions on a needs-led basis for service users in CTTs but it is hoped to offer this to all service users in due course.
Leaflets	Yes	Yes	Yes

Table 6.2 *Continued*

Model	NWBH	NHFT	CNTW
Care coordination	No, but link workers can work with people who don't fit in pathway	Partial and determined based on factors impacting on engagement	Yes, all service users are allocated a care coordinator or lead professional who is usually also a group facilitator.
EBE involvement in programme	Partial	Limited to education sessions	Partial and developing for resource development, training, and evaluation
Linkworker	Yes	Yes	Yes, between the hub and CTTs
Effective medication management	Partial—could have more integration with psychiatry	No and in development	Partial—more integration with SCM and adherence to prescribing guidance needed
Graduation	Yes	No	Yes
Encourage active participation from SU	Yes	Yes	Yes
Easy in, Easy out	Partial due to capacity but want to achieve this	Yes	Partial Yes, for those enrolled on the programme. Capacity issues mean there are potentially people who would like to be enrolled on the full programme receiving individual SCM only.
Systemic therapy	No – looking to pilot this	No	Partial but not available to everyone
Focus on occupational/vocative outcomes	More needs to be done on this aspect	Yes, in the form of early referral to locality-based Employment Specialists	Yes, through relationships with partner organizations and more recently employment specialists based in CTTs

Table 6.3 Organizational Enablers: Three SCM-UK Pathways

Organization enablers	NWBH	NHFT	CNTW
Organizational support	Yes	Yes	Yes
Operational support	Yes	Yes	Yes
Key systematic operational direction for the pathway	Yes, it was a high Trust objective	Yes, operational direction supported by Senior Managers and Commissioners	Yes
Transformational support	Had transformational support as part of a Trust transformational project— protected time from lead clinician	Partial	Yes, but not initially accepted as part of wider transformational project, until it was later 'owned' in collaboration with operations
Strong clinical leadership (clear vision and model) with designated role	Yes	Yes	Yes
Specialist personality disorder lead/service	Yes	Yes	Yes
Positive engagement with service users	Yes, Trust has a comprehensive involvement programme	Yes	Yes
External training	Yes, SCM, MBT, and DBT	Yes	Yes
Established specialist treatment (MBT/DBT, etc.)	Yes	Yes	Yes, but new to MBT
Multidisciplinary involvement	Yes	Yes	Yes
Specialist roles	Yes (specialist protective roles rather than generic)	Yes	Yes
Clear job plans for staff working on pathway	Yes, clear linkworker and SCM practitioner job plans	Yes, and requires ongoing maintenance in general services	Yes, but requires further clarification and protection of roles
Pragmatism in approach implementation	Yes	Yes	Yes
Co-produced and co-owned pathway	Yes	Yes	Yes, mostly

Table 6.4 Governance Enablers: Three SCM-UK Pathways

Governance enablers	NWBH	NHFT	CNTW
Governance board for monitoring the pathway	Yes, monthly governance board meeting and local implementation teams	Yes, bimonthly Trust-wide co-attended meeting with themed implementation subgroups	Yes, monthly Personality and Complex trauma (PACT) Network and bimonthly Trust-wide SCM Implementation Group
Engagement with service users in governance	Yes	Yes	Yes
Regular training, internal and external	Yes, SCM training in house plus biannually updates in assessment/SCM pathway work	Yes	Yes, SCM training in-house, with basic plus group training and 1-day training for Managers and Pathway Leads
Supervision system	Yes—weekly peer	Yes, weekly peer supervision and monthly SCM supervisors meeting	Yes, weekly peer supervision or 'Share, Learn, and Do' groups and monthly SCM supervisors meeting
Audit process	Yes—POD	Yes, POD and service utilization data analysed	Yes, but ad hoc. Inconsistent measures used. Aiming to use POD and collect further service utilization data.
Personality Disorder Policy/procedure	Yes, Personality Disorder Pathway Procedure	Partial, a range of Standard Operating Procedures across the pathway	Yes, pathway procedures and guidance in place.

Conclusion

The three pathways presented in this chapter are examples of what an SCM-based pathway can look like. What is evident from these programmes are the similarities in the 'key enablers' that appeared to have helped with their successful implementation. These enablers came from many areas within the three organizations and across the wider health and social care system. Of key importance is the organizational support, transformation assistance, strong clinical expertise and leadership, a non-protectionist approach to care, a 'team' approach to model development, a culture of working 'with' rather than 'to' service users, and having people who believe in the model and service users' ability to change delivering the care.

SCM was central to all these programmes and provided a helpful framework in which to facilitate whole system cultural change for working with people diagnosed with BPD/complex relational and emotional needs.

SCM enables organizations to develop an organized structured care pathway that can provide clear direction to both practitioners and service users. The experience of these three UK mental health organizations has been that the structure that SCM provides with its relational focus and empowerment of generalist mental health practitioners not only improves the care offered to people diagnosed with BPD but also leads to developments in other areas of organizational change, such as diagnosis, care coordination, and safety planning and management.

References

Dale, O., Sethi, F., Stanton, C., Evans, S., Barnicot, K., Sedgwick, R., … Moran, P. (2017). Personality disorder services in England: findings from a national survey. *British Journal of Psychiatry Bulletin, 41*(5), 247–253.

Davies, J., Sampson, M., Beesley, F., Smith, D., & Baldwin, V. (2014). An evaluation of knowledge and understanding framework personality disorder awareness training: can a co-production model be effective in a local NHS Mental Health Trust? *Personality and Mental Health, 8*(2) 161–168.

MIND. (2018). *The consensus statement for people with complex mental health difficulties who are diagnosed with a personality disorder.* London: MIND.

NICE. (2009). *Borderline personality disorder: treatment and management.* London: NICE.

7

Models of SCM Implementation: Europe

Helga Aalders, Peder Björling, and Niki Sundström

Introduction

It is well known that specialized treatments for borderline personality disorder (BPD), such as dialectical behaviour therapy (DBT) and mentalization-based treatment (MBT), are not widespread enough to provide treatment for all people presenting to services with that diagnosis (Ileakis, Sonley, Lagan, & Choi-Kain, 2019). Generalist approaches to treating service users diagnosed with BPD, such as structured clinical management (SCM) and good psychiatric management (GPM), demand less training, are more flexible in how treatment is delivered, and can be adapted to local conditions more readily. In this chapter, we will describe how implementation and adaptation of these generalist approaches was made in a Dutch and a Swedish setting. In both countries, the SCM treatment caters for people diagnosed with personality disorder, not exclusively BPD, and have integrated SCM into a range of treatments provided.

SCM in Sweden

The Personality Disorders Program at Karolinska Huddinge

The Personality Disorders Program (PDP) is one of the programmes at the Psychiatric Clinic of Karolinska University Hospital of Huddinge in Sweden. The clinic is situated in south-west Stockholm and has a catchment area of 250,000 inhabitants. The clinic's programmes are based on diagnostic groups such as affective disorders, anxiety syndrome, psychosis, trauma, and obsessive-compulsive disorder.

The PDP's mission is to assess and treat people with suspected or diagnosed personality disorder, provide expert support to the other programmes, and to collaborate with the in-patient ward specialized in treating diagnosed personality disorder. The PDP aims to provide effective evidence-based care and treatment for a large number of service users diagnosed with personality disorder. When there is no evidence-based treatment available, treatment comes from a sound theoretical framework and expert consensus. The treatment is aimed at increasing functioning and reducing distress and emotional suffering.

The PDP currently has about 250 ongoing service users and receives about 150 referrals yearly. Since demand for the PDP is greater than its capacity, there is a waiting list for the program. The PDP is staffed by 20 people and is open during office hours. The SCM clinical team consists of two psychologists, two counsellors, two case managers, a nurse, and two psychiatrists.

Implementing SCM at a Swedish psychiatric clinic

Until 2016, the only specific care for service users diagnosed with personality disorder was an MBT team consisting of six people who treated about 45 service users. Prior to the reorganization of the whole mental health services into diagnosis-based programmes, plans were developed to organize an out-patient service user clinic for people diagnosed with BPD. However, it was agreed to extend the assignment to cover service users diagnosed with any personality disorder because boundaries between personality disorder–not specified and BPD are vague and people diagnosed with personality disorders other than BPD can also benefit from structured investigation and treatment.

In the years preceding the start of the programme, we had been interested in generalist treatment of BPD. In particular, service users treated in SCM and GPM were noted to show positive changes in research studies when compared to MBT (Bateman & Fonagy, 2009) and DBT (McMain et al., 2009, McMain, Guimond, Cardish, Streiner, & Links, 2012). Since evidence for treatment for personality disorders other than BPD and antisocial personality disorder (ASPD) is limited, a generalist method, based on personality disorder general criteria and utilizing existing expertise at our clinic, was chosen. The aim was to utilize the expertise that active practitioners already had, help them develop it further, and adapt it to the service user group.

An important factor in obtaining resources to start an SCM team was generating a structured and deliberate proposal for management. The proposal contained several parts. First, it contained a summary of the current state of evidence regarding the treatment of personality disorder. Second, a rationale for generalist treatment being a good complement to pre-existing specific treatment (MBT) was presented. Third, a description of SCM for BPD was based on the first manual (Bateman & Krawitz, 2013). Fourth, an overview of the prevalence of personality disorders at our clinic and a description of how an SCM team of eight practitioners could be responsible for about 125 service users diagnosed with personality disorder was offered. The clinic management team approved a budget for our choice of SCM as method of treatment.

In order for the internal organization of the SCM team to function, support from clinical management was needed. The SCM team needs to have a clearly formulated mission and at the same time be given time to develop its internal organization and methods based on the needs, evidence, and the experience and competence of the staff members. The combination of a clear framework and flexibility is important not only in the SCM team but in the whole programme. As the organization within which the SCM team operates undergoes change, it was important for the SCM team management to highlight to management how the SCM work is affected by changes. This included, for example, changes in remuneration models, assessment methods, working methods, or meeting work schedule-related guidelines.

When hiring staff, we sought out individuals with both the interest and the capability to treat service users diagnosed with personality problems and from the start of this diagnosis; SCM was to be delivered by a multidisciplinary team. There were no other SCM teams in Sweden on which to base the model. The training before the start-up of the SCM team consisted of 2 days with SCM practitioners from the United Kingdom. Further skill development uses internal training time to self-educate in the method, both from the SCM manual and from scientific articles or literature when needed, and visiting experts to discuss SCM development. New staff learned about SCM from working with co-therapists and by internal training and supervision.

In-patient ward staff who specialized in the treatment of personality disorders are offered training by the SCM team. The course teaches basic information about assessing personality disorder, the therapeutic stance, how to work in teams, and using a care plan and a safety plan. The aim is for in-patient staff to recognize and understand people diagnosed with personality disorder and for them to integrate the in-patient admission with the SCM therapeutic approach being delivered by the SCM team when service users are admitted to the ward. The ward now integrates their safety plan and care plan with those of the SCM programme.

Key factors in implementing SCM

When planning implementation of SCM a number of key factors were identified. The first is a common approach to personality disorders. The second is the organization of the programme. The way the programme is organized must create conditions for service users to receive effective treatment. There needs to be a level of competence and stability in the staff and a distinct structure for the practitioners to work within if they are to be able to use their expertise skilfully.

Several elements supported the structure and working of the SCM-team. The PDP has a flat organizational structure including managers who have years of experience working with specialized treatment for people diagnosed with BPD.

Having available senior team members to act as leaders is important both for developing staff skills and for maintaining team morale in difficult situations. Teamwork is an important part of how the work itself is structured. Working in teams allows the practitioner to ask for help when needed. Teamwork can also serve as a platform for independent therapeutic work and provide the opportunity to learn from others. Decisions within the SCM team are made at the treatment multidisciplinary team level and conference. This applies to all treatment-related decisions. An important aspect is that multiple professions participate. Knowing that decisions about treatment need to be reconciled at a treatment conference provides the practitioner the chance to examine aspects of important decisions with the service user, and increases the opportunity for practitioners, also the less experienced, to work independently and learn from more experienced staff. Finally, a distinct treatment structure is offered to service users. Diagnostic investigation, psycho-educational course, care plan, emergency plan, and treatment are well described to both practitioners and service users. This creates predictability and prepares service user and practitioners for the end of treatment. A clear structure also makes it easier to discover when and how individual adjustments need to be made.

Experience of implementing SCM in a Swedish context

The PDP started in 2016. In addition to the existing four MBT groups, there are now four SCM groups that provide 12 months of SCM according to the manual (Bateman & Krawitz, 2013).

A brief 3-month version of SCM that service users can choose or be assigned to has also been developed. For example, a pregnant service user could get a full 3-month treatment rather than having to interrupt a longer treatment due to childbirth. The shorter treatment can also be chosen by or suggested to highly motivated service users with less severe problems. It may also be offered to those with low motivation and those whose clinical assessment suggested were unlikely to be able to stay in treatment for 12 months such as service users who had unstable psychosocial conditions, such as housing problems or ongoing domestic violence. In such cases, the goal can be for them to enter SCM or MBT after their social problems are more stable. For the majority of the service users, however, the goal of SCM for 3 months is for the service user to receive a programmed intervention that allows discharge from the psychiatric services upon completion. The 3-month version of SCM contains the same modules as 12-month SCM. The main difference is that the group is closed, meaning service users start and finish treatment at the same time. A general impression from practitioners is that the 3-month version is more intense, although the frequency of visits is the same as the 12-month version. Since the experiences of service users and practitioners were generally positive, the service has continued. So far, eight 3-month SCM treatments have been completed. A small number of those service users have later entered a 12-month SCM treatment or MBT.

An SCM 'summer group' runs over the summer holidays. In this group, individual contact is not necessary. The summer group is used to provide a structured treatment for service users who for various reasons are not in MBT or SCM and have difficulties managing when their regular practitioner is on holiday. This group has also allowed a few service users who study/work in other areas of Sweden to have treatment while they are back in Stockholm during the school/university break.

About 100 service users have completed either the long or short version of SCM treatment. Since the start of the programme, one service user has committed suicide. The service user was in assessment and had not yet entered treatment. Raw data on hospitalization show that service users had six times more days as an in-patient the year before treatment started compared to after starting SCM treatment.

The SCM programme method works as expected for service users diagnosed with BPD. The clinical impression is that treatment in SCM is helpful, that service users tend to like the method, and describe that they can use different aspects of the treatment. They are positive about the combination of group and individual therapy, meeting other service users, the content of the psycho-education, and reflective discussions on themes. We see similar results for service users diagnosed with other personality disorders. SCM is easier to implement for BPD since the method and the manual was developed for this service user group. Adjustments to the content is required to fit a wider group of service users.

Experience so far has been that there are advantages to having groups with mixed diagnoses. All service users diagnosed with personality disorder have difficulty in relationships and managing emotions, expressed in different ways. It is rewarding for service users to share the experience of others; for example a service user diagnosed with avoidant personality disorder wishes they could express affect in the same way as another group member diagnosed with BPD. A service user who routinely gets into problems because of impulsivity might envy the avoidant group member who withdraws in a conflict. Many service users have in common that they have difficulty mentalizing others when they are under stress. When it comes to problem-solving skills, different perspectives can help service users dare to try things that other service users suggest.

The theme of impulsivity has been more complicated to adapt. Many service users diagnosed with avoidant personality disorder do not recognize the typical examples of impulsivity. Our solution has been to talk about impulses and behaviours. Service users who present as avoidant can often give examples of withdrawing or avoiding something in an impulsive way such as cancelling an activity, skipping a social event, or going the other way when seeing an acquaintance in the street. That can be a common ground for conversation in a group where others have impulses to do or say something.

By having mixed groups some difficulties are avoided. Having mostly service users who are avoidant in the same group is difficult. There can be long silences that can be difficult to break. Several service users diagnosed with Narcissistic Personality Disorder (NPD) present other challenges; for example, they gravitate towards being the 'perfect' service user. This affects the climate in the group and makes it difficult for other perspectives to be allowed. It can also be difficult to share time and focus between service users in a group when many of them are diagnosed with NPD.

Another experience of SCM is the focus on work or employment early in the treatment. In Swedish psychiatry, there has been a tendency for long and sometimes quite undefined support contacts which is rarely helpful for service users diagnosed with personality disorder. There has been a clear risk of medicalization and a risk of service users being adversely affected by the care provided. A focus for service development and SCM implementation has therefore been how to work with ending treatment.

It is important that service users are aware of the timed (time-limited) nature of treatment from the very beginning and that it is planned that most people will be able to manage without specialist psychiatric contact when treatment has been completed. Service users are informed that they can re-refer later if a major threat to safety appears or if a situation arises where they may need psychiatric intervention again. The aim at the start of the programme is that all service users should have an end date set when they started treatment. This is an ambitious goal, which has not been fully met, but there is a steady in-flow and out-flow of service users. Fewer service users than anticipated return after completion of treatment. This applies both to service users who terminated after 3 months and 12 months of treatment. In accordance with a focus on ending treatment, practitioners work hard to ensure that service users have a comprehensive and useful safety plan following discharge. The idea is that the safety plan promotes self-agency and a sense of security as the service user is discharged from psychiatry.

Returning service users

When the programme started, it was anticipated that a proportion of service users who were discharged after 12 months of SCM would return fairly soon in connection with a safety issue or comorbid mental illness, particularly because many of them had been in services for a considerable time before commencing SCM. However, few service users have returned. Nor have they applied for other programmes at the clinic. Those service users who telephoned reception were offered quick appointments at the clinic for two to six 'safety visits' where the safety plan was used and updated. In some cases, this could be done solely by phone. For a few service users who had shown significant improvement from SCM or MBT at the end of treatment, the gains were not maintained and safety interventions were not enough, so they were assigned to a 3-month SCM group and were again discharged after that. In general, service users who complete SCM for three or 12 months do well after treatment. Service users who are re-referred to the programme after being discharged are the ones that never entered SCM treatment due to lack of motivation, comorbid substance abuse, or other factors.

SCM in the Netherlands

From SCM to GIT–PD (Guideline-informed Treatment–Personality Disorders)

Similar to other countries, in recent years in the Netherlands attempts have been made to develop generalist treatment for personality disorders. This has resulted in GIT–PD (Guideline Informed Treatment–Personality Disorders), developed in 2015 by the Dutch Expertise Centre Personality Disorders (ECPD) (Kaasenbrood, Hutsebaut, & Bunningen, 2015). The ECPD was founded in 2010 by 12 general mental health institutions in the Netherlands with the goal of enhancing the treatment of personality disorders.

GIT–PD is not a manual but a framework very much in line with and partly based on SCM (Bateman & Krawitz, 2013) and GPM) (Choi-Kain & Gunderson, 2019), both of which have been shown to be effective. The ideas of Andrew Chanen (Chanen, 2009) and John Livesley (Livesley, Dimaggio, & Clarkin, 2017) on effective treatment for personality disorders in general have influenced the GIT–PD framework (Kaasenbrood et al., 2015). The reason the ECPD chose a GIT–PD framework and not a manual is to allow the mental health institutions to develop and implement the guideline in line with their own organization's 'culture' and history. At the time of writing, already 20 institutions have their own variety of GIT–PD. Of course, there are significant dangers to this approach as services may adapt treatments to make them fit a pathological service culture so the GIT–PD framework requires services to meet essential non-changeable criteria for implementation.

In this section, we will describe how the Department of Personality Disorders of Mental Health Institution Altrecht developed GIT–PD into a manual and the implementation of this in six GIT–PD teams in different regions of Utrecht (with a total of 1,200 service users and 75 practitioners). The GIT–PD manual is mostly based on SCM principles, supplemented with already known modules in Emotion-Regulation (STEPPS), Self-Esteem (COMETT), and mindfulness-based treatments. In the book *GIT–PD in de Praktijk* (*GIT–PD in daily practice*), the manual and the process of implementation are described (Aalders & Hengstmengel, 2019).

The Position of GIT–PD within the Total Treatment Programme of the Department of Personality Disorders Altrecht

In the region of Utrecht there are a lot of institutions and independent practitioners who offer treatment to service users diagnosed with personality disorder. Mental Health Institution Altrecht is aimed at service users with a broad spectrum of severe personality problems and referral there thus is usually as a last resort. The service users in our department already have had one or more treatments that were not effective, mostly due to multiple comorbidities and a high level of dysfunction. Most of the service users suffer from (chronic) suicidality and/or self-harming patterns of coping.

In our department of personality disorders (2,500 service users and 180 practitioners), we divide care into three forms of treatment. There are two out-patient programs: AMBIT (adaptive mentalization based integrative treatment: Bevington, Fuggle, Cracknell, & Fonagy, 2017) for service users with the most severe forms of personality disorders (very low epistemic trust and disorganized attachment), and GIT–PD for quite severe forms of personality problems (low to medium epistemic trust and anxious-ambivalent and avoidant attachment). The in-patient user programs (intensive/time-limited) based on schema-focused therapy (service users diagnosed with borderline/narcissistic problems) and affect phobia therapy (avoidant and obsessive-compulsive personality disorders) are for service users who can tolerate and need high-intensity treatment.

The GIT–PD manual

The GIT–PD treatment is divided into four phases:

- The pre-treatment phase
- The contract phase
- The treatment phase
- The 'outflow' phase

The pre-treatment phase

Service users who are referred are invited to make use of our pre-treatment e-health platform. On this platform they can find psycho-education about personality disorders, information about the different treatment programmes, and self-help modules on, for instance, sleeping disturbances, lifestyle, and addiction. They can also find contact details for social care services, information for family members, and a pre-intake form.

The contract phase (6–12 weeks)

The most important goal of the contract phase is to get to know the service user and his/her problems. The establishment of a relationship of trust and safety is of paramount importance. All practitioners are well trained in relation management and the specific treatment attitude (clinical stance) for personality disorders.

The contract phase also serves the purpose of developing an integrated view of the mental, somatic, and social problems of the service user. A diagnosis is made including an evaluation of severity, and an assessment made of the service user's functional deficits, level of risk, social environment, status of work, personal history, longitudinal course of the disorder, and treatment history. Finally, a case conceptualization from a multidisciplinary perspective is drawn up along with treatment goals, all based on shared decision-making.

Treatment goals are formulated around SMART goals: Specific, Measurable, Achievable, Realistic, and anchored within a Time frame. Problems are linked to repetitive patterns of maladaptive behaviours. In the treatment plan, goals are prioritized, interventions are described, there is a description of 'who is doing what', and of how treatment is to be evaluated, for example which instruments are used when. Psychological treatment goals are specified using the most important characteristics of personality disorders: emotion regulation, self-esteem, impulsivity or lack of it (e.g. suicidality versus sudden withdrawal), and interpersonal sensitivity.

The treatment phase (12–24 months)

In the treatment phase, at least two practitioners from the multidisciplinary team (psychologist, psychiatrist, caseworkers, art therapist, or psychomotor therapist) are involved. They choose a specific strategy to treat the complaints and symptoms of the service user. In fact, it does not matter which strategy is chosen as long as it is a well-described, generally accepted intervention that is agreed with the service user and executed systematically with fixed points of evaluation. When it is possible, there is a preference for group treatment over individual treatment. The group offers members the opportunity to learn from each other, the notion they are not the only individual with these kind of problems, and a healing environment to develop awareness of unhelpful patterns and to practise change behaviour.

A substantial part of the treatment is also to work with important others like family and friends and with social organizations to support living, work, and social relationships. The transfer and generalization of treatment effect to the service user's own life needs ongoing attention and support.

During treatment there is a permanent focus on monitoring the therapeutic relationship. Ruptures of the relationship are repaired before continuing therapy.

In fact, the repairing itself may be considered therapy (Kaasenbrood et al., 2015). Practitioners also have to monitor treatment progress at pre-agreed set times, preferably together with important others such as family members. In case of treatment impasse and/or no change, reasons are sought and analysed. If necessary, the treatment plan is adjusted.

Termination of treatment ('outflow') phase

Termination is not the easiest part of the treatment. Both service users and practitioners experience the termination of treatment as complicated. The difficulty of stopping treatment is generally related to three factors: attachment, hope, and trust. It is important to take time and attend to the specified elements of this last part of the treatment. In GIT–PD, we developed a module aimed specifically at this difficulty. First, by starting this module we are setting the scene/stage and emphasizing that the treatment will stop at a set time, and second, in meeting's attention is paid only to those topics that make the ending of treatment a success. No new treatment goals are added at this point.

The module contains elements of relapse prevention training, acceptance and commitment therapy, and working together with the network. An offer of short booster sessions is available if necessary.

Implementation of GIT–PD

Over a decade ago, services were increasingly confronted with many service users diagnosed with severe personality disorders in daily mental health practice, with no appropriate treatments available. The most important reasons for this were limited capacity of care and strict entry criteria to include service users for psychotherapy. Service users who could not easily commit to specialist treatment standards were often excluded from the four available psychotherapy treatments (solutions-focused therapy (SFT), MBT, DBT, transference-focused psychotherapy (TFP)). To address these issues, an SCM pilot team was formed called 'On Board'. Service users diagnosed with severe personality disorders who were excluded from the standard psychotherapy treatments joined the 'On Board' programme. After a few months it turned out to be a success. Service users, their close relatives, and also the team members of the On Board team were very enthusiastic. The result was that many service users were quickly registered with the On Board team. The team was almost unable to handle the influx of service users.

In 2015, this development led to a decision to transform all the regional outpatient teams for personality disorders into an SCM team. The On Board name was changed to SCM. In the same period the ECPD developed a specific GIT–PD train-the-trainer programme (<http://www.kenniscentrumps.nl>). We sent ten practitioners on this train-the-trainer programme and started to train every practitioner in the clinical service.

To manage this process a strategy was developed based on the ideas of the eight-step-change model of Kotter (Kotter, 1996). The first step is to underline the sense of urgency. The urgency was very clear: too many service users didn't get the treatment they needed (Hermens, van Splunteren, van den Bosch, & Verheul, 2011). A leading coalition of staff members was formed consisting of the medical director and six (one from each team) early adopters. Their assignment was to develop a treatment programme based on the principles of SCM and to implement this programme in six teams, all of which historically had very different backgrounds and cultures. The leading coalition met every month to discuss substantive developments, strategic choices, and staff issues. The first year of implementation was difficult. Not all practitioners were equally enthusiastic about the transformation. The psychotherapists who were used to working alone found it especially difficult to work within a team (due to a larger, shared caseload) and to support the nurses and case managers in dealing with difficulties in relationship management and safety intervention. Some professionals struggled with integration of the new principles and chose to leave the GIT–PD team. The management team addressed the underlying tensions that led to people leaving and supported the remaining professionals with extra workshops, supervision, and training.

After 6 months, a book was written summarizing the ideas and programmes that had been developed. This was crucial in clarifying our views and defining the pathway for clinical implementation. The programme was a variation on SCM but with clear differences and so it was rebadged GIT–PD, a generally applicable name for the treatment programme in the Netherlands.

After 5 years, six well-functioning GIT–PD teams are running it effectively in the clinical service. The leading coalition still meets every 6 weeks to evaluate the programme and make it more attuned to service users' needs. At this moment, for instance, the coalition group gives specific attention to working with service users who have comorbidity with trauma and post-traumatic stress disorder (PTSD).

Experiences of implementing SCM (GIT–PD) in the Netherlands

In the Netherlands, GIT–PD is currently an established therapy programme. The ECPD has succeeded in developing a framework for good care for service users diagnosed with personality disorder. The GIT–PD training has been incorporated in the regular education programmes for psychologists and psychiatrists in residence.

What makes the GIT–PD programme distinctive in relation to the 'old school' of working with personality disorders in generic mental health services? First, treatment is phase-oriented and timed (time-limited). In the past, after the clinical interview, service users were offered treatment without a clear framework and pre-determined time span. Since implementation of phase-oriented and timed treatment, the mean total duration of treatment has decreased.

Second, in the contract phase there is more focus on an integrated and comprehensive view of the service user and their problems. The contract phase manual requires the practitioner and service user to look carefully at the problems, link them coherently, and create a shared view of both the problems and ways to solve them, and the manual supports them in doing so. Mental health treatment has therefore become part of a larger package of interventions integrated in a network which includes support from other community organizations. In the past, a group of service users were excluded from psychotherapy because of the severity of their social problems. Service users, community organizations, and voluntary sector services as well as practitioners and mental health staff report considerable satisfaction with these changes in working method.

A final characteristic and valuable part of our GIT–PD programme is the GIT–PD group. The GIT–PD group is a treatment programme consisting of three parts: a psychotherapy group (a mix of mentalization-based and CBT), a problem-solving group, and a non-verbal therapy group like creative therapy or psychomotor therapy. Every week, there is a specific focus (in total, six) running through the whole treatment programme. After every 6 weeks the focus is repeated. Service users participate for at least 3 months and when indicated have the opportunity to repeat the program a total of six times. The programme stops after 18 months.

This GIT–PD group is specifically developed for vulnerable service users with high interpersonal hypersensitivity who in the past have often dropped out of group programmes. Attention is given to safety, acceptance of problem behaviours and level of distress, and engagement and hope for change. When necessary, there is individual coaching to support the group programme. Again, service users report high acceptance of the group and practitioners are enthusiastic in being able to offer something specific for this vulnerable service user group.

In the GIT–PD group, the teams offer specific programmes for emotion regulation, self-esteem, PTSD, or impulse control. The GIT–PD teams also offer treatments like schema-focused (group) therapy or affect phobia (group) therapy for service users when appropriate. Four years after the introduction of GIT–PD, it has become an indispensable form of treatment of personality disorders in local mental health services and is now being implemented in other mental health institutions in the Netherlands. It forms the missing link in the treatment programmes of personality disorders.

Most of the mental health workers acknowledge the importance and value of an integrated and accessible treatment programme for people diagnosed with personality disorder. Serious concerns were expressed by experienced psychotherapists who were concerned that the dilution of specialist individual therapy might undermine its effectiveness, but most psychiatrists and nurses were enthusiastic from the start and were eager to help setting up the programme. However, after a year, most other psychologists and psychotherapists discovered the value of the GIT–PD programme, particularly when experiencing the work according to the GIT–PD method as less difficult and less solitary.

Service users also report being satisfied. They praise the service user and encouraging attitude of the care workers and the intensity of the (group) programme. The collaboration with important others and network partners is also considered important to them in order to reach the treatment goals.

Reflection on the implementation process

Reviewing the development and implementation of the GIT–PD programme, it can be concluded that it was a success in terms of service development, staff and service user satisfaction, integration of community social services with mental health services, and positive outcomes. What made it successful? The most significant ingredient was the initiative of the ECPD to develop a clearly written GIT–PD framework, based on well-documented and evidence-based knowledge. Second, the urgent realization that care programmes had to be reorganized acted like a catalyst. The gap between supply and demand had led to ineffective treatment programmes for personality disorders.

Another factor that assisted implementation was the clinical and strategic support of senior practitioners and management. For example, the medical director was and is a practitioner with a lot of experience in working with personality disorders; knowledge, authority, and management worked hand in hand. The majority of the early adopters were respected practitioners blessed with enthusiasm and diplomacy. Strategic action had a place on the agenda every month in the meetings of the leading coalition.

GIT–PD has two aspects in financial terms. Importantly for health economics, the teams cost less than earlier treatment options. This is mainly due to a change in the balance of disciplines in the teams, with more social workers and nurses in addition to psychologists and a psychiatrist. Second, the GIT–PD treatment programme was initially more expensive because of the higher intensity of the treatment compared to previous treatment but this was counterbalanced by shorter duration of treatment. Therefore, with little financial cost service users receive effective treatment instead of 'papering over the scratches'. The Board of Directors of Altrecht and the health insurance providers are following us critically but with interest.

Conclusion

In conclusion, we have outlined how two European clinical SCM-based services are implementing SCM in adapted form. We consider that SCM is a good model of providing assessment and treatment for people diagnosed with BPD. In both countries, SCM is also used to treat people diagnosed with other personality disorders and it coexists well alongside other treatments, such as MBT or schema-focused therapy. It is a popular treatment model that is liked by all mental health professional using it and has been shown to be highly effective with service users diagnosed with a broad range of personality problems, not just BPD. The key experiences of implementing SCM from the Swedish and the Dutch experience are shown in Box 7.1.

Box 7.1 Key Factors in SCM Implementation in Sweden and Netherlands

- The Dutch GIT–PD has written a manual; the Swedish SCM team have written a manual for SCM group therapy. Local adaptation of SCM is one of its strengths and local manuals support team function and service implementation.
- SCM is well-liked by staff of various psychiatric and psychotherapeutic backgrounds.
- Introducing practitioners to SCM is through supervision, pairing experienced and less experienced practitioners, reading the manual together.
- Early adopters or senior practitioners play an important role in developing and maintaining the SCM model and SCM approach and in creating an SCM team. This is done by leadership, supervision, co-practitioner sessions, and integrated clinical presence. For example, in the Swedish SCM team has an administrative and medical director who also work as practitioners for part of the week.
- SCM targets all service users with problems with personality functioning rather than only those with emotionally unstable personality disorder (EUPD). This is helpful when adapting the treatment for other personality disorders or psychiatric conditions.

References

Aalders, H., & Hengstmengel, M. (2019). *GIT–PD in de praktijk. guideline-informed treatment for personality disorders.* Amsterdam: Hogrefe.

Bach, B., & First. M. (2018). Application of the ICD-11 classification of personality disorders. *BMC Psychiatry, 18,* 351.

Bateman, A., & Fonagy, P. (2009). Randomized controlled trial of outpatient mentalization-based treatment versus structured clinical management for borderline personality disorder. *American Journal of Psychiatry, 166,* 1355–1364.

Bateman, A. & Krawitz, R. (2013). *Borderline personality disorder: an evidence-based guide for generalist mental health professionals.* Oxford: Oxford University Press.

Beckwith H., Moran P. F., & Reilly J. (2014). Personality disorder prevalence in psychiatric outpatient users: a systematic literature review. *Personal Mental Health, 8,* 91–101.

Bevington, D., Fuggle, P., Cracknell, L., & Fonagy, P. (2017). *Adaptive mentalization based integrative treatment: a guide for teams to develop systems of care.* Oxford: Oxford University Press.

Chanen, A. (2009). Borderline personality disorder. *Personality and Mental Health, 3*(2), 116–119.

Choi-Kain, L., & Gunderson, J. (2019). *Applications of good psychiatric management for borderline personality disorder: a practical guide.* Washington, DC: American Psychiatric Association Publishing.

Hermens, M. L., van Splunteren, P. T., van den Bosch, A., & Verheul, R. (2011). Barriers to implementing the clinical guideline on borderline personality disorder in the Netherlands. *Psychiatric Services, 62*(11), 1381–1383.

Ileakis E.A., Sonley, A.K.I., Lagan, G. S., & Choi-Kain, L. W. (2019). Treatment of borderline personality disorder: is supply adequate to meet public health needs? *Psychiatric Services, 70*(9), 772–781.

Kaasenbrood, A., Hutsebaut, J., & van Bunningen, N. (2015). *Guideline informed treatment-personality disorders.* Retrieved from <http://www.kenniscentrumps.nl>.

Kotter, J. P. (1996). *Leading change.* Boston, MA: Harvard Business School Press.

Livesley, W. J., Dimaggio, G., & Clarkin, J. F. (Eds.) (2017). *Integrated treatment for personality disorder: a modular approach.* New York, NY: Guilford Press.

McMain, S., Guimond, T., Cardish, R., Streiner, D., & Links, P. (2012). Clinical outcomes and functioning post-treatment: A 2-year follow-up of dialectical behavior therapy versus general psychiatric management for borderline personality disorder. *The American Journal of Psychiatry, 169*(6), 650–661.

Torgersen S. (2014). Prevalence, sociodemographics, and functional impairment. In J. M. Oldham, A. E. Skodol, & D. S. Bender (Eds.), *Textbook of personality disorders* (pp. 109–30). Arlington, VA: American Psychiatric Publishing.

8

Teamworking, System, and Service Interfaces in SCM

Stuart Mitchell and Julia Harrison

Introduction

Integration of clinical teams and services within a comprehensive healthcare system is an essential part of the care and treatment of people diagnosed with personality disorder, yet there are many different elements of treatment teams or services which do not always work in synchrony or follow agreed care plans and strategies. Many teams, services, and healthcare systems are under intense pressure and scrutiny to achieve targets within tight financial envelopes and limited resources, which can lead to a loss of service user focus and clinical needs-led practice (Baker et al., 2010; Muller, 2018;). For the service user, this may be experienced as inconsistent, neglectful, or even harmful clinical practice, even if it is mostly well intentioned (Linehan, 2015). Inconsistency, reactivity, over focusing on certainty and general non-mentalizing within teams and across systems can leave the service user feeling lost, misunderstood, lacking in clear direction, or even re-traumatized, all of which mitigate optimal recovery (Bateman & Fonagy, 2016; Bateman & Tyrer, 2004; Livesley, 2019; NICE, 2009). The National Institute for Health and Care Excellence (NICE) guidance recommends that key principles are followed and services develop comprehensive assessments, safety and treatment plans, and work closely with other services, such as in-patient services, crisis teams, and specialist teams where present (NICE, 2009). Other experts emphasize how practitioners and services or teams need to structure, coordinate, and integrate the service provision for all service users diagnosed with personality disorder (Bateman & Krawitz, 2013; Gunderson, 2014; Livesley, 2019; Paris, 2008; Zanarini, 2008).

There are many areas where the service may interface with the wider system of care. This covers teamworking itself, the range of services with which service users comes into contact, the cultural aspects of organizations and the system, the pathway of care, and the system of families and carers. Each of these will be discussed within this chapter. In terms of teamworking, the word 'TEAM' may signify that 'Together Everyone Achieves More'. However, without effective and reflective leadership, the motto can just as easily be that 'Together Everyone **Argues** More'. Every team is made up of a number of individuals, with their own perspectives, belief systems, preferences, skills, and character traits. Interface issues can occur not only when different teams come together to provide joint or sequential aspects of care for an individual but can also arise in intra-team differences.

Due to the complex nature of their difficulties, a service user diagnosed with personality disorder may engage with a wide range of services, within both the statutory and non-statutory sector. Within these there will be further service division, for example within the National Health Service (NHS) a person may receive care simultaneously from primary, secondary, acute, and specialist services. Often these services have significantly different processes, policies, and procedures that can at times cause frustration and confusion for the service user.

Cultural interface issues occur when there are significant differences between the core ethos, attitudes, and the underpinning 'spirit' of organizations. The organizational culture provides the foundations for all the resulting processes, policies, and working procedures of its service provision. In health and social care, organizational culture clashes can occur when differences exist relating to attitudes towards risk management, leadership styles, cultures of blame versus support, etc.

In terms of the pathway of care, service users have at times referred to their progress towards recovery or better well-being as a 'journey'. Though this involves a great deal of personal resilience and effort, the service pathways they access will inevitably influence their progress. Parts of a pathway may work in isolation, with poor communication and connection with others. Waiting lists, referral criteria, and processes can be problematic, and perceptions of the individual's 'readiness' to engage can differ. In terms of interfaces, a service user's 'journey' between parts of a pathway can either involve smooth, timely, well-planned transitions that aid recovery or be reminiscent of stressful long-distance travel with extensive delays and missed connections.

The final system that we consider is the system of families and carer support. In addition to the healthcare system, service users are usually part of a wider support network of family, friends, and carers. There can be issues of consent and information sharing, carer needs, and engagement. A number of interface issues can occur and present both challenges and simultaneously opportunities for better integration of care and treatment effectiveness

This chapter will outline how services can ensure effective integrated team and service interface working within a structured clinical management (SCM) pathway for personality disorder. It will then review some of the problems experienced across the whole healthcare system and how these can be understood within the SCM approach. Finally, it will illustrate this with several practical examples of service-related problems and suggest practical solutions based on the SCM approach.

Typical interfaces occur between community-based services, including the clinical team and the service user's General Practitioner (GP), or other services such as children and young people. Other third sector services, such as Recovery Colleges, may become involved at different points in the service user's pathway.

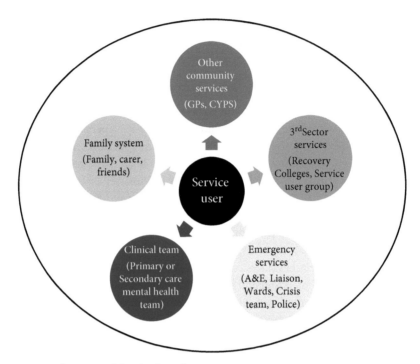

Figure 8.1 System and Service Interfaces

Emergency services may be used when the service user is in crisis and presents with high-risk behaviours. The clinical team will usually work closely within the service user and act as a point of safety and attachment from which all other contact points are organized. Finally, the service user will interact with their wider social network which may also be a part of the care and treatment plan, subject to negotiation and consent from the service user. A summary of typical interface issues is provided in Figure 8.1.

Teamworking

Whilst having a clear and structured personalized approach to care with an individual service user can in itself be effective, once a team is involved in the overall care plan then this may rapidly become more problematic as service users experience more intense attachments to their practitioners or the service to which they are connected. These intense attachments create reciprocal responses from team members, driven by their own attachment processes, thereby eliciting different responses that, if not reflected on and carefully managed, can lead to inconsistent or disorganized care. Every team is made up of a number of individuals, with their own perspectives, belief systems, attachment style and preferences, skills, and character traits. Each member's attachment style may be concordant or discordant with that of the service user. When it is concordant, such as if both service user and practitioner have an anxious preoccupied attachment pattern, it may be harder for the practitioner to remain calm and reflective when similar anxieties are engendered in them. This will affect how the team functions as a whole. In this context, Bateman and Krawitz (2013) have suggested that it is useful to have a united team and agree a common language as a focus for the work in order to prevent or overcome the problems just described. They suggest a focus on 'mentalizing' as a basis for good teamwork. Mentalizing refers to the ability to attend to mental states in ourselves and others and to work out the bases for one's actions explicitly. Mentalizing may act as a 'common factor' (Bateman & Fonagy, 2019) which underpins effective teamwork, whilst practitioners work within their own particular model of therapy, whether it is SCM, dialectical behaviour therapy (DBT), mentalization-based treatment (MBT), or cognitive analytic therapy (CAT). Mentalizing may assist practitioners when they feel lost, overwhelmed, or detached from their service users or colleagues and help them rediscover their way of working so it is balanced, reflective, and in tune with their service users' needs. A mentalizing team will show:

- A united mind with a common purpose, whilst also maintaining respect for each member of the team and valuing of different perspectives.
- An ability to develop and adhere to coherent clinical plans.
- Good team morale through validation, understanding, and compassionate self-care.
- Effective leadership through adherence to agreed protocols, shared responsibility, and effective reasoned decision-making.

Bateman and Krawitz (2013) offer some suggestions for structuring clinical meetings so they work more effectively and remain balanced and focused. The structure is based around four steps:

1. **Identifying and marking the task.** The practitioner states succinctly what problem, question, or concern is that they want help with resolving.
2. **Stating the case.** The practitioner briefly presents material about their issue or problem without interruption, whilst staying focused on the task.
3. **Team discussion and mentalizing the process.** All team members are invited to offer their views and perspectives, whilst one practitioner not directly involved helps to keep the process balanced, dialectical, and reflective.
4. **Returning to the task to link the discussion to the identified task.** This may start with an integrated or synthesizing summary of the views presented and linking it to the identified problem or concern.

It is helpful to use this to structure all clinical meetings where service users are discussed within the SCM team.

Service Interfaces

Due to the complex nature of their difficulties, a service user diagnosed with personality disorder may engage with a wide range of services within both the statutory and non-statutory sector. Within this there will be further service division; for example, within the NHS a person may simultaneously receive care from primary, secondary, acute, and specialist services. Often these services have significantly different processes, policies, and procedures that can at times cause frustration and confusion for the service user because services can appear to be inconsistent and not joined up in their approach. This is a reciprocal relationship, with the system affecting the service user, and vice versa. For example, a service user may present to emergency services following self-harm and seek medication as a remedy to their distress, while the SCM care and safety plan would not necessarily be to prescribe further medication in a crisis. Staff in emergency services may feel unsure about how to proceed and may take a cautious approach to risk and safety which does not align with the SCM plan. This inevitably means frequent communication not only between service users and services but also between the services themselves. In this sense, services inevitably both affect and are affected by the care provision. Box 8.1 provides a case example illustrating the many services from which clients receive care and which may be involved in this process.

With the potential and actual involvement of many different services, there is also potential for divided care and disagreement about the best approach to take in the interest of the service user. In line with the UK NHS Care Programme Approach (CPA), it is best practice for the primary team who are coordinating care or who are designated primary case managers to provide the leadership and coordination on how different services collaborate over the details of the service user's actual SCM care pathway. The onus is on the primary practitioner, with the support of their team, to scaffold or consult with the relevant services and teams on the approach being used in order to influence the way they deliver their component of the pathway. This is not an easy task because different services and treatment teams may have different models of care and styles of delivery which conflict with the SCM approach. They may even wish simply to 'hand over' the service user's care and treatment so they do not have to contain the anxiety engendered by the work with a service user presenting with high levels of risk. The primary task is to agree a common pathway and the strategic steps for all to follow (Bateman & Krawitz, 2013). Chapters 6 and 7 provide detailed descriptions of some different pathways.

A key point of potential risk in service interfacing is when a service user is being considered for transition to another service, such as from an in-patient ward to a

---

Box 8.1 Case Example—Interfaces When Multiple Services Are Involved

---

Due to their complex difficulties and frequent incidents of self-harm, a service user received combined care from a GP, a consultant psychiatrist, supported housing, and a specialist tertiary personality disorder service, with the latter also providing care coordination. In addition to the regular care from these services, the person frequently attended acute services, where they engaged with departments, both within the healthcare Trust and at times travelling to hospitals many miles away.

Increasing numbers of staff from various services, disciplines, and organizations became involved. Communication across services was difficult at times, particularly when the service user presented out of hours, or to a service within another Trust. Decision-making around risk became increasingly complex and at times was understandably reactive, due to levels of anxiety engendered. There were different perspectives and opinions on use of the Mental Health Act, and complex discussions about capacity and informed consent.

In order to resolve such interface issues, the principles of SCM were drawn upon, specifically that case management, guidance, and leadership should primarily lie with the care coordinating team. This was important because again, as SCM principles had been utilized soundly in this person's care, the care coordinator had developed a comprehensive formulation with the service user. The formulation had explored in depth the likely functions of risk-related behaviours, and the factors that were likely to enhance or mitigate risk.

What followed was a resource-intensive piece of work as the care coordinator methodically engaged the many agencies involved. As the person most familiar with the service user, she consistently invited other services to communicate their perspectives to develop the formulation further and use this to create collaborative guidance. The resulting Emergency Health Care Plan was a significantly collaborative piece of work, shared with and contributed to by the client and heavily influenced by the teamworking, proactive, and reflective approaches recommended within SCM.

---

community service or from a children and young people's service to adult services. See Chapter 11 for details how to ensure transitions are handled well, with some in-depth reasoning and examples of best practice. Suffice to say, problems emerge when services either refuse to adapt their way of working, decline to work alongside others, or fail to collaborate over the work during an agreed transition period.

For example, some young people are referred from children and young people's services (CYPS) to adult services very close to their 18th birthday. This may be for a variety of reasons including time pressures and constraints. These same demands can often lead to difficulties in delivering transitional joint work. For the service user this can feel like a huge loss of contact and structure to which they are accustomed, with a resulting loss of epistemic trust (Bateman & Fonagy, 2019) with the adult receiving team.

Another interface issue often encountered is when services provide treatment according to evidence-based models (such as DBT or MBT), but an individual service user clearly is not responding well to this. On occasion, despite this being identified and discussed by a multidisciplinary team (MDT), there are difficulties in adjusting the treatment approach. This may relate to the knowledge and training base of the practitioners or the preferred models of the service. However, this at best can be ineffective for the service user and frustrating for the practitioner, and at worst can lead to iatrogenic failures of care. This can occur when the care pathway and service or system response has been shown that it cannot adapt adequately to the service user's clinical needs and has remained too rigid in its application of its model. Within SCM, this is a target of intervention itself so the team and system interface becomes more integrated, flexible, stable, and can mentalize the service user's problems across the whole system (Steele, Boon, & Van Der Hart, 2017). This is much more difficult if the treatment team is provided by another organization, with different management structures and cultures, rather than when this is within the same organization and more influence and scaffolding is possible. An example of a case where different therapeutic models were applied is shown in Box 8.2.

System and Cultural Interfaces

The organization or healthcare system as whole may be a source of helpful or unhelpful influences in being able to implement an effective SCM pathway. When this is working well, the 'system' or broader organization supports the SCM pathway through supporting its practitioners to deliver the treatment with fidelity and provide appropriate dedicated time and supervision support, including ongoing attendance at supervision and trouble-shooting meetings. This will include a culture of appreciation, growth, innovation, and change (Schein, 2017; Seddon, 2008).

The culture of the organization and the associated organizational structures and processes may sometimes be detrimental to effective implementation of SCM. Culture is best defined as simply the 'organization's way of doing things' which is embedded in the fabric akin to the 'DNA' of the organization, and includes their values, beliefs, behaviours, and general implicit assumptions about how things are done (Schein, 2017). A 'clear and sustained culture' is often the most important factor in leading to organizational success (Collins & Porras, 2004), but some

---

Box 8.2 Case Example—Interfaces When Different Therapeutic Models Are Applied

---

Within one UK NHS service the primary treatment model for individuals diagnosed with personality disorder is SCM. SCM can be used as a discrete piece of therapeutic work or as a preparatory stage, after which the person may engage with more specialist psychological therapies (such as CAT, eye-movement desensitization and reprocessing (EMDR), solutions-focused therapy (SFT)).

An interface issue occurred when one NHS service found themselves providing care coordination for service users living in a therapeutic community that implemented its own (psychoanalytic) treatment model over a lengthy period. There were some clear benefits in this provision, due to the NHS service's experience and skills in working with the risk issues presented, however the models of both services were significantly different.

This raised a number of interface issues. One difficulty was in the NHS service staff having clarity of role and not confusing the service user with conflicting models of treatment. Another difficulty that emerged was that the treatment model used by the non-NHS service was effective in targeting many of the interpersonal dynamics and emotional difficulties of the clients but did not address some of the underlying trauma contributing to presentation. This resulted in service users at times completing a lengthy piece of work, and then requiring a considerable period of trauma stabilization work, which raised issues in regard to timescales and resources for the NHS service.

As with many of the other interface issues described, these can intensify in isolation or be mitigated by good communication, an open and curious approach, and the desire to be reflective and flexible in developing goals. In this situation, both services showed a high level of commitment to collaborating, communicating, and addressing the interface issues without defensiveness. When this worked well, this was noted by the clinical teams to lead to a greater sense of safety and containment for service users

As a result, ideas about appropriate point of referral, shared formulations, joint working, and a review of trauma stabilization provision were all generated, and at this time are being further developed

---

cultures, such as a blaming or controlling culture, can lead to poor performance and harmful practices (Schein, 2017).

Management structures may also have an effect on the implementation and delivery of the SCM pathway. With a move towards locality management organization, it may be increasingly difficult to obtain consensus from all areas of an organization on their implementation of the SCM model. Even with an organization-wide implementation group to oversee implementation and ensure consistency and fidelity to the model, there are still differences according to local practitioners' preferences and the capacity and ability of teams to embed the model in full. Due to this, a flexible approach was adopted to assist teams to implement what they can according to the model, and later move towards full implementation. Again, this may involve an element of slow-drip cultural change to fairly rigid ways of working.

Within UK NHS organizations there may often be complex case panels established which aim to provide expert consultation on cases where clinical teams may be unsure or divided on the best clinical approach. These structures are intended as additional clinical governance and assurance, but they do not always actually lead to better understanding or clinically useful decisions being made. For example, some organizations describe their complex case panel discussions as purely 'advisory' and the clinical team do not have to follow the advice of the panel. This is of questionable effectiveness when many of the clinical teams at these panels are seeking some guidance and assurance on what to do and for this to have some authority, especially when disagreement in the team was one of key reasons behind the referral to the complex case panel. An example of a case where cultural aspects of the system were slowly addressed is shown in Box 8.3.

The Family System

In addition to the healthcare system, there is also a system which surrounds the service user involving the family, carers, friends, and others who are important to them and may be involved in supporting recovery. The service user often lives at home with family members and carers, which may be a source of financial, psychological, and emotional support to them. The family system may be neglected. Family members become distressed, often with a sense of burden through taking responsibility for their relative, and may need support or assistance themselves (Bateman & Krawitz, 2013). NICE recommends that families are involved in the treatment of people diagnosed with BPD so they are not overlooked, their own needs are attended to, and they are offered information and support where needed (NICE, 2009). More will be said about how this support can be structured and provided in Chapter 12. This is a key additional system which needs to be incorporated into the treatment plan for the benefit of the service user overall, and to facilitate effective use of the SCM pathway for the service user. It has been found that greater family involvement in treatment predicts better outcomes for service users (Bateman & Krawitz, 2013). Various brief intervention packages have been developed for working with families and carers (Carter & Gordon, 2015; Flynn et al., 2017; Liljedahl et al., 2019; Pearce et al., 2017; Porr, 2010).

Box 8.3 Case Example—Cultural Interfaces

Due to a number of factors, including deaths of service users during admission, and the subsequent investigations, one UK NHS organization developed a highly anxious culture, particularly in relation to risk management, and a fear of being blamed if things 'went wrong'. This culture appeared to be pervasive and affected staff in a range of services across the organization, from those in senior leadership positions to newly qualified staff working for the Trust.

The anxious blaming culture manifested in a variety of ways; complaints at times were handled in a reactive, 'teleological' (reactive, action-driven) way. The communication between corporate services and clinical teams when investigating complaints was limited to concrete actions that would try to eliminate all areas of risk. Outcomes often included recommendations that the clinical team continued to offer increasing amounts of interventions or input, when from the latter's perspective this would likely prove to be ineffective, or even iatrogenic. The cultural environment also engendered conflicted interface issues between community and in-patient services, with both feeling a heavy burden of 'managing' service user risk, and the service user's own autonomy and personal control getting lost. Service users were often admitted to acute wards for extended periods of time or sent out of area for treatment.

During this time a specialist team was set up to model and lead on implementing SCM principles within a personality disorder pathway. Initially the team met with some resistance and struggled to retain its autonomy and implement its evidence-based approaches to positive risk management and the promotion of self-safety.

It was possible over a number of years, however, to modify and shape this culture gradually by being sensitive to, but not condoning, the prevailing culture, promoting and demonstrating an alternative model of care and treatment, consulting widely with colleagues, service users, and carers, and by asking that the senior management team place trust in the new specialist team to do things differently. Along with this approach, a change in leadership at the top of the organization promoted a desire to embed a culture that moves away from blame and encourages self-reflection and responsibility. In conjunction with the team's presence being felt across several community teams, this led to a slow change from the previous anxious culture to one that was more accepting of risk and change.

SCM Pathway Interfaces

SCM is the cornerstone of effective evidence-based practice for service users diagnosed with personality disorder and should underpin most, if not all, generic
mental health services. The SCM practitioner strives to provide structure, coordination, and integration of a wide range of services involved with the service user.
These are the core principles of SCM. For this reason, and the fact that most service
users are likely to receive generic rather than specialist treatment and management,
a care pathway for personality disorder where SCM is a first-line treatment option
is often appropriate (Mitchell, 2015). The various components of the pathway from
initial assessment through to discharge and transition into other services or recovery-focused community services need to be identified and supported by clear
guidance. The clarity of a pathway enables more consistency within what can be
a fragmented system. Without an elaborated care pathway that identifies the different aspects of care and treatment and how they fit together, service users may
not receive consistent or high-quality generic care, and instead receive whatever is
available, usually care coordination or psychological therapy that may or may not
be influenced by the background, training, or preferred model of the individual
practitioner.

The role of the care coordination is integrated within the SCM programme so
that the tasks of care coordination may be undertaken by the nominated SCM
practitioner, whilst the strategic tasks and process of SCM are also followed and
implemented according to the model. This requires careful separation of the care
coordination and SCM tasks and processes, so that one does not detract from implementation of the other. It is worth noting that other SCM pathways work outside care coordination using a case management approach. Both approaches are
appropriate as long as the pathways are clearly structured, organized, and key functions delivered. Chapters 6 and 7 provides illustrations of different but effective
pathways.

Conclusion

An effective clinical team needs to be integrated and coordinated with a range of
services within a healthcare system, including the family system of care that might
support the service user. Different elements of a treatment team or service may not
always work in synchrony or follow agreed care plans and strategies. Services can
ensure effective integrated team working through agreeing a common language.
In SCM the common language is that of problem solving. The 'team' and systemic
approach is all about helping the service user to become a 'better' problem-solver
with an emphasis on building their confidence to manage their internal mental

distress and increasing their abilities to harness effective mental, interpersonal, and behavioural skills.

It is recommended that the clinical team which is coordinating care and managing a case provides the leadership and coordination on how different services collaborate over the details of the service users actual SCM care pathway. Any movement or transition in care is a point of potential risk for problems to emerge when services either refuse to adapt their way of working, decline to work alongside others, or fail to collaborate over the work during an agreed transition period.

Iatrogenic failures of care and treatment occur when the care pathway and service or system response has not shown enough flexible adaptation to the service user's clinical needs and has remained too rigid in its application of its model. Within SCM, this is a target of intervention itself so the team and system interface becomes more integrated, stable, and can mentalize the service user's problems across the whole system (Steele et al., 2017).

A 'clear and sustained culture', such as blaming or controlling, is often a limiting factor in leading to organizational success (Collins & Porras, 2004). It is possible to modify and shape such cultures gradually in a number of ways: by doing the new evidence-based work that is mandated; by being sensitive to, but not condoning, the prevailing culture; by promoting and demonstrating an alternative model of care and treatment; by consulting widely with colleagues, service users, and carers; and by asking that the senior management team put some trust in any new specialist team and their approach to doing things differently.

It is helpful to integrate the role of the primary practitioner or care coordinator within the SCM programme so that the tasks of care coordination may be undertaken, usually by the same SCM practitioner, whilst the strategic tasks and process of SCM are also followed and implemented according to the model.

Finally, in addition to the healthcare system, there is also a system which surrounds the service user involving the family, carers, friends, and others who are important to them and may be involved in supporting recovery in some way. It is recommended to the use a brief SCM intervention package for working with families and carers as illustrated in Chapter 12, which have been found to be effective for practitioners who have little time, as this enhances the SCM pathway through working at this level of the system

References

Bateman, A., & Fonagy, P. (2016). *Mentalization-based treatment for personality disorders.* Oxford: Oxford University Press.
Bateman, A. W., & Krawitz, R. (2013). *Borderline personality disorder: an evidence-based guide for generalist mental health professionals.* Oxford: Oxford University Press.
Carter, C., & Gordon, C. (2015). Evaluation of borderline personality disorder awareness workshops for service users and carers. *Mental Health Practice, 19*(2), 26–31.

Collins, J., & Porras, J. (2004). *Built to last: successful habits of visionary companies.* London: Random House Business Books.

Flynn, D., Kells, M., Joyce, M., Corcoran, P., Herley, S., Suarez, C., ... Groeger, J. (2017). Family connections versus optimised treatment-as-usual for family members of individuals with borderline personality disorder: non-randomised controlled study. *Borderline Personality Disorder and Emotion Regulation, 6,* 14. <https://doi.org/10.1186/s40479-017-0069-1>.

Krawitz, R., & Jackson, W. (2008). *Borderline personality disorder: the facts.* Oxford: Oxford University Press.

Lester, G., Wilson, B., Griffin, L., & Mullen, P. (2004). Unusually persistent complainants. *British Journal of Psychiatry, 184,* 352–356.

Liljedahl, S. L., Kleindienst, N., Wangby-Lundh, M., Lundh, L-G., Daukantaite, D., Fruzetti, A. E., & Westling, S. (2019). Family connections in different settings and intensities for underserved and geographically isolated families: a non-randomised comparison study. *Borderline Personality Disorder and Emotion Regulation, 6,* 14. doi.org/10.1186/s40479-019-0111-6

NICE. (2009). *Borderline personality disorder, clinical guideline 78.* London: NICE.

NICE. (2009). *Antisocial personality disorder, clinical guideline 77.* London: NICE.

NICE. (2015). *Personality disorders: borderline and antisocial. NICE Quality Standard 88.* London: NICE.

NICE. (2015). *Transition between inpatient hospital settings and community or care home settings for adults with social care needs. Clinical Guideline 27.* London: NICE

NICE. (2016). *Transition from children's to adults' services for young people using health or social care services. Clinical Guideline 43.* London: NICE.

Pearce, J., Jovev, M., Hulbert, C., McKechnie, B., McCutcheon, L., Betts, J., & Chanen, A. M. (2017). Evaluation of a psychoeducational group intervention for family and friends of youth with borderline personality disorder. *Borderline Personality Disorder and Emotion Regulation, 4*(5). doi.org/10.1186/s40479-017-0056-6

Poor, V. (2010). *Overcoming borderline personality disorder: a family guide for healing and change.* New York, NY: Oxford University Press.

Schein, E. H. (2017). *Organizational culture and leadership* (5th Ed.). NJ: Wiley.

Seddon, J. (2008). *Systems thinking in the public sector: the failure of the reform regime ... and a manifesto for a better way.* Axminster: Triarchy Press.

Steele, K. (2016). Attachment, dependency and collaboration in the psychotherapy of complex developmental trauma. *ESTD Conference*, Amsterdam, 15 April 2016.

Steele, K., Boon, S. & Van Der Hart, O. (2017). *Treating trauma-related dissociation: a practical integrative approach.* New York, NY: Norton & Co.

9

Prescribing in SCM: United Kingdom and Europe

Rajesh Nair, Peder Björling, Muhammad Abdul-Rahman, and Gordon Turkington

Introduction

This chapter provides guidelines on how to integrate pharmacological treatment for service users diagnosed with borderline personality disorder (BPD) in structured clinical management (SCM) treatment. We examine current international and national guidelines on pharmacological treatment, discuss the importance of service user–practitioner alliance, distinguish between crisis-driven symptoms and co-occurring disorders, setting goals, and evaluating any pharmacological interventions. Integrating clinical decisions on drug treatment into the SCM team model is also discussed. BPD is characterized by a pervasive pattern of unstable relationships, marked affective instability, impulsivity, a distorted sense of self, or chronic sense of emptiness, and often presents with a high rate of self-harm and suicide attempts (Zanarini, Schmahl, Linehan, & Bohus, 2004). Self-harming behaviour for people diagnosed with BPD is associated with a variety of different goals for the person, including relief from acute distress and reconnecting with feelings after a period of dissociation. Substance use, depression, and eating disorders are commonly associated with a diagnosis of BPD.

How Service Users Present to Services

Service users diagnosed with BPD commonly present in late adolescence to early adulthood to mental health services. Many are likely to have sought treatment via their General Practitioner (GP) and, having found little success in treatment with antidepressants, are referred on to secondary care services. Although low mood, self-harm, and suicidal ideation are common presenting themes, it is equally common for service users or practitioners to believe that their condition is better explained by a diagnosis of bipolar disorder, and service users will often attribute their emotional difficulties to this. Others often come to the attention of services via the criminal justice system or drug and alcohol services (Kaess, Bruuner, & Chanen, 2014).

In clinical practice, the high levels of emotional distress experienced by some people diagnosed with personality disorder, together with a perceived need to offer rapidly effective treatments when service users present in crisis, mean that drug treatments are often used despite the lack of research evidence underpinning this approach. Often feelings of helplessness in service users evoke strong responses in practitioners making an initial assessment, which can lead to anxiety-led prescribing. It is equally common for service users diagnosed with BPD to be misdiagnosed, with up to 40% of service users noted to have been previously been diagnosed with bipolar affective disorder (Cloninger & Svarkic, 2016). The implications of misdiagnosis are that this often leads to a delay in accessing effective psychological treatment. Further complications for effective prescribing often arise over the course of treatment itself with high rates of non-attendance and complications arising from co-occurring substance misuse and ruptures in the therapeutic alliance between service user and practitioner.

Existing Prescribing Guidance

No psychotropic drug has specific marketing authorization in the United Kingdom, the Netherlands, or Sweden for the treatment of people diagnosed with BPD.

UK guidance

In the United Kingdom, the National Institute for Health and Care Excellence guidance (NICE, 2009) recommends:

- Drug treatment should not be used specifically for BPD or for the individual symptoms or behaviour associated with the disorder.
- Antipsychotic drugs should not be used for the medium- and long-term treatment of BPD.
- Drug treatment may be considered in the overall treatment of comorbid conditions.
- Review the treatment of people diagnosed with BPD who do not have a diagnosed comorbid mental or physical illness and who are currently being prescribed drugs, with the aim of reducing and stopping unnecessary treatment.

US guidance

In the United States, the American Psychiatric Association guidelines (APA, 2001) for BPD endorse a symptom-targeted approach and provide pharmacological algorithms for treatment of 'affective dysregulation symptoms', 'impulsive-behavioural dyscontrol symptoms', and 'cognitive perceptual symptoms'. All three algorithms are noted to have no empirical trials to support their effectiveness beyond the first phase, of which the first two symptom clusters suggest using a selective serotonin reuptake inhibitor (SSRI), and the last suggesting an antipsychotic.

Cochrane review guidance

Cochrane review guidelines for BPD (Lieb, Völlm, Rücker, Timmer, & Stoffers, 2010) conclude that there is weak evidence for treating overall severity of BPD but lists studies showing some effect in treating some of BPD core symptoms. The guideline lists 27 randomized controlled trials (RCTs) for BPD and rates overall evidence for treating target symptoms as weak due to few studies and variations in outcome measures. They suggest that mood stabilizers and neuroleptics might reduce affective dysregulation and that aripiprazole has beneficial effects on overall impulsivity but it should be noted that the published data for this drug were rejected in the NICE guidelines due to concerns about the research methodology. Nevertheless, the Cochrane review recommends aripiprazole and olanzapine for cognitive-perceptual symptoms but adds that there are conflicting results on olanzapine and its effects on suicidality and self-mutilation. The guidelines clearly state that the APA guideline's suggestion of using SSRIs for core BPD symptoms can no longer be recommended.

Maudsley prescribing guidance

Maudsley prescribing guidelines suggest that open studies show some benefit from first- and second-generation antipsychotics. However, in contrast, placebo-controlled studies only demonstrated a modest improvement for active drug over placebo (Lieb et al., 2010). Clozapine is noted to have shown a reduction in numbers of hospital admissions with people diagnosed with BPD. In relation to antidepressants, it was noted again that where open studies suggested that SSRIs reduce impulsivity and aggression in BPD, these findings have not been replicated in RCTs (Lieb et al., 2010). The guidelines suggest that there is some evidence that mood stabilizers reduce impulsivity, anger, and affect dysregulation in people diagnosed with BPD (Ingenhoven et al., 2010).

There is currently no guidance published by the British Association of Psychopharmacologists (BAP).

Swedish guidelines

In Sweden, the Swedish Association of Psychiatrist's guideline for personality disorders (Ekselius, 2017) states that medication is never a first line of treatment and that evidence for pharmacological treatment in BPD is lacking. The Swedish guideline suggests pharmacological treatment for comorbid syndromes and as an adjunct to other interventions in specific situations. The guideline cautions against polypharmacy as it puts the service user at risk of side effects and adverse drug interactions. The guideline also cautions against use of benzodiazepines. Finally, the guideline recommends careful deliberation on the goal of medication, how medication will be evaluated, and how long it is meant to continue.

Regional guidelines for BPD in Stockholm (Sahlin, 2017) advise that psychological treatment is preferred, and pharmacological treatment is appropriate in comorbid disorders after careful differential diagnostic assessment. The guideline also strongly advises against the use of benzodiazepines.

Conclusion on international and national guidelines on pharmacological treatment

UK NICE guidelines and Swedish guidelines are decidedly more conservative than APA and Cochrane guidelines. It is interesting that whilst more recent guidelines are based on roughly the same RCTs, their conclusions differ perhaps because of the way the data are merged and processed. More recent evidence discussed below also suggests that the guidelines need further reviewing and updating. Most guidelines do not take into account whether the service user is in structured psychological treatment for BPD or not when considering prescribing recommendations. Whilst the summary above is about UK and Swedish guidelines, a review of all European national guidelines for the treatment of people with BPD also showed some differences in recommendations for prescribing but remarkable uniformity around recommending psychological treatments as the primary intervention (Simonsen et al., 2019).

For service users in SCM treatment, we suggest a conservative approach to prescribing in line with UK and Swedish guidelines. The primary treatment for people diagnosed with BPD is psychological treatment, not medication. Other interventions available within SCM should be considered first. Consider treating comorbid disorders when appropriate and avoid off-label treatment for core BPD symptoms.

Clinical Practice and Polypharmacy in the Treatment of Service Users Diagnosed with BPD

In spite of the fact that national guidelines all suggest careful and conservative use of drugs when treating service users diagnosed with BPD, the use of antidepressants, mood stabilizers, and antipsychotics in the treatment of people diagnosed with BPD is common in clinical practice. Such treatment is often initiated during periods of crisis and the likelihood of placebo response in this context is high; the crisis is usually time-limited and will resolve itself irrespective of drug treatment. Regardless of rapid improvement, the prescribed drug is often continued in an attempt to protect against further transient, stress-related symptoms and when these occur, another drug from a different class is commonly added (Paton, Crawford, Bhatti, Patel, & Barnes, 2015).

By this time adherence to medication, reported as low in people diagnosed with BPD as a result of their chaotic lifestyles, may complicate any assessment of symptom response to prescribing and frequent changes of dose and class of drug make it difficult to see which drug, if any, has been helpful.

Polypharmacy

It is common for service users diagnosed with BPD to be prescribed multiple medications to address their mental health symptoms. In a controlled cohort study of mental health service use in the United States with a 6-year follow-up, it was found that over 50% were taking two or more drugs concurrently, over 36% taking three or more drugs, over 19% were taking four or more, and over 11% were taking five or more at 6 years (Zanarini et al., 2004). This was consistent with a subsequent audit undertaken by the Prescribing Observatory for Mental Health (POMH) in the United Kingdom, where it was found that of 1,054 service users diagnosed with personality disorder alone, 82% were prescribed at least one psychotropic medication (Paton et al., 2015).

Results of a recent local audit in the United Kingdom

Within a sample of 20 clients diagnosed with BPD and/or mixed personality disorder (emotionally unstable and antisocial) who had been referred for a standardized assessment of personality disorder, 14 (70%) did not have any other comorbid diagnosis. However, even though only one person had a diagnosis of drug-induced psychosis, 14 (70%) were on antipsychotic medication. Similarly, even though no-one had a comorbid diagnosis of depression, 14 (70%) were prescribed an antidepressant. Fifteen (75%) of them were noted to have been prescribed multiple classes of drug to a level of polypharmacy, with the most usual combination being a mood-stabilizing and antipsychotic drug along with an antidepressant.

Decision-making in pharmacological treatment in SCM

Establishing and maintaining a positive and strong therapeutic alliance is a key element in SCM. When a service user or practitioner suggests that pharmacological treatment should be considered, a positive working alliance between the practitioner and the service user is important. The quality of the alliance will help the service user make informed decisions regarding drug treatment, and is likely to improve compliance and evaluation of pharmacological treatment.

In the practitioner–service user alliance there are some particular aspects to consider. Service users sometimes see doctors as authority figures in the health-care system and may have previous experiences of doctors who adopt an 'expert stance' and are more directive than a typical SCM-trained practitioner. In the case of Sweden, doctors are also responsible for admitting service users to in-service user units for treatment, deciding on sick-leave and on detention under the Mental Health Act for in-patient user treatment. The service user response to prescribed medication may depend on how they react to this power differential. Some service users, possibly those who have more anxious insecure attachment styles, may show good adherence whereas those with greater self-agency or detachment trait expression are likely to be less compliant. This is not necessarily a bad thing.

The practitioner's stance, as described in Chapter 3 in this book, about prescribing needs to be the same as it is for all other aspects of the SCM programme. The prescribing practitioner should adopt a curious and interested attitude, using validation regularly to help the service user regulate affects and reduce the risk of prescribing becoming a 'proof of caring' for the service user.

The prescribing practitioner aims to be reflective and stimulate problem-solving instead of being expert and taking over responsibility or reacting to the service user's anxieties. When the practitioner feels pressured by their own worry about the service user or by demands from the service user, he/she enlists support from SCM team members. They are careful to discuss medication as one non-primary aspect of the SCM-treatment that is integrated into the overall care plan rather than something that occurs separately from the treatment. They will also support the service user in making their own choices in a collaborative manner and be transparent about the limitations of and expectations about medication.

When the service user is in SCM treatment, the practitioner also needs to consider how pharmacological treatment will affect the psychosocial aspects of treatment; for example, treating attention deficit hyperactivity disorder (ADHD) can reduce missed appointments or increase the service user's ability to focus in sessions, and medication with mild cognitive side effects might reduce attention in therapy. It is therefore important that major pharmacological decisions are discussed within the SCM team as a whole and considered in the context of the whole treatment plan, rather than being taken in haste to manage symptoms or anxiety in a current crisis.

In a well-functioning SCM team, the prescribing practitioner will have information from practitioners providing individual and/or group sessions, including reports of any major changes in the service user's mood, behaviour, and psychosocial situation. For example, a service user with increasingly depressed mood and suicidal ideation will be discussed in a team conference and the team may conclude that the prescribing practitioner assesses the service user for comorbid depression and whether medication is an option for this. Ideally, the prescribing practitioner works within or close to the SCM team so that they will have a well-informed basis for any prescribing and follow-up can be shared by all members of the treating team.

Often demand for medication arises during a crisis. For example, the service user may present after a difficult situation and ask for medication to help with anxiety, irritability, and low mood. The prescribing practitioner needs to be careful to be reflective and containing rather than reactive in assessing the situation and to coordinate their response with the SCM team. The service user will have a SCM safety plan that contains strategies for the service user and the SCM team and in most cases, many, if not all of those strategies should be tried before considering medication. In some cases, the plan may already have specific advice on drug treatment, usually with a specifier that medication can only be used in the short term and has to be reviewed within a week of commencement. The aim will then be reducing and stopping the medication over an agreed time frame (e.g. short-term use of medication is acceptable to improve sleep in a crisis or the use of non-addictive anxiolytics may be used when SCM strategies are insufficient in reducing distress, providing these are withdrawn after a few weeks of use).

Talking about and discussing pharmacological treatment with the service user

In some SCM treatments, the service user will already have attended a psycho-educational or socialization phase at the start of treatment when relevant information on pharmacological treatment was provided. In the Swedish SCM team, the psycho-educational course includes a summary of guidelines on prescribing, common side effects of the major medication groups, and a discussion among service users about their experience with medication.

The prescribing practitioner should be transparent about their stance regarding medication; for example, pharmacological treatment can be helpful when comorbid disorders are present but careful assessment and follow-up is vital. Starting long-term medication in a crisis with a worsening of problems related to a diagnosis of BPD is not recommended. The prescribing practitioner should also facilitate realistic expectations on what to expect from medication, and the likely withdrawal effects and time scales needed for withdrawal from different types of drugs. Once the service user has had this opportunity to think about their experiences with medication, the problems in its use, and what recommendations there are for its use in people with a diagnosis of BPD, this information can be used during treatment to discuss whether drug treatment is relevant and likely to be helpful.

If the prescribing practitioner and the service user conclude that there is a comorbid disorder where pharmacological intervention can be helpful and common side effects can be tolerated or managed, pharmacological treatment and follow-up for review of the pharmacological treatment are added to the SCM care plan. The service user and prescribing practitioner should agree on individually defined targets for the medication and how to evaluate the effect of treatment; for example, target problems could be low mood, fatigue, reduced motivation resulting in social withdrawal and reduced self-care, and recurrent self-harm. The service user and prescribing practitioner should then have a strategy agreed on how to evaluate the effects of medication over time; is evaluation to be undertaken with a standardized instrument or is it monitoring a behaviour? For example, is their mood improving on a mood questionnaire given weekly? Does the service user see friends more often? Have they started buying and preparing food again? Did they get back to college work again? Did self-harm decrease in frequency or severity? Administering a standard questionnaire for depression is likely to be less informative than exploring wider social and interpersonal outcomes unless there is a clear comorbid depression. The key problems indicating severity of BPD include social and interpersonal disruption and the characteristics of depressed mood in BPD are different from those of depression in people without personality disorder as they commonly are dominated by feelings of emptiness and despair rather than low mood.

Treating a crisis with medication

Generally, the prescribing practitioner should be conservative in their decision to use medication to treat a short-term worsening of problems. It does not make sense to treat a 4-day episode of anxiety and low mood with long-acting and drugs such as antidepressants, which require up to 2 weeks to have an effect on mood. If the strategy in a crisis is to use short-acting anxiolytics or even short-term use of neuroleptics, the service user might miss the opportunity to utilize non-pharmacological strategies, already agreed and stated in the safety plan.

Nevertheless, there are situations when prescribing a medication where no clear comorbid disorder is present might be helpful. For example, short-term treatment with anxiolytics or sleep medication (non-tolerance inducing) can make problems seem less intractable, a placebo effect perhaps, build service user–practitioner alliance, and facilitate the use of other aspects of crisis and safety management. For example, the use of sleep medication over the weekend, practise self-care skills from the safety plan, enlist help from others to manage thoughts on self-harm, and socialize with family as positive distraction. When prescribing medication outside the prescribing licence, the prescribing practitioner should choose a medication with low toxicity and few side effects and start with a low dose such as omega-3, fluoxetine in BPD.

Stopping or withdrawing from medication

At the start of treatment with SCM, the service user's need for medication should be assessed and this should include details of their response to any previously prescribed drugs. As previously stated, polypharmacy is very common (Zanarini et al., 2004) and it is therefore appropriate for the practitioner to discuss and even suggest discontinuation of unhelpful and unnecessary medication. Particular care should be given to side effects (e.g. drowsiness, cognitive side effects) that might affect the service user's ability to benefit from the psychological aspects of SCM treatment. In the Swedish SCM team, benzodiazepines are discontinued or withdrawn before the start of SCM treatment, that is during the 'socialization' phase. Since some service users are taking four or more medications at the same time and have tried many more for years, evaluating the costs and benefits from medications can be difficult. Often medical records can be used to remind the service user why medication was started and what the target symptoms were and whether there was any positive response.

Some medications are known to cause powerful and long-lasting discontinuation side effects (Wilson & Lader, 2015) so the prescribing practitioner and the service user should plan careful follow-up and the SCM team should be consulted.

Medication within in-patient settings

In the Swedish SCM team, service users are usually admitted to the same ward within our psychiatric hospital. The SCM practitioner and the consultant psychiatrist on the ward have video conferences weekly. To facilitate developing a common view among the SCM team and ward-based practitioners it is helpful if the ward practitioners linking with the SCM team are part of the permanent staff. During their stay on the ward, service users will use their safety plan together with ward staff. The safety plan, rather than an anxiolytic, is the primary tool used to handle short-term crises. Despite these efforts to maintain the basic SCM principles and strategies related to a diagnosis of BPD, the ward psychiatrist may still have reason to act unilaterally and start the service user on antidepressants or a low-dose neuroleptic. When medication has been started whilst the service user is on the ward, the SCM practitioner should make sure it is a relevant intervention and that the service user was involved collaboratively in the decision-making process. The medication can then be integrated into the SCM formulation and treatment plan. It is common that the problems driving the prescribing, the service user's opinion on medication, and an agreed way of evaluating the medication is not well described in service user records. One service user described their experience of in-patient treatment and medication as follows: 'every time I am admitted, the doctor adds something. They add more than they take away and the list of drugs just grows.' This situation indicates that greater integration of prescribing into the overall SCM treatment and care plan is required.

SCM practitioner's role in pharmacological treatment

In the SCM team, there should be a common understanding of the biopsychosocial model of personality disorders and an agreement on the strategy underpinning prescribing for people diagnosed with BPD. SCM practitioners will often be asked questions about medication by service users and, at times, they will be first to raise the issue because of increasing problems of comorbid disorders. Practitioners should maintain their therapeutic stance when issues concerning comorbid disorders and medication arises. Collaborative exploration of problem areas, the service user's reasons for considering medication, and discussion of alternative strategies to regulate affects or behaviours during a crisis are all necessary prior to any decision to prescribe. The practitioner has an important role in giving information about medication and in preparatory discussions before the service user sees the prescribing practitioner, especially if that practitioner is not part of the SCM team. Prescribing practitioners need to avoid making major medication decisions independently from the SCM team and non-prescribing practitioners need to avoid playing into this separation of physical and psychological treatments and not treat medication as an isolated issue that they leave to the prescribing practitioner. Instead, all practitioners should have some knowledge about both the psychopharmacological and the psychological interventions and educate themselves if needed, ideally agreeing an integrated treatment plan.

Current Evidence on Pharmacological Treatment for Service Users Diagnosed with BPD

Mood-stabilizer medication—Valproate, Carbamazepine, Lamotrigine, Lithium. Although mood stabilizers are commonly used in the treatment of bipolar disorder and some investigators have suggested an overlap between affective disorders and BPD, studies show little evidence to suggest they are helpful in the treatment of BPD (Harpur, Harris, & Masson, 2018). Although valproate and carbamazepine have historically been used in the treatment of BPD to manage anger-related problems specifically, there has been little evidence to suggest this is actually helpful (Soloff, 2000). Furthermore, prescribing guidance now suggests that valproate cannot be used in women of child-bearing age who represent a large proportion of service users diagnosed with BPD (MHRA Guidance). Carbamazepine is a potent hepatic enzyme inducer which interacts with many other drugs—for example, it interacts with many oral contraceptives and raises the risk of unwanted pregnancy—and it is teratogenic. The recent LABILE study looking at lamotrigine in the treatment of BPD equally found this to show no superiority compared to placebo (Crawford, Sanatinia, Barrett, et al., 2018). While lithium is licenced for the treatment and prophylaxis of aggression and self-harming behaviour, it could be lethal in an overdose and could cause problems with thyroid and renal function. Furthermore, the need for regular compliance and monitoring makes it rather impractical to use in treatment of service users who have a chaotic lifestyle.

Antipsychotic drugs

NICE (2009) states that antipsychotic drugs are not advised over the medium or long term but may be beneficial for brief psychotic episodes which are known to be associated with a diagnosis of BPD. However, there is no evidence that they are helpful beyond this indication. Although antipsychotics are also used in the treatment of bipolar affective disorder to stabilize mood, there is little to suggest that they serve a similar function in the treatment of BPD. Equally, most antipsychotic drugs are associated with weight gain with increased risk of heart disease and diabetes (Correl, Detaux, De Lepeleine, & De Hert, 2015). Weight gain is likely to compound issues of self-esteem and self-image, which are already compromised in people diagnosed with BPD. Of note, however, is that within the class of antipsychotic drugs, clozapine, one of the medications used for treatment-resistant schizophrenia, is suggested to lower rates of self-harm markedly in people diagnosed with schizophrenia and may have a similar effect on people with BPD (Taylor, Barnes, & Young, 2018). The evidence for the latter, however, is confined to a few case reports. Equally it should be noted that clozapine itself is associated with risks of agranulocytosis and severe cardiac conditions such as myocarditis and cardiomyopathy and can be fatal in overdose (Merrill, Dec, & Goff, 2005). In the United Kingdom, clozapine is not licenced for treatment of BPD. Furthermore, undertaking this approach requires stringent monitoring with regular blood tests in view of the risk of agranulocytosis.

Antidepressant drugs

Antidepressant drugs are commonly prescribed for the treatment of depression, eating disorders, and anxiety disorders such as obsessive-compulsive disorder, post-traumatic stress disorder, and panic disorder, all of which are common co-morbid conditions of BPD. Unsurprisingly, they are therefore frequently pre-scribed for service users diagnosed with BPD. However, most antidepressant drugs that act on serotonergic pathways can increase suicidal ideation in the initial phase of treatment (Friedman and Leon, 2007), making their frequent use concerning in service users with BPD who are at risk of suicide and self-harm. Nevertheless, there is evidence for them to be used in BPD when comorbid disorders are identi-fied (Taylor, Barnes, & Young, 2018), although subsyndromal depression responds poorly to antidepressant therapy, with or without a comorbid diagnosis of person-ality disorder (Dobrzynska, 2017). It is important that when antidepressants are prescribed, the anticipated effects are made clear; is it expected that the depressive symptoms such as persistent low mood, poor sleep, reduced appetite, inability to concentrate, will improve or the symptoms of BPD will change, for example inter-personal volatility, self-harm, chronic thoughts of suicide, and impulsivity, or are both to be monitored? Current evidence suggests that BPD reduces the respon-siveness of depressed mood to antidepressants and unless the BPD is treated, the depression is likely to continue unabated.

Others

Naltrexone and naloxone, both opioid antagonists, were speculated to have a role to play in reducing rates of non-suicidal self-injury (NSSI) which can be used by service users with BPD to manage tension and mental pain partly because they have deficits in physical pain perception (Bekrater-Bodmann et al., 2015). NSSI releases endogenous opioids during the act itself leading to a reduction in ten-sion and an experience of tranquillity. This may reinforce the behaviour, which quickly becomes the most effective way of managing tension. Opioid antagon-ists might block this positive reinforcement and so make the action itself inef-fective. However, studies have not confirmed this (Hancock-Johnson, Griffiths, & Picchioni, 2017) although their use has increased (Timäus et al., 2019) and there may be some effect on dissociative symptoms (Schmahl et al., 2012). It is possible that NSSI reduces mental pain via a range of mechanisms. It may shift attention away from unpleasant emotions or thoughts. It may change cognitions about the self via self-punishment or transformation of the self from higher-order to lower-order awareness or even activate the parasympathetic nervous system, as a way of modulating emotional response However, further research into this area is re-quired before firm conclusions can be drawn.

In one non-randomized study (Prada et al., 2015), service users diagnosed with both ADHD and BPD treated with methylphenidate had better response on measures of anger, depression, and motor impulsivity than untreated service users. Given there is some overlap between the diagnostic criteria for ADHD and BPD (Deberdt et al., 2015), future research on medication for ADHD may indicate further avenues of research for prescribing in BPD. Finally, it is also important to note that electroconvulsive therapy (ECT) was found to be ineffective in the treatment of BPD (Black, Goldstein, Nasrallah, & Winokur, 1991; Pfohl, Stangl, & Zimmerman, 1984; Zimmerman, Coryell, Pfohl, Corenthal, & Stangl, 1986).

Conclusion

Any prescribing for service users diagnosed with BPD should be integrated into the SCM framework, be done in collaboration with the SCM team, and follow the principle of collaborative decision-making, which is central to SCM. The current evidence for medication for the treatment of BPD is not there and despite medication having the appeal of providing a quick and easy fix, it should never be first choice as a treatment for people with a diagnosis of BPD. Evidence for targeting specific core BPD problems is weak and should be avoided. Treating comorbid disorders such as depression, bipolar disorder, or ADHD can be beneficial for the service user's problems and functioning. Relevant medication of comorbid disorders can increase the service user's ability to benefit from SCM treatment.

The prescribing practitioner needs to be careful in distinguishing treatable comorbid disorders from variations in core BPD problems. This is achieved by collaboratively exploring whether the service user's problems align with the problems of BPD or relate more to comorbid disorders. Dialogue with all practitioners involved in the treatment programme will provide valuable information. The prescribing practitioner should build an alliance with the service user to provide the basis for making decisions about medication and to improve outcomes of prescribing. The prescribing practitioner should help the service user develop realistic expectations on what to expect from medication and identify indicators for reducing or withdrawing the medication.

The role of medication use should be carefully considered and discussed in a way that is planned and integrated into the overall SCM care and safety plan. Managing a crisis with a prescription should never be used in place of psychological strategies identified in the safety plan. For example, an extra telephone call, focused on helping a service user to use the crisis plan, might be more appropriate than short-term anxiolytic treatment. Ideally, medication is used only when it enhances SCM treatment outcome.

Non-effective or harmful medication should be discontinued in a carefully negotiated and gradual way. Polypharmacy should be avoided. If off-label medication is used then the prescribing practitioner should choose drugs with low toxicity and few side effects. Implementation of practice based evidence such as frequent measuring (via questionnaires) of comorbid symptoms in BPD can help prescribing practitioners evaluate the effectiveness of pharmacological treatments. This reduces the risk of polypharmacy and aids effectiveness of symptom-based prescribing.

References

American Psychiatric Association. (2001). *Practice guideline for the treatment of service users with borderline personality disorder.* Washington, DC: American Psychiatric Association.

Bekrater-Bodmann, R., Chung, B. Y., Richter, I., Wicking, M., Foell, J., Mancke, F., ... Flor, H. (2015). Deficits in pain perception in borderline personality disorder: results from the thermal grill illusion. *Pain, 156*(10), 2084–2092.

Benedetti, F. et al. (1998). Low-dose clozapine in acute and continuation treatment of severe borderline personality disorder. *Journal of Clinical Psychiatry, 59*, 103–107.

Black, D. W., Goldstein, R. B., Nasrallah, A., & Winokur, G. (1991). The prediction of recovery using a multivariate model in 1471 depressed inpatients. *European Archives Psychiatry Clinical Neuroscience, 241*, 41–45.

Cloninger, R., & Svarkic, D. M. (2016). Personality disorders. In S. Fatemi Hossein, & P. J. Clayton (Eds.), *The medical basis of psychiatry* (pp. 471–483).

Chengappa, K. N. et al. (1999). Clozapine reduces severe self-mutilation and aggression in psychotic service users with borderline personality disorder. *Journal of Clinical Psychiatry, 60*, 477–484.

Correl C. U., Detaux J., De Lepeleine, J., & De Hert, M. (1991). Effects of antipsychotics, antidepressants and mood stabilizers on risk for physical diseases in people with schizophrenia, depression and bipolar disorder. *World Psychiatry, 14*, 119–136.

Crawford, M. J., Sanatinia, R., Barrett, B., et al. (2018). The clinical effectiveness and cost-effectiveness of lamotrigine in borderline personality disorder: a randomized placebo-controlled trial. *American Journal of Psychiatry, 175*(8), 756–764. doi:10.1176/appi. ajp.2018.17091006.

Deberdt, W., Thome, J., Lebrec, J., et al. (2015). Prevalence of ADHD in nonpsychotic adult psychiatric care (ADPSYC): a multinational cross-sectional study in Europe. *BMC Psychiatry, 15,* 242

Dickens, G. L., et al. (2016). Experiences of women in secure care who have been prescribed clozapine for borderline personality disorder. *Borderline Personality Disorder Emotional Dysregulation, 3,* 12.

Dobrzynska, E. (2017). Are service users with emotionally unstable personality disorder overmedicated? *European Psychiatry, 41*, 256.

Ekselius, L. (2017). Personality disorders. Clinical guidelines for assessment and treatment. *Swedish Association of Psychiatry.*

Friedman, R. A., & Leon, A. C. (2007). Expanding the black box—depression, antidepressants, and the risk of suicide. *New England Journal of Medicine, 356*, 2343–2346.

Frogley, C., et al. (2013). A case series of clozapine for borderline personality disorder. *Annals of Clinical Psychiatry, 25*, 125–134.

Hancock-Johnson, E., Griffiths, C., & Picchioni, M. (2017). A focused systematic review of pharmacological treatment for borderline personality disorder. *CNS Drugs, 31*(5), 345–356.

Harpur, C., Harris, L., & Masson, N. (2018). Mood instability versus bipolar disorder. *The Journal of Prescribing and Medicines Management,* 17–23.

Ingenhoven, T. et al. (2010). Effectiveness of pharmacotherapy for severe personality disorders: meta-analyses of randomized controlled trials. *Journal of Clinical Psychiatry, 71,* 14–25. (12)

Kaess, M., Brunner, R., & Chanen, A. (2014). Borderline personality disorder in adolescence. *Official Journal of The American Academy of Pediatrics, 134*(4), 782–793.

Kaptchuk, T. J., Kelley, J. M., Conboy, Roger, L. A., Davis, B., Kerr, C. E., ... & Lembo, A. J. (2008). Components of placebo effect: randomised controlled trial in service users with irritable bowel syndrome. *British Medical Journal,* 999.

Lieb, K., Zanarini, M. C., Schmahl, C., Linehan, M. M., & Bohus, M. (2004). Borderline personality disorder. *The Lancet, 364*(9432), 453–461.

Lieb, K., Völlm, B., Rücker, G., Timmer, A., & Stoffers, J. M. (2010). Pharmacotherapy for borderline personality disorder: Cochrane systematic review of randomised trials. *British Journal of Psychiatry, 196,* 4–12

Merrill, D. B., Dec, W. G., & Goff, D. C. (2005). Adverse cardiac effects associated with clozapine. *Journal of Clinical Psychiatry, 25*(1), 32–41.

Paton, C., Crawford, M. J., Bhatti, S. F., Patel, M. X., & Barnes, T. R. E. (2015). The use of psychotropic medication in service users with emotionally unstable personality disorder under the care of UK mental health services. *Journal of Clinical Psychiatry, 76,* 4.

Pfohl, B., Stangl, D., & Zimmerman, M. (1984). The implications of DSM-III personality disorders for service users with major depression. *Journal of Affective Disorders, 7,* 309–318. [B]

Prada, P., et al. (2015). Addition of methylphenidate to intensive dialectical behaviour therapy for service users suffering from comorbid borderline personality disorder and ADHD: a naturalistic study. *Attention Deficit Hyperactivity Disorder, 7,* 199.

Sahlin, H. et al. (2017). *Regional care program for BPD.* Council of Psychiatry, Stockholm medical advice and Regions Stockholm drugs Expert Committee on Mental Health.

Schmahl, C., Kleindienst, N., Limberger, M., Ludäscher, P., Mauchnik, J., Deibler, P., ... Bohus, M. (2012). Evaluation of naltrexone for dissociative symptoms in borderline personality disorder. *International Clinical Psychopharmacology, 27*(1).

Simonsen, S., Bateman, A., Bohus, M., Dalewijk, H. J., Doering, S., Kaera, A., & Mehlum, L. (2019). European guidelines for personality disorders: past, present and future. *Borderline Personality Disorder and Emotion Dysregulation, 6*(1), 9. doi:10.1186/s40479-019-0106-3

Smith, K., Shah, A., Wright, K., & Lewis, G. (1995). The prevalence and costs of psychiatric disorders and learning disabilities. *The British Journal of Psychiatry, 166*(1), 9–18

Soeteman, D. I., Roijen, L. H. V., Verheul, R., & Busschbach, J. J. V. (2008). The economic burden of personality disorders in mental health care. *Journal of Clinical Psychiatry, 69*(259), 265.

Soloff, P. H. (2000) Psychopharmacology of borderline personality disorder. *Psychiatric Clinics of North America, 23*(1), 169–192.

Taylor, D. M., Barnes, T. R. E., & Young, A. H. (2018). *The Maudsley prescribing guidelines in psychiatry* (13 Ed.). London: .

Timäus, C., Meiser, M., Bandelow, B., Engel, K. R., Paschke, A. M., Wiltfang, J., & Wedekind, D. (2019). Pharmacotherapy of borderline personality disorder: what has changed over two decades? a retrospective evaluation of clinical practice. *BMC Psychiatry, 19*(1), 393.

Wilson, E., & Lader, M. (2015). A review of the management of antidepressant discontinuation symptoms. *Therapeutic Advances in Psychopharmacology, 5*(6), 357–368.

Zimmerman, M., Coryell, W., Pfohl, B., Corenthal, C., & Stangl, D. (1986). ECT response in depressed service users with and without a DSM-III personality disorder. *American Journal of Psychiatry, 143*, 1030–1032. [B]

10

SCM and In-patient Care

Elaine Swift, Louise Roper, Genevieve Quayle,
Kathryn Strom, and Jill Everett

Introduction

Although structured clinical management (SCM) was developed as a community-based treatment for people with a diagnosis of borderline personality disorder (BPD), the pragmatic organization of SCM lends itself well to providing a containing therapeutic framework for in-patient environments. This chapter will illustrate how applying SCM in in-patient settings can both enhance an effective whole care programme whilst also describing how SCM itself can provide a model to support in-patient environments. The chapter uses acute in-patient wards for adults and a female low secure unit as examples.

In-patient Care and People with Borderline Personality Disorder

In-patient treatment is not recommended as a primary treatment or treatment of choice for people diagnosed with BPD (NICE, 2009). Furthermore, one of the primary aims of SCM within community settings is to enhance autonomy, coping, and reduce the need for hospital admissions to help service users diagnosed with BPD (Bateman & Krawitz, 2013).

So, why would we consider in-patient care and BPD when clinical experts have questioned the appropriateness of any in-patient environment for the care and treatment of people with BPD, stating the milieu is not an appropriate setting for somebody who struggles with attachments, trust, and emotional regulation (Coyle, Shaver, & Linehan, 2018)? Although this view is widely held, actual empirical data supporting this position are not conclusive. The National Institute for Health and Care Excellence (NICE) guidance in 2009 did not find any evidence for or against in-patient care. In fact, Fowler et al.(2018), following their naturalistic longitudinal study of extended in-patient treatment for BPD, cautioned against making blanket assumptions on the harmful effects of in-patient care for people diagnosed with BPD in part because of the well-known heterogeneity of the disorder.

Weighing up the current evidence regarding in-patient care, the general consensus is that 'less is more'. A decision to admit a patient should be based on the needs of the service user and result from an assessment by a practitioner independent of, but informed by, the current treatment team who takes into account the service user's individual characteristics, current problems, and stressors.

Although in-patient care is generally not recommended or in fact designed for people diagnosed with personality disorder and related difficulties (even if they are not the primary cause of the admission), they still make up at least 50% of all in-patients (Evans et al., 2017). The clinical reality is that for BPD in particular, hospital admission may be necessary at times, particularly when risk to self or others is increased (e.g. suicide), or where there is the onset of severe depression and other comorbidity or when a clinical review or rationalization of medication is required.

Despite the high prevalence of personality-related difficulties on in-patient wards, many wards do not have a clear model of care for personality-related difficulties and/or service users with complex relational and emotional needs. It could be argued that the lack of a clear rationale for in-patient care for people diagnosed with BPD has not helped in the establishment of clear in-patient care approaches/ pathways.

Encouragingly, there are now an increasing number of in-patient units which recognize trauma and personality disorder as part of their 'core business'. They are more focused on 'how' they can be more effective for people with complex emotional and relational needs/BPD. The ambiguity or sometimes stigma around personality disorder has prevented adaptations to the ward environment that might be beneficial to staff and service users alike.

SCM is one approach that can help provide a framework for the 'how'. Implementing SCM within in-patient settings provides a therapeutic framework which enables all aspects of the service user's hospital experience to become part of a therapeutic intervention and a whole systems pathway approach to BPD from community to in-patient care.

SCM, In-patient Care, and Personality Disorder

Despite the different functions of acute and low secure wards,[1] admission to either may be necessary to reduce the risk to self and others in people diagnosed with personality disorder.

---

[1] Low secure services provide care for those who pose a significant risk to others and require physical security that impedes escape from hospital. Some will have been in contact with the Criminal Justice System and will have either been charged with or convicted of a criminal offence.

All patients admitted to low secure in-patient services will be detained under the Mental Health Act and the decision to admit will have been based on a comprehensive risk assessment and detailed consideration of how the risks identified can be safely managed whilst in hospital.

The core objectives for secure services are to assess and treat mental disorder, reduce the risk of harm that the patient exhibits to others, and to support recovery and rehabilitation (Adult low secure care NHS England Service Specification). Acute wards admit the general population needing mental health related admissions.

NHS England (2018). Service specification: Low secure mental health services (Adult). (Service specification No. 170041S). Retrieved from https://www.england.nhs.uk/publication/ service-specification-low-secure-mental-health-services-adult/

SCM and the admission process

Key strengths of SCM are its adaptability, its accessibility to practitioners in terms of understanding the model, and its straightforward, problem-focused approach. SCM provides a containing guiding framework to help with the admission process as well as clarifying and unifying the approach of the practitioners working on the ward.

A person diagnosed with BPD admitted to an in-patient ward should have a clearly defined purpose and realistic goals agreed for the admission. Although in practice this can be difficult to achieve when the person is in acute distress, this should not prevent discussion about goals and identification of the purpose of the admission with the service user and the ward team. The SCM-CV or clinical stance (see later) with its emphasis on curiosity and validation can provide a helpful model for the assessing practitioner to 'hold in mind' during the assessment and admission process. The SCM clinical stance can help the practitioner sensitively explore with the service user the purpose of the admission. Validating how the service user feels and curiously exploring the demands of the service user can generate a therapeutic alliance between the service user and the ward staff, reduce the level of anxiety and atmosphere of panic, and give an opportunity to explore the pros/cons and purpose of admission.

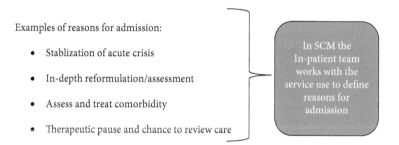

Examples of reasons for admission:

- Stablization of acute crisis

- In-depth reformulation/assessment

- Assess and treat comorbidity

- Therapeutic pause and chance to review care

In SCM the In-patient team works with the service use to define reasons for admission

SCM and in-patient environments

A challenge for any in-patient unit is to agree a coherent approach to the care of people diagnosed with BPD and/or complex trauma. SCM is a pragmatic solution. Implementing SCM within in-patient settings provides a framework within which all aspects of the service user's hospital experience is considered so the setting itself becomes an important part of the therapeutic intervention.

Box 10.1   Core Components of SCM Informed In-patient Care

- A coherent, pragmatic organized team model that all members of the unit can sign up to and deliver.
- SCMs uses enhanced problem identification and problem-solving as a core approach. It is about doing the basics of care well with greater emphasis on defining the problem in terms of internal mental states as well as focusing on external behaviour.
- SCM provides a clinical stance ('how to be') for the team to hold onto especially at times of high stress. In particular, there is considerable emphasis on curiosity and validation when interacting with service users with BPD/complex trauma.
- An approach that always aims to build self-agency and autonomy and thus supports least restrictive practice.
- Encourages active participation from the service users in their care and treatment.
- The approach stresses the importance of building trusting relationships and relational security, seeing attachments and relationships as the core to effective risk management.
- Provides a base for structured organized care prioritizing reliability and consistency.
- Multi-modal therapeutic offer of structured core treatment strategies delivered within individual and group therapy (tolerating emotions, mood regulation, impulse control, and sensitivity, and interpersonal problems)

Box 10.1 illustrates core components in SCM that can help in-patient environments.

With its emphasis on autonomy, SCM recommends that any hospital admission should be time-limited, structured, and have specific aims including helping the person to understand the nature of their crisis.

SCM and the ward milieu

SCM is a pragmatic and readily understood model in which general mental health professionals can become proficient with relatively limited additional training. This makes it an ideal model for in-patient environments practically and financially. SCM can bring clarity and containment to in-patient environments with a focus on defining the problem and thus ensuring more effective defined in-patient care. The next section of the chapter illustrates how SCM principles can underpin many in-patient approaches to care.

Non-specific and Specific interventions and In-patient Care

Interventions within SCM are categorized as non-specific or specific (Bateman & Krawitz, 2013). Both are deemed equally important and both require implementation within the ward setting to provide a coherent therapeutic process (see Chapter 3 on the clinical stance). The core interpersonal and communication skills of active listening, validation, genuineness, authenticity, and warmth among others are seen as central to effective care for people diagnosed with BPD, especially when delivered by all staff (including healthcare support workers) in all interactions with the service user.

At times, these fundamental skills can be undervalued in in-patient environments with too much emphasis being given to specific skills and behavioural management. SCM refocuses attention on the non-specific components, placing greater emphasis on these as an essential component of the care and treatment on the ward. Putting greater emphasis on these can empower all staff and enable all conversations to be potentially therapeutic. Embedding non-specific skills into all interactions on the ward provides a platform for exploring when things go wrong. SCM encourages a non-judgement approach and would curiously explore reasons for any slips in high-quality communication. These could be due to the tension of the ward 'environment', team dynamics, staff emotional capacity, and/or the intensity of the service user's interpersonal and emotional reactions. All these are likely to impact on the staff's ability to maintain therapeutic levels of communication and interaction with service users. Having an agreed and a clear model about factors that encourage good communication provides a useful foundation for reflective practice and staff supervision groups. Without a model of care ('what we are aiming to do'), in-patient team discussion and supervision can feel unclear, unfocused, and subsequently unhelpful for staff. As with all aspects of SCM, supervision would be clearly structured and organized whilst also being relationally focused. The four Rs can be a useful model/framework for the supervision.

SCM supervision:

- Revisit—model/goals
- Reflection—how are we delivering care?
- Recognize—define and understand challenges to implementing care effectively.
- Reboot and Refresh—re-energize and refocus on the care, model, and goals.

In SCM, how to interact with service users is seen as a whole team approach with every interaction valued and seen as a chance to facilitate recovery. As mentioned above, at times there can be too much importance and an overemphasis placed on formalized psychology/SCM sessions. SCM argues that every interaction counts and staff are valued as part of the overall psychological approach on the ward so it is vital that all staff are trained, given that most direct care in in-patient settings is delivered by healthcare support workers, who are also in the front line of managing service users' distress or frustrations with the system. This doesn't mean that planned sessions are not important. The formalized or planned SCM sessions are helpful but in a different way. In these structured sessions, the SCM practitioner/key nurse uses specific interventions aimed at identifying and defining problems for the service user and exploring solutions collaboratively.

Table 10.1 Values, Structures, and Equipment Needed for In-patient SCM

Values and core principles	Structures	Equipment
Wanting to be proactive as a whole MDT	Nursing teams including health care assistants offer pre-planned appointments two to three per week Active pathways such as a self-harm pathway, recovery pathway and behaviours which challenge pathway. All with simple bespoke interventions, training, and governance	Wide range of psycho-educational materials Distress tolerance materials Emotional regulation materials Problem-solving 'Surfing the urge' material Safety plans grown dynamically and person-centred.
Valuing least restrictive approaches that empower, give patients a sense of agency and control	Collaborative person-centred care planning Risk assessment histories up to date Least restrictive practice groups locally and organization-wide Governance structures that audit and review data to inform practice. Patient safety structures that fully understand least restrictive practice Peer reviews of services	Staff trained in dynamic risk assessment guiding our MDT decision-making understanding the function of risk within the in-patient setting for each individual patient and individual episodes of risk behaviour. Asking the patient and ourselves 'what is the person communicating?'

Table 10.1 *Continued*

Values and core principles	Structures	Equipment
Seeing the person, not the diagnosis	Understanding the function of the individual's behaviours and emotions in the context of their life experience, current difficulties, and previous and current relationships with services Daily communal meeting with patients to collaboratively plan the day and hold in mind the patient voice	Staff trained and working within a biopsychosocial model. Staff trained to understand the function of behaviours, not to just see behaviour or diagnosis
To want to offer reliable care so that the patient feels 'held in mind'. Valuing activity over passivity. Planned sessions including MDT reviews.	Knowing what to expect, when, and with whom Scheduling sessions with the MDT ahead of time, scheduling groups and individual sessions	Collaborative goals and care plans Collaborative leave and discharge plans If a person doesn't want to engage, we keep gently offering the structure
To be friendly but professionally boundaried	Mutual expectations of how we work together in a proactive and least restrictive way	Pathway leaflets Daily community meetings MDT formulation Group and individual supervision for reflection
Activities with our patients are considered to be everyone's business. Team buy-in including full-time activities coordinators who support other staff to deliver interventions throughout the shifts	Access to a 7-day per week activity programme Daily mindful breathing and or relaxation group Access to relaxation equipment 24 hours a day Weekly skills-based therapy groups along with diversional groups	Quick grab boxes full of therapeutic activities to aid communal observations and quick delivery of groups. Nurse led mindful breathing; nurse-led problem-solving groups Relaxation equipment Sensory equipment, e.g. weighted blankets Activity workers and peer support workers in dedicated roles.
Curious responses and active listening	Values a 'you said, we did' culture	At least weekly reflective practice/group supervision for staff, daily meetings with patients, staff meetings Gathers patients' views, shows thanks and appreciation to patients and staff via regular meetings The use of soft language

Continued

Table 10.1 *Continued*

Values and core principles	Structures	Equipment
Adherence to the model	Challenging others gently to stay on model Local structures to support the governance and support of the staff Daily patients meetings	Using shared IT portals to share video examples of skills and pathway materials Structures around once or twice weekly group supervision Audits of named nurse team interventions to ensure governance. Staff training being offered routinely Post-incident support for staff and patients
Staff and patients feeling empowered and valued	Staff being trained and having a whole team model allows staff to feel contained which in turn act as a positive impact on patient care	Safety huddles Feedback actively sought from patients Peer workers employed Gender informed care Access to relaxation equipment 24 hours a day,
Patients leaving with core skills appropriate to the length of stay Valuing structure and containment over firefighting and unboundaried, inconsistent care	The whole pathway structure which is multimodal (individual and group) and within the therapeutic milieu Also promoting the use of skills and 'in the moment' application to support in-between the structured session	Building a therapeutic alliance is seen as a central task Cultures that support least restrictive practice and model-driven care

Table 10.1 provides guidance on what is needed to implement SCM on a ward. Like supervision, it is an opportunity for the service user to revisit, reflect, recognize, and reboot.

SCM and the Core Functions for Effective In-patient Care

Below are six key areas for in-patient care.

- Understanding service user safety and least restrictive practice
- Trauma and gender-informed care

- Therapeutic systems: recognizing and challenging invalidating and harmful environments
- Structures to implement and embed the pathway
- Staff well-being
- Governance and practical elements

Understanding service users' safety and least restrictive practice

The challenge around caring for people diagnosed with BPD in a 'safety first' in-patient environment is complex. In-patient environments have to strike the delicate balance between a safety first approach whilst simultaneously trying to avoid being drawn into overprotective, defensive, and sometimes controlling models of care to manage high-risk behaviours. This is not easy.

Generally, with the 'less is more' approach to in-patient care and BPD, the aim is to have least restrictive care and shorter admissions, acknowledging that the main treatment will be delivered in a community setting. Therefore, in order to support in-patient environments as part of a care pathway it is essential that there are responsive, well-established community interventions for BPD.

Even with a clear community pathway and a focus on briefer admissions with seamless transitions, service users diagnosed with BPD can become trapped within the hospital system due to social issues. Such issues include accommodation, safeguarding concerns, their lack of confidence to manage their mind states and emotions, and/or lack of agreement between colleagues about the pathway to discharge and the most appropriate way to manage risk within the community. It is not uncommon for in-patient teams to interpret the safety first principles (Department of Health, 2015) literally and be drawn too far into a risk-averse approach which conflicts with the higher-risk approaches recommended in most evidence-based treatments for BPD. Consequently, in-patient environments are in danger of taking over the service user's autonomy, potentially interfering with the promotion of greater self-agency, which is at the centre of SCM and other evidence-informed community approaches.

In secure services, the process of hospital admission and detention becomes even more challenging. Secure hospital care, often for prolonged periods, may be enforced on the service user where risk to others is the primary clinical concern. Therefore, ensuring service users receive a structured approach to care and treatment over the long term that underpins all therapeutic contact, including treatment when they are detained against their will, becomes essential.

'Safety' first is a core principle of in-patient work and any approach to risk (Department of Health, 2015; NICE, 2015, 2019). However, safety requires staff to empower service users to take control of their behaviour even if it could be life threatening (e.g. empower service users to untie a loose ligature themselves and actively supporting them to use a safety plan to manage their distress). Relationships are central to this way of managing risk; the ward team works hard to form a trusting working alliance with the service user and focuses on offering them control and empowerment. It is crucial for ward staff and service users to have regular conversations about what is being done and why. It is worth noting that a 'least restrictive care' approach can feel dismissive and uncaring to the service user and be challenging for in-patient staff who often have to make decisions rapidly regarding risk to self and others. In-patient environments, like all community evidence-based interventions for BPD, should socialize the service users to the approach and philosophy of care. The principles of SCM provide a structured approach to enhancing service user autonomy through effective problem-solving and this can be applied when addressing risk and increasing safety (more on this later). However, if safety dictates, a restrictive intervention may be needed to manage imminent risk safely when proactive and least restrictive approaches do not work. If a restrictive intervention is necessary, a clear/revised support plan is immediately re-developed collaboratively to empower the service user to take back control gradually for managing the overwhelming and complex emotions that increased their risk. High levels of nurse observation during restrictive care can give the service user a feeling of being cared for in safety but this can quickly lead to the service user feeling inadequate, intruded upon, neglected, and rejected, resulting in further self-harming behaviour.

Restrictive practices are often easily recognized but sometimes may be more subtle. They may be part of a carefully developed care plan or a reactive response to an unforeseen emergency. Examples of restrictive practices include the use of 'blanket' rules such as the routine locking of doors, bedtime curfews, increased observation levels, use of seclusion, restraint and removing personal items including clothing or possessions. Restrictive practice also includes treatments such as medication which can inadvertently cause excessive sedation. Repeatedly accessing or being prescribed additional medication without time being taken to consider alternative psychological and self-management skills prevents their acquisition as an effective method of self-care. Restriction becomes part of control and restraint rather than a temporary intervention and inevitably leads to 'counter-control' responses from service users which may include self-harm and aggression and hostility and other expressions of resentment and frustration. Service users diagnosed with BPD and complex trauma may be particularly sensitive and reactive to coercive approaches. The interaction that unfolds in the dynamic of restraint and counter-control allows the service user to abandon self-control over complex emotions they themselves cannot manage and to submit to external control (e.g. punishment can become soothing over time). They may experience a sense that they have some degree of control over acts of 'power' that other people are imposing on them (Sweeney & Taggert, 2018). Powerlessness becomes power in behavioural action terms and the dynamic interaction with others is activated whenever the service user feels misunderstood or controlled by others and struggles to verbalize their predicament. SCM with its focus on building autonomy, curiosity, relational focus, and effective defining of problems provides a framework that can minimize a natural 'threat- (risk-) based' pull to restrictive care.

Adhering to the use of least restrictive principles has a number of effects:

1. It ensures that staff within the in-patient service remain flexible and open to managing creatively the dynamic risks that in-patient care presents to themselves and the service users;
2. It fosters a service user's increased sense of agency, control, and responsibility for their own recovery and well-being.
3. It helps both practitioners and service users avoid being pulled into mutually defensive oppositional-type actions in a system that may be experienced by both staff and service users as unsupportive, harmful, or blaming.

The self-harm pathway—an example of a SCM informed intervention

It is not uncommon for service users diagnosed with BPD to engage in self-harm and suicidal behaviour in an in-patient environment. The challenge for in-patient staff is 'how' to respond effectively to such a service user. The underlying drivers of self-harm are complex and often include a mixture of emotional dysregulation (difficulties around intensity, tolerance, and regulation confidence) and problems with interpersonal communication. Any approach to risk needs to address both functions.

Self-harm and self-destructive behaviours cause considerable problems on in-patient wards and implementing SCM as the building block of the therapeutic environment allows a coherent approach to managing self-harm. In-patient environments are based on nurse-led care and include a full professional team, all of whom have the aim of empowering and building service user strengths, skills, and resilience. Implementation of SCM provides support, structure, consistency, and a therapeutic stance including active collaboration, curiosity, validation, and personalized care. The self-harm pathway is an example of this. On the self-harm pathway, every opportunity to cope in less harmful ways is encouraged with service users 'at every turn', that is in all interactions on the ward, to promote the learning of skills to reduce self-harm and to enhance personal resilience. The approach is by necessity multimodal offering individual structured sessions and access to skill-orientated groups focusing on emotional management, impulsivity, and interpersonal skills to support the self-harm pathway. Table 10.2 describes elements of the self-harm pathway.

It is important that both the service user and staff are fully aware of the structure and function of the self-harm pathway. Clarity is central to this. SCM recommends

Table 10.2 Elements of a Self-harm Pathway

Clinical intervention	Clinical stance	Tools
Named nurse team sessions. This includes qualified and support staff	Structured, pre-planned. If cancelled by the nursing team there is an apology to the patient, a rescheduling, and a rationale placed in the patient's notes	Patient given dates and staff names of expected sessions. Name nurse session audits. Description of the pathway leaflet. Evaluation tools
Safety plans aim to help patients understand their triggers, explore patient's resources, and identify skills they might benefit from using/learning/ accessing to help them stay safe when faced with often overwhelming emotions. If the patient is expecting bad news use 'bad news mitigation', an idea from Safe Wards (Bowers, 2014) that helps the patient and team hold in mind the patient's support needs ahead of time	Grows dynamically and reviewed frequently, patient-centred, curious, and empowering. Is used actively within the system in between structured to encourage the use of the plan in a supportive manner. At a time of crisis, encourage the person to identify a strategy and feedback on its usefulness so we are reinforcing any approximation towards resisting the urge to self-harm. This is easily done within daily conversations and it is not time-consuming	The key is to take the time to encourage patients to reflect and come up with their own ideas. This is to be developed in named-nurse sessions and used proactively ahead of self-harm and after self-harm by the patient and the whole team. Values can be helpful in safety care planning; for example if someone values creativity or helping out, these can be used to think how they may help in a ward situation
Understanding what the patient is communicating in their behaviour	Curious, person-centred, authentic	Tools which understand behaviour such as self-harm and what triggers it, what the function is at the time, what helps
Chain analysis helps us break down the antecedents (interpersonal, physical, emotional, or cognitive), actions, and consequences to learn to break the cycle of self-harm	Curious, validating, and problem-solving	Chain analysis basic sheet to links thoughts feelings, behaviours, and exits. Helpful for those who self-harm or those with substance misuse to link the pattern of events leading up to the behaviour

Table 10.2 *Continued*

Clinical intervention	Clinical stance	Tools
Distraction skills Self-soothing skills Grounding skills Surging the urge Problem-solving steps	Curious, empowering, skills-based, and requires practice Helps build emotional tolerance, regulate distress, and manage poor impulse control around often complex emotions such as numbness, anger, shame, and guilt	Leaflets on the different ways to distract yourself Any materials are used and are collaboratively discussed not just given out Can be used within one-to-one psychology, nursing, or OT sessions
Substance misuse	Motivational stance looking at the pros and cons, problem-solving curious, goals and values discussed	Psycho-education, signposting information, motivational rating sheets
Recovery	Hope In control, educative, curious, collaborative problem-solving	Psycho-education on a range of difficulties such as hearing voices, depression, anxiety, personality disorder, domestic violence Goal setting, discharge road maps.
Activity programme	Offers opportunities for a wide range of group activities including exercise, psychological skills groups, and relaxation and fun groups	Staff in place to coordinate this MDT that contributes to the programme Daily patient meetings that embed the active stance and collaborative planning
Specific therapeutic groups	Offer the multimodal element of SCM being both individual and group	Standalone sessions of managing emotions, recovery, breaking the substance misuse patterns, mindful breathing
Communal observations and intervention	Driven to help promote a sense of relational safety and can offer easy interventions using the grab boxes	Plan the shift's communal observation rota Use grab boxes with pamper, quizzes, films, karaoke, and games options
Daily communal meeting	Gives a sense of agency and control in the system. Helps us plan and structure the shifts for the day	Led by healthcare support staff and supported by activity staff

Continued

Table 10.2 *Continued*

Clinical intervention	Clinical stance	Tools
Eating together	Safety and collaboration	Breaks down barriers
Non-specific skills	Interviewing skills; attitudes and values, empathy, compassion, validation, positive regard, and advocacy Therapeutic relationships have been shown to be a good predictor of positive outcomes for our patients All the skills and structure need attention to alliance building	A reflective team whose members can sensitively challenge each other to stay on model when we invariably experience emotional pulls and pushes to enact over soothing or punitive responses
Evaluation	To highlight progress with the patient To evaluate our practice	Staff confidence measures Subjective Units of Distress Scale (SUDS) that targets several emotions rated on a scale of 1 (not strong at all) to 10 (extremely strong). The In-patient Treatment Alliance Scale (Blais, 2004) that measures the quality of the therapeutic relationships between service users and the team. The Mental Health Confidence Scale that measures the service user's sense of confidence and self-control (Markowitz, Pease, Knight, & Carpinello, 2000). Individualized patient experience evaluation form at the end of the pathway to enable service users to provide valuable feedback.
Reasonable adjustments for those with mental and physical impairments and to aid thinking when emotions feel overwhelming	Asking what works for patients and holding in mind any extra scaffold that may be needed.	Coloured paper, pictorial safety plans; use the audio version of self-help materials Use of sensory equipment such as weighted blanket: use of aromatherapy smells; a safety box with tactile items in or food items that help in times of crisis Use shorter sessions if needed

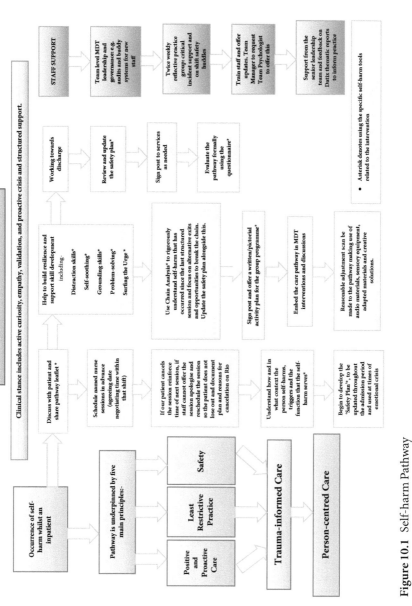

IN-PATIENT SELF-HARM PATHWAY

Clinical stance includes active curiosity, empathy, validation, and proactive crisis and structured support.

STAFF SUPPORT

Team level MDT leadership and governance e.g. audits and buddy systems for new staff

Twice weekly reflective practice group: critical incident support and on shift safety huddles

Train staff and offer updates. Team Manager to request Team Psychologist to offer this

Support from the senior leadership team and feedback on Datix thematic reports to inform practice

Working towards discharge

Review and update the safety plan*

Sign post to services as needed

Evaluate the pathway formally using the questionnaire*

Help to build resilience and support skill development including:-

Distraction skills*

Self-soothing*

Grounding skills*

Problem-solving*

Surfing the Urge*

Use Chain Analysis* to rigorously understand self-harm that has occurred since the last structured session and focus on alternative exits and opportunities to break the chain. Update the safety plan alongside this.

Sign post and offer a written/pictorial activity plan for the group programme*

Embed the care pathway in MDT interventions and discussions

Reasonable adjustment scan be made to the pathway making use of audio materials, sensory equipment, adapted materials and creative solutions.

Discuss with patient and share pathway leaflet *

Schedule named nurse sessions in advance (agreeing date negotiating time within that shift)

If our patient cancels the session reinforce time of next session, if staff cannot offer the session apologise and reschedule the session so the patient does not lose out and document plan and reasons for cancelation on Rio

Understand how and in what context the person self-harms, triggers and the function that self-harm serves*

Begin to develop the 'Safety Plan*, to be updated throughout the admission period and used at times of emotional crisis

Occurrence of self-harm whilst an inpatient

Pathway is underpinned by five main principles:-

Safety

Least Restrictive Practice

Positive and Proactive Care

Trauma-informed Care

Person-centred Care

- Asterisk denotes using the specific self-harm tools related to the intervention

Figure 10.1 Self-harm Pathway

Self-Harm Pathway

Working on Improving Self-Harm

... Ward

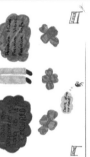

Mental illness is not a choice but... Recovery IS!

Positive feedback from women who have been on the pathway...

The pathway allowed me to be more involved with my care. I was able to develop my own care plan.

The pathway helped me to understand my feelings and learn how to self-soothe by using coping strategies.

Between sessions I was encouraged to keep a diary. I found this helpful as in the sessions me and my named nurse would reflect on my mood and feelings.

I found the structured sessions really beneficial. I always knew in advance who and when I would be seeing someone from my named-nurse team and knew I would be getting time.

I have been able to use my safety plan in times of difficulty and I will be taking these skills home with me. The pathway has helped me to think about things differently and will help me in the future when I am in crisis.

Groups and Activities

You can meet our activity coordinator(s) who will explain what groups we have on the ward and together we will come up with a timetable of activities you would like to attend each week. We encourage you to get involved in the activities on the ward, and ask that you please consider attending our daily community meeting.

Access to our gym

Anxiety management

Arts and crafts

Cooking and baking

Exercise groups

Managing emotions

Mindfulness

Pet therapy

Problem-solving

Psychology run groups

Sensory/relaxation groups

Peer support

You can also meet our peer support worker, who can offer one to one work focused on your recovery journey

Your Feedback Matters

We would greatly value your feedback on the pathway and we will give you the opportunity to complete a questionnaire; this is to help us develop the pathway further. Thank you.

Figure 10.2 Self-harm Pathway Leaflet

Principles of our pathway

The aim of our pathway is to provide a structured and consistent approach for people who self-harm.

We aim to support you through this difficult time by helping you understand why you self-harm, support you in using skills when feeling overwhelmed (such as distraction / self-soothing), and guide you in developing your own safety plan, which you can use on the ward and when you leave.

During your work on the pathway, you will have the opportunity to develop your own personal pack of resources for coping with your emotions, which you will then be able to use both on the ward and once you progress from here.

Understanding

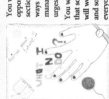

We want to be able to gain a full understanding of why you self-harm.

If we all have a good understanding it will help us to support and offer guidance on how we can try and help you.

Some women have reported that, at times, they have been unsure themselves of the reasons for their self-harm. They have reported that using the tools in this section has been beneficial to them in gaining an understanding of their own difficulties. One of the tools we use within the pathway is called chain analysis; your named nurse team will explain this fully to you. This tool gives you the opportunity to break down cycles of self-harm by identifying triggers, thoughts, feelings, and ways of coping. You would then have the means to explore what you might do differently if the same trigger were to arise again.

Developing distraction / self-soothing skills

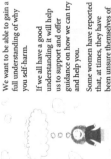

You will have the opportunity within this section to look at other ways in which you can manage and cope with urges to self-harm.

You will probably find that some techniques will work well for you and some won't; everyone is different. Together, we want to identify what suits you and works for you.

Safety planning

The skills you will have learnt through the pathway will help you when developing your own personalized safety plan. We will promote and encourage you to actively use your safety plan on the ward and beyond. We have different tools which can be used for this section depending on what you feel works best for you.

We ask that you are actively involved in creating and developing your own care plan with your named-nurse team. Your care plan will reflect what you have been discussing within your sessions; identifying what works for you in crisis.

What to expect from the ward?

You can have three structured sessions per week with your identified named-nurse team members. If you choose not to attend your session you will have missed that particular session for the week. Appointments will be organized with you giving you advance notice.

If you have been in hospital before, the way we now respond to self-harm may feel a little different at first. If you have the urge to self-harm, staff will offer you support to practise the skills you have been developing in your named-nurse and group work sessions. Together we will refer to your safety plan within your care plan.

If you self-harm you will find that staff respond in a least restrictive way. This will be individualized to each person and your named-nurse team will discuss this further with you; making sure it is documented within your care plan so that you have a full understanding and hopefully won't feel dismissed or uncared for, and rather feel in control and empowered.

It may also feel different if you have been used to being put on high levels of observations after self harm in the past. We now promote the development and practise of skills and understanding by engaging in the structured sessions and empowering you to use your own safety plan. Again your named-nurse team will discuss this least restrictive approach with you within a care planning session.

If you are actively self-harming this will be discussed and reflected on using the chain analysis tool during your next planned structured session. We also really want to reinforce and give praise when you have been able to 'surf the urge' and use the skills and techniques you have learnt on the ward.

Figure 10.2 continued

clarity around what the team and staff members are expected to do, and what is expected from the service user. Consequently, information leaflets about self-harm and repeated discussions around the model of care are important. As with all leaflets and pathways, these should be co-produced and ideally co-governed with service users.

Figure 10.1 illustrates a self-harm pathway and Figure 10.2 illustrates a leaflet. Table 10.2 provides guidance to staff on how to implement the self-harm pathway.

Trauma and gender-informed care

Like trauma-informed care (TIC), SCM is about treating the individual and taking into account the environment in which they live, the effects of their past trauma, and their coping strategies. Practitioners aim to be proactive about creating a safe physical and emotional environment for service users, visitors, and staff. The SCM clinical stance with its emphasis on curiosity about what has happened to service users over time and how adversity and trauma have affected them, what sense they have made of it, and what they do to survive or cope in their current life can be particularly helpful. Consideration is given to the impact that in-patient culture can have on well-being, including the risk of being re-traumatized by the system. By understanding, validating, and showing authentic interest in their problems, practitioners increase the opportunities of working collaboratively with service users to build their strengths, skills, and resilience whilst avoiding judgemental and punitive attitudes. Practitioners aim to empower service users to feel in control of themselves and their lives and to help them build on their strengths and become compassionate towards themselves. Staff aim to reduce any reinforcement of trauma experiences by being continually aware of the behavioural and mental effects of trauma and adversity as they play out in the symptoms of the service user and in their interactions with staff, and by showing compassion whilst using least restrictive care and proactive intervention. A biopsychosocial and cultural understanding of the person and the healthcare system is vital.

Gender-informed care is necessary when considering the impact of how services offer care and deciding who delivers it. An example of this is avoiding the use of male staff to undertake close nursing observations of a woman with a trauma history of domestic violence or sexual abuse as this might trigger traumatic memories and flashbacks. Teams may also need to consider how single gender or mixed gender groups are organized.

Therapeutic systems—recognizing and challenging invalidating and iatrogenic environments

SCM enables mental health in-patient teams to 'hold in mind' their core values and what they want to consistently deliver and in what manner. Service users coming into hospital are invariably at points of crisis in their life and teams need to help them to stabilize their emotions and maintain or develop new their links with community services to access further support at the point of discharge, which is integrated with their in-patient treatment. Having a clear therapeutic model driving care helps busy wards, which can at times have an atmosphere of anxiety and tension, to be less reactive. A model or framework can provide the anchor to help the ward staff see things from the service user's perspective (mentalize them), thereby bringing therapeutic structure and focus to clinical engagement with the service user.

In-patient wards attempt to create warm, bright, welcoming environments that actively encourage and enable service users to engage collaboratively in understanding and reflecting on their mental health, symptoms, triggers, and assumptions held in others' minds. Mentalization (holding one's mind and curiosity of others' minds in mind) underpins many aspects of SCM. An SCM informed ward is one in which the practitioners are asked to implement problem solving skilfully. In essence, SCM, albeit in the language of problem-solving, exhorts the practitioner and service user to reflect on their own mind and get a better understanding of their assumptions of others' minds to make sure that everyone becomes an effective problem-solver.

In-patient staff formulate service users from biological, social, psychological, and cultural perspectives. Values shared by the team and the system within which they work are at the heart of what is delivered. The aim is to offer open, engaging, and transparent care which is predictable—for example, having the same bed to sleep in every night—but also at the level of interaction, with consistent responses from staff to their problems. There is a focus on personal skill development, and a 'say' within the system and their treatment; for example, developing plans and goals for leave from the ward to enhance personal responsibility for managing risk and impulsivity.

By rejection of others, distrust, seeking care, and emotional responses, submission, self-blame, interpersonal violence, hoarding, appeasement, self-silencing, self-punishment.

Invalidating environments—assessing your environment

Many in-patient wards can become invalidating environments so far as they inadvertently trigger or reinforce difficult emotions for service users that link to past trauma. In doing this, the ward becomes a harmful environment causing service users to self-harm or engage in other risky behaviours in order to cope. This works against effective treatment and service users will have difficulty developing skills to manage emotions and abilities to build personal resilience.

Staff may become insensitive to the intensity of interactions between all service users on the ward and between service users and staff. Intense interaction will trigger the hyper-responsive attachment processes of service users, which then undermines their ability to make sense of what is in their own and others' minds. This can result in activation of abandonment fears, increased self-harm, and proximity-seeking behaviours with demand for increasing care from staff. Dismissal or criticism of a service user's insistent demands can be experienced as invalidating and shaming. Examples of this are dismissing or disregarding the service user's self-harm with statements such as 'it is just a superficial cut' or 'you are not even bruised', or failing to understand the underlying emotional distress of the service user and making personally invalidating statements such as 'you shouldn't feel like …' or 'that's unhelpful. Why did you do that?' Inadvertent invalidation and shaming as a result of staff attitudes may also occur when behaviour is categorized and labelled as being the result of an impersonal diagnosis; 'it's their BPD'. Within a framework of the 'boundary see-saw' (Hamilton, 2010), staff may counter a pull towards an invalidating and rejecting attitude by engaging in a pacifying and over-soothing stance, with unclear personal or professional boundaries being enacted within the therapeutic relationship. For example, staff can be drawn by the interpersonal pulls to see the service user as 'special' and extend favours to them in the belief that this will show the service user that they are cared for and that the team understand the service user and their needs.

Attention also needs to be paid to systematic invalidation within an in-patient setting whereby the in-patient team struggle to create a system that promotes reflection on therapeutic relationships with service users and team culture. In effective in-patient environments staff accept, acknowledge, and name the pulls (these are often extremely strong internal and external pressures) that lead to, for example, giving in to service user demand for a quiet shift, and recognize and address restrictive interventions that are being used without adequate consideration of the consequences, for example over-reliance on additional medication demanded by the service user. The team can easily drift into a failure to offer the safety, structure, and personal skills a service user needs if they are to develop abilities to function in the world. For example, teams may not fulfil agreements around named-nurse sessions organized to promote the service user's understanding of themselves, fail to validate the service user's positive achievements, and even neglect the focus on emotional management and interpersonal skills. This is more likely when the team do not have a consistent model that they all follow. Obviously, ensuring an effective space to re-address implementation of a model that is losing traction in the team is important. The supervision process in the form of the four Rs is one structured approach that provides a way to address such harmful dynamics.

Staff well-being

SCM practitioners report that the structure of SCM helps them by providing a framework within which they work and by giving them clarity about appropriate intervention (see Chapter 17), both of which reduce their anxiety and enhance job satisfaction. Having a clear model of care and a clear rationale for what you are doing and why helps in-patient staff and their well-being. With its greater emphasis on the importance of all interactions and giving equal value to input from all members of the team, SCM helps the whole team feel valued. The use of structured group and individual clinical supervision/reflective practice is vital for individual casework, teamwork, and ultimately staff well-being. SCM can also provide a framework for staff training/team-building days, which are essential for in-patient ward teams.

Structured team meetings are essential to embed reflective practice with a frequency of at least once a week; twice a week may be necessary to ensure equal access for staff who work on variable shifts.

Team meetings are best supported by SCM psychologically informed practitioners who are ideally senior practitioners in the team. The aims of the meeting are to provide time for staff to reflect on the emotional pulls and pushes of working on the ward with service users who engage in challenging interpersonal interactions and self-destructive behaviours, to ensure agreement and consistency in treatment approach, to support the well-being of the staff, and to offer review and learning from incidents. In addition, compassion-focused reflective time can be used as a forum to discuss how the team care for themselves—what helps and hinders functioning as a team.

Governance and practical elements of in-patient SCM

Ensuring that an in-patient team adhere to the SCM pathway requires governance procedures to be fully embedded and a stable in-patient leadership team that may include nurse leads, psychologists, psychiatrists, and occupation therapists (OTs). Furthermore, commitment to the pathway by the senior leadership team including senior leaders and executive team is important to ensure support from the whole organization. This is particularly important when applying SCM to managing service users exhibiting high-risk behaviours on the ward and the potential for serious untoward incidents.

Practical steps in supporting safe discharge

In acute psychiatric wards, discharge should ideally be planned over a period of time and at least 48 hours prior to discharge. Ward teams work with each service user to develop clear criteria for discharge starting from the point of admission. SCM, with its structured approach, can lead to further developments in the team, for instance emphasis in the named-nurse/practitioner sessions developing discharge plans with stepped goals and using problem-solving to address any barriers to discharge embedding the whole process within a clear, well-organized pathway.

The team reviews progress daily towards the stepped goals leading to discharge. They may include stabilization of risk, agreement on community-based intervention or social care support, reduction in symptoms, and ability to manage life stressors. If self-harm increases as a result of admission then the team need to consider a high-risk approach with discharge home rather than imposing more restricted care in low secure rehabilitation wards. Collaborative discussions with service users combined with recognition that risk is to some extent contextual and in-patient risk does not necessarily translate to the same risk in the community is key. Successful discharge of service users is more likely if the process is collaborative, the service user's perspective is taken into account, and there is negotiation around the discharge plan. The criteria for discharge can be set as an advance directive on how best to use admission to hospital along with a dynamic risk assessment. If the service user and in-patient team cannot use the hospital admission effectively, and if agreed in the advance directive and treatment plan, discharge procedures are activated. Actively discussing transitions and endings is important and often overlooked (or sometimes avoided), but open discussion can validate service user's mixed feelings and uncertainty in practitioners about leaving the ward. If a service user has been on the unit for a long period, therapeutic goodbye letters from the practitioner can be used to acknowledge progress and to outline hopes for the future and identify difficult feelings raised by the transition and the new beginning. This is particularly useful in a low secure setting where a service user may also be invited to send a similar letter to the named-nurse team.

Conclusion

Although SCM was initially developed within community settings, it can be integrated usefully in hospital settings. It is an effective intervention for a range of clinical problems encountered in in-patient treatment facilities and not just those presented by people diagnosed with personality disorder.

Although SCM is an 'atheoretical' model, the principles of attachment informed care, reliability, and structure, combined with a clinical stance of curiosity and validation (SCM-CV), provide a 'model of care' that supports in-patient care and dynamic clinical decision-making and buffers these against the potentially harmful impacts that acute crisis/distress can have on a care system. Through the implementation of SCM as the guiding framework for the ward environment, every interaction between staff and service users can become therapeutic and be part of the overall treatment. This enhances the therapeutic milieu and encourages effective teamworking. Following an agreed and coherent model allows all staff to act therapeutically in all their discussions with service users and between themselves.

SCM interventions were designed to be within the competence of generalist mental health practitioners or require only limited additional training (Bateman & Krawitz, 2013). This makes SCM easy to implement in services and it can be done at low cost with limited additional training time. Staff experience SCM as an intuitive model that 'makes sense' for service users and staff alike.

Further research is required to assess the efficacy of SCM within acute and low secure in-service user settings and with service users with a diagnosis other than BPD. In addition, other specialist in-patient settings, such as those treating people with substance use disorder who have core difficulties of impulsivity and poor problem-solving, may also benefit from SCM. Finally, the lived experience of engaging in a SCM ward for service users and staff alike is a further area for investigation.

References

Bateman, A. W., & Krawitz, R. (2013). *Borderline personality disorder: an evidence-based guide for generalist mental health professionals*. Oxford: Oxford University Press.

Coyle, T. N., Shaver, J. A., & Linehan, M. M. (2018). On the potential for iatrogenic effects of psychiatric crisis services: the example of dialectical behavior therapy for adult women with borderline personality disorder. *Journal of Consulting and Clinical Psychology, 86*(2), 116–124.

Department of Health. (2015). *The Mental Health Act 1983: Code of Practice, 2015. Annex 2*, pp. 269–273, paragraph 14.78. London: Department of Health.

Evans, S., Sethi, F., Dale, O., Stanton, C., Sedgwick, R., Doran, M., . . . Haigh, R. (2017). Personality disorder service provision: a review of the recent literature. *Mental Health Review Journal, 22*(2), 65–82.

Fowler, J. C., Clapp, J. D., Madan, A., Allen, J. G., Frueh, B. C., Fonagy, P., & Oldham, J. M. (2018). A naturalistic longitudinal study of extended inpatient treatment for adults with borderline personality disorder: an examination of treatment response, remission and deterioration. *Journal of Affective Disorders, 235*, 323–331.

Hamilton, L. (2010). The boundary seesaw model: good fences make for good neighbours. Chapter 13 *Using Time, Not Doing Time: Practitioner Perspectives on Personality Disorder and Risk Using Time*. Wiley and Sons.

NICE. (2009). *Borderline personality disorder: recognition and management. NICE Clinical Guideline CG78*. London: NICE.

NICE. (2015). *Violence and aggression: short-term management in mental health, health and community settings NG10*. London: NICE.

NICE. (2019). *Restrictive interventions for managing violence and aggression in adults*. London: NICE.

Sweeney, A., & Taggert, D. (2018). (Mis)understanding trauma-informed approaches in mental health. *Journal of Mental Health*, 1–5.

PART 3
SPECIAL ADAPTATIONS

11

Managing Transitions and Endings

Genevieve Quayle and Stuart Mitchell

Introduction

Managing endings and transitions in care for people who have experienced trauma and who are diagnosed with personality disorder is a key aspect of the structured clinical management (SCM) pathway in order to promote safe and effective care and treatment. It is important for practitioners to become aware of and anticipate that service users are likely to show strong emotions and reactions to any changes in care and treatment. This will include changes to who provides it, particularly as ending of an episode of care or changing a treatment approach may trigger fears of abandonment and sensitivity to rejection (NICE, 2009, 2015). The National Institute for Health and Care Excellence (NICE) recommends that for all people diagnosed with personality disorder a structured and phased approach is used before their services are changed or withdrawn (NICE, 2015). This approach should not be limited to people with borderline personality disorder (BPD) and many of the principles below are central to any trauma-informed pathway.

These points of change or movement between services become important for the service user as their attachment system is activated and they may experience anxious, avoidant, or disorganized reactions as the change in their current care episode may partially match their internal working attachment model or system (Bateman & Fonagy, 2016).

The practitioner also needs to be aware of their own attachment style and how this affects their interactions with the service user. As described in Chapter 3, it is incumbent on the practitioner to provide care and treatment that does not overly stimulate the service user's already insecure attachment system but instead promotes a collaborative shared sense of safety and goal-focused therapeutic work (Steele, 2016; Steele, Boon, & Van Der Hart, 2017). Care that is too intimate or close can cause distress to service users and lead to a loss of the service user's ability to understand and manage their mind (mentalizing and reflective capacity). This can lead to a harmful anxious dependency on the practitioner or the service (Bateman & Fonagy, 2016; Steele, 2016; Steele et al., 2017). Too little attention to the therapeutic relationship and the service user is likely to feel ignored, misunderstood, angry, and rejected. So getting the balance of attention to this is key (Steele et al., 2017).

Similarly, reaching the ending of an episode of care or treatment can stimulate feelings of loss, abandonment, and rejection in the service user, as well as in the practitioner. These reactions should generally be seen as normal and do not directly indicate an impending crisis but are elements of vulnerability the service user should have worked on within the SCM therapeutic individual and group work. During these times, the practitioner would spend more time working with the service user on the thoughts and feelings around the ending phase. It is important that both the practitioner and the service user can see the change and separation as a point of growth and learning rather than a sign of deterioration and need for further care or treatment, which might risk fostering dependency (Steele et al., 2017). This chapter will discuss how transitions and endings fit into the SCM treatment pathway, the key factors in the ending and transition process, and the therapeutic implications of these for what makes a good or poor transition or ending. Clinical examples of good and poor transitions will be used to illustrate principles.

Where Do Transitions and Endings Fit into the SCM Pathway?

Transitions and endings within the SCM pathway are events or processes of clinical significance to consider at all points along the pathway, from the initial referral through to completion of care and treatment and follow-up. Traditionally, it has been common for standard psychiatric care to pay less attention to this process than currently recommended as they have often been problem- and outcome-focused, with different services or teams operating independently, each with its own operating procedures and policies. However, clinically it is crucial for the service user that all services and practitioners involved in a care package consider the service user's unique experiences of attachment, change, insecurity, and loss. This is treated with the seriousness it deserves in SCM and should be carefully managed by the SCM practitioner, service user, and the care team as a whole. This enables safe and effective care and treatment where the service user feels truly understood (mentalized) by the clinical team.

From the service user's perspective, they may experience 'transition' or 'ending' at several junctures, as shown in Box 11.1

All these potential points of transition or change in the SCM pathway need to be carefully considered and taken into account within the planning of care and treatment and in their delivery. Without this, service users are likely to make limited progress, find themselves seeking out further care and treatment, and feel misunderstood and disgruntled about having received 'poor care'. So the practitioner and care team are responsible for providing care and treatment that fosters trusting, secure attachment. The care team attempts to strike the right balance between not overactivating the (insecure) attachment system by being too intense, for example treating the service user as fragile, or too underactivating by being too distant and remote. It is important that practitioners and the care team focus on fostering the

---

Box 11.1 Type of Transition Experience within the SCM Pathway

---

- **Transitions within the organization**—When being referred from children's to adult services, from community in-patient teams to community (generalist) services to specialist treatment teams, and so forth.
- **Transitions out of the organization**—When being discharged out of the care and treatment of the organization, or to other agencies, health, or social care providers.
- **Transfers between or within other agencies**—Such as from one health-care provider to another; to a voluntary organization, or from supported to independent housing.
- **Transitions within teams**—When having a change of practitioner or care coordinator; change of shifts or different level of engagement (e.g. observation levels whilst an in-patient).
- **Personal transitions**—For example, when experiencing the transition from young person to adult, or becoming a parent, or losing a parent.
- **Changes in status**—such as through becoming more independent, less in need of services, more able to live independently.

---

collaborative motivational system of the service user so that goals can be worked on, with minimal attention to the attachment-seeking system (Mitchell & Steele, 2020; Steele et al., 2017). By maintaining a focus on mentalizing, the care team can be clear about what they are trying to do with the service user, without getting into 'doing too much' (e.g. 'rescuing') or 'too little' (i.e. avoiding) (Bateman & Fonagy, 2016; Mosquera & Gonzalez, 2012).

The Ending and Transition Process

As discussed above, the experience of transitions and ending may be felt by the service user at any point along their journey in the SCM pathway. The service user may feel anxiety or threat at points of potential connection, change, or disconnection. They may then use attachment-based strategies, such as proximity seeking, aggression, avoidance, and dissociative shutdown. These attachment strategies are based on a wish to re-establish security and a felt sense of current safety (Steele et al., 2017). When the service user is experiencing high levels of anxiety and threat triggered by the action system of defence rather than daily life functioning, there is less mental capacity available to observe, reflect, and manage their mind and the assumptions they make of others' minds (Bateman & Fonagy, 2016; Mitchell & Steele, 2020). In this mode of functioning, service users are more likely to use

---

Box 11.2 What Happens Mentally at Points of Transition—Client Perspectives

---

- Attachment system stimulated
- Strong emotions often arise
- Mentalizing capacity reduces
- Window of tolerance narrows
- Defence system activated: 'quick-fix' behaviours may escalate
- Suicidality may increase

---

drastic 'quick-fix' actions in order to attempt to restore mental and emotional stability and felt safety, such as through self-harm, suicidal behaviours, or substance misuse (see Box 11.2).

For example, a young person was referred to child mental health services aged 13, then to the Early Intervention for Psychosis Service 1–2 years later, and then at 18 to adult mental health services. The service user felt that she couldn't trust all these different professionals owing to her early experiences and that it was 'terrifying' to be expected to let someone in emotionally. She felt misunderstood as she didn't understand why she was in those particular services and developed a belief that 'if I misbehave, I will be transferred again'. She also felt that no-one stayed with her long enough to help her change, and with each change of worker, her internal mental defences and attachment strategies became stronger and her self-harm and mood got worse. When she felt the workers from different services were working together and working with her, she felt safe and ready to work on her recovery. This illustrates the importance of how increased awareness of the whole team with respect to focusing on understanding the service user's mind and the team's actions and assumptions related to this can foster epistemic trust in the service user (Bateman & Fonagy, 2016).

Therapeutic Care and Treatment Implications

Understanding the meaning of transitions and change for the service user has important implications for the SCM pathway of care and treatment. There are things as practitioners we will strive to avoid and issues we will attempt to provide in more consistent and structured ways throughout the pathway of care. It helps to think of providing care that is *planned*, *includes* the service user, *links* up different services or practitioners' and is *personalized* to the service user (Planned Inclusive, Linked, and Personalized, PILP).

Planned

When a transition is *planned*, the professionals involved from both services consider the service user's perspective, how they will experience the transition, and how their history and attachment difficulties might unfold. They should not expect the service user to go over the whole of their history again with the new worker but instead will discuss what are the key headlines and significant events and meanings that the new worker needs to know. The fuller history will emerge as the new worker builds a relationship with the service user, and epistemic trust develops (Bateman & Fonagy, 2016). This planning needs to happen at a pace that the service user can manage: not too fast and not too slow. Too fast, and the service user will feel outside of their window of tolerance and overwhelmed; too slow, and they will feel frustrated and under-stimulated, or that the practitioner is acting too cautiously. What is key is that there is continuity of care and the service user's feelings are considered and validated, and the impact of the transition on them is appreciated by everyone. It can often be helpful to check in with the service user regularly and ask, 'is this working for you, how is it feeling, are we going at the right pace, involving the right people … ?' Arising from this work, there should be an action plan, with a series of clearly written steps to help the transition go smoothly. An example of a good transition plan is provided in Table 11.1.

Inclusive

A transition that is *inclusive* should involve the service user at every stage of the proposed transition in a collaborative manner and style (Steele et al., 2017). It is important to foster adult autonomy, self-agency, and independence so the service user feels empowered to make the transition and not so alone that they feel unsupported or forgotten in the midst of significant change. It is important to treat the service user as an equal partner in the process, ensuring that processes and decisions are collaboratively made and choices are provided.

Transition plans and processes should be inclusive of the person's strengths and internal resources. They should include a focus on what or who has helped to date, alongside what is possible to achieve. Any transition should include attention to what is developmentally or cognitively appropriate to the individual; for example, paying attention to the person's developmental stage, cognitive abilities, communication needs, or carer's responsibilities.

It can help to provide written information, such as service or therapy information leaflets, a care or safety plan, or even a therapy contract as it is developed with the person during the initial few weeks of the transition. Visual maps of services and the links, pathways, or steps between them, or a 'who's who' guide to the new service, can be useful.

Table 11.1 Example Transition Plan

Overall goal: To have a positive transition from children's to adult services	
Specific goal	**Plan**
For the right information to be shared with the right people, at the right time	My CYPS worker Sam will contact adult services when I'm 17½. There will be a professionals meeting where they identify who from adult services will be my named worker. I will be told their name after the meeting. Sam will share my formulation with X and give them my 'getting to know you' booklet. I will write down my story for my new worker. Sam and I will develop a list of all the people who will remain involved in my care and those people who I do NOT consent to share information with or don't want involved.
To get to know my new worker and manage the transition in a phased way	Sam, the new worker, and I will develop a schedule of appointments which will span 3 months either side of my transfer at 18. This will involve a gradual decrease in appointments with Sam and increase in ones with my new worker.
To know where my new appointments will be before having to go for my first appointment alone	Sam will take me to meet my new worker at their base. We will go together, have a look around. I will meet the receptionist, find out where I can get a coffee, and where I will see my new therapist. I'll note some safe anchors and develop a mental map of what felt good. I can tell Sam about any of my worries or concerns afterwards. I will work out which bus I need to get and plan it in my head.
To say goodbye to Sam in a way that can give me a good memory	I will have a card-making appointment with Sam and will write her a goodbye note on the card we make during the appointment. Sam will write an ending letter that will identify the positive journey I've been on over the last 15 months.
To feel safe and not have sudden changes to my care if I do use self-harming strategies	Sam and I will have made sure my crisis plan, Safety Wellness Action Plan, and WRAP plan are all up to date and accessible on my records. I can use burning impulsively when I feel distressed. This can lead to acute care input which at times leads to Mental Health Act review. I don't believe admissions help me and they can cause me more distress. If I do burn, the care team and I should work out what this is in response to and prompt me to use the strategies I've learnt. If I'm really low then the care team will consider increased input such as home-based treatment via the crisis team.

It may also be prudent to involve key people who provide support in the person's social network, with the service user's consent, such as family members, partners, or friends. Such individuals can provide much needed support to the person at times of crisis, and can benefit from understanding what SCM is, how it works, who does what, and what they can do to support the person on their SCM journey. More detailed 'family work' is described in the next Chapter. In addition to family and carers, remembering the value of community inclusion can also be of benefit. Ensuring that any key individuals from the person's social and/or vocational network are included, with the service user's consent, can not only help the person feel that their support network and personal world has been considered but also help reduce the intensity felt of the change from one worker to another.

Linked

During the process of managing the transition, practitioners from both services involved need to be named to the person, with their role explained, so it feels *linked*. There should be some agreement about contact details and frequency of appointments. For a young person transitioning from children and young people's to adult mental health services, there may be a sense of a huge change from a protective sort of care, where less is expected of them, to one where they are seen more as an adult and more is expected of them. This may feel like a dramatic loss of care to the person. In this situation, the practitioners from both services need to be aware the impact of this on the service user and find a way to manage the differences in care and treatment received so that the change does not feel so dramatic but more gradual and manageable. It will also help if the practitioners involved facilitate visits to new services to enable the person to familiarize themselves with the setting, venue, layout, etc. Finally, it is important that all professionals adopt a shared approach to the work and do not express a view that the service user is 'now someone else's concern'. The task of helping the service user through transition needs to be truly joint and focused on the service user's needs, so that consistency and compassionate care is felt by the service user during the process, and they don't feel mentally 'dropped'. Joint multidisciplinary team meetings, clinics, and assessments may facilitate this joined up process. Good teamworking is essential in this regard.

Personalized

The final aspect of a good transition is to make it *personalized*, or bespoke, to the individual. Practitioners from both services, the old and the new, need to act in flexible ways so that they are responsive to the service user's needs, without a rigid adherence to maintaining structure or processes which distance the service user or make them feel ignored or forgotten in the process. Flexibility with firm boundaries and structure is what is needed, with services focusing on the primary clinical needs of the service user rather than the needs of the service. An example of bespoke, flexible working around a transition could be helping the service user find ways to make the change so they can adjust to the change gradually. The use of transitional objects (Winnicott, 1953) such as letters, postcards, collage, or painting could be used here as a mental 'bridge' to the new service and worker. The service user could be asked to write a personal introduction to themselves, such as a 'this is me' information sheet, within their transition plan so the new worker gets an immediate sense of them and doesn't miss important elements. It may be helpful also to design a way of saying goodbye when finishing in treatment or ending one phase of therapy and moving to another service or into another stage of treatment. For example, writing a goodbye letter, having a graduation certificate, or arranging a follow-up meeting can facilitate the emotional upheaval involved in the change. All these aspects of a good transition are summarized in Box 11.3.

What Makes a Less Positive Transition?

It is worth reflecting on what makes a transition less positive for a service user so that we may then be able to avoid or limit the things we do which lead to reinforcement of this process or iatrogenic harm. Of course, an absence of PILP factors discussed previously will be unhelpful, but in particular minimizing or dismissing the importance of the transition, having little or no time dedicated to reflection, planning, and sharing of information between services with dedicated staff is likely to be unhelpful or even harmful. Frequent changes of worker and an inability to make clear decisions about the transition will also foster insecurity and anxiety about what is going to happen. It is important that the team also does not act in ways that appear to be fixed or rigid, such as 'no-one with a personality disorder should be admitted for more than 72 hours', or 'it's just behaviour and personality, not a real crisis'. These judgements and reactions are understandable, given the anxiety and pressure staff often feel when working with service users (Kernberg, 2007). However, they reflect how staff can resort to non-mentalizing language and states of mind; for example, certainty about what the service user needs, rigid assumptions about the services user's motives, and losing the core stance of curiosity when they themselves are overwhelmed or struggling to comprehend the service user or their own reactions (Bateman & Fonagy, 2016). These sorts of reactions are shorthand ways of trying to understand the service user and their behaviour, but they do not really get to the heart of the range of mental states, especially affective states and attachment status, currently felt by the service user.

Box 11.3 What Makes a Positive Transition (PILP)?

- Planned
  - o Holds in mind the person's mind, their history, and attachment difficulties
  - o Doesn't make the person repeat their history
  - o Paced and timely
  - o Provides continuity of care
  - o Clearly laid out steps/actions into a written transition plan
  - o Visits to new people and services
- Inclusive
  - o Involves the person at every stage collaboratively
  - o Involves key people in the person's life with consent
  - o Provides appropriate written information about the transition and after care arrangements
- Linked
  - o Named individual staff members—link people from each service
  - o Visits to meet new people and services
  - o All professionals involved identified, named, and their roles clearly explained and linked up
  - o Joint multidisciplinary teams (MDTs), clinics, and assessments to ensure consistency across and within teams
- Personalized
  - o Bespoke (mentalized) transition planning with the person
  - o Flexible services according to clinical need
  - o Use of transitional objects considered for some young people to 'bridge' to new service and staff member
  - o Appropriate endings, managed safely
  - o 'This is me' information sheet developed with the person

---

There may be a lack of openness and curiosity to establishing mental states that have led to a crisis and a need for admission, such as a new worker triggering a traumatic reaction based on previous changes of worker which have been traumatic. There are often concerns and disagreements within the team about fluctuating capacity of a service user to give consent and understand the risks associated with their behaviour and states of mind. These issues are best reflected upon as a team in a balanced and reasoned way so as to promote curiosity and mental awareness (mentalizing) within the team as whole, whilst focused on the service user (Bateman & Fonagy, 2016; Bateman & Krawitz, 2013).

On an individual practitioner level, the worker may have formed some attachment and understanding of their service user (Holmes, 2010), and be reluctant to let them leave the service, fearing that others may not be able to help or provide the same level of service that they provided. They may even worry that the receiving service will not be as good, and the service user will suffer and then blame them for any problems experienced within the new service. This is a natural response and one to be accepted and supported by consultation with a senior colleague, or with the team as a whole. It is important that responsibility ultimately lies with the service user themselves for managing the transition, which practitioners facilitate in moderate ways by being present, consistent, reflective, and supportive, and not too distant or unavailable.

At a systemic level, each service may have a different language, system, and pathway process it uses. There may be different foci in terms of commissioning, targets, and outcomes for services. Services for children and young people may have age cut-offs. Staff may be trained only within their own speciality and not within the speciality to which the service user is being transferred, so they may not have the appropriate skills. Care may be limited by time or number of sessions, so that a longer term pathway is not considered and needs are left unaddressed. Case loads can also be high, with pressure from managers to produce outcomes and flow within the system. When this is felt too strongly, there may be a focus away from the needs of the service user towards service level needs. This can all be confusing for the service user. These factors are summarized in Box 11.4.

Box 11.4 Factors Leading to Less Positive Transitions

- An absence of a Planned, Inclusive, Linked, and Personalized (PILP) approach
- Multiple changes of decision-making or workers within the transition
- Use of different language by services and workers
- Rigid or poorly understood reactions to service user's difficulties
- Workers own attachment patterns which affect how they manage the transition
- Different system, language, pathways, and processes
- Age cut-off variations
- Worker skill and lack of training
- Systemic pressure—for example, case load size, outcomes, targets, finance, capacity, and resource limitation

Ending Therapy Phase

Therapy in SCM usually takes 12 to 18 months and occasionally longer if other issues are being addressed concurrently, such as psychological trauma, substance misuse, or housing problems. First, it is important that the practitioner and service user jointly maintain an awareness of time and monitor of progress throughout the whole period of SCM therapy and at each review point. This will ensure that the ending is not only considered when it appears but is a consistent theme, with different points of emphasis throughout the therapy period. However, for at least the last 6 months of therapy, the practitioner helps the service user move into an ending or completion phase. This is where they will focus on consolidating progress made during SCM in terms of applying more of what they have learned in SCM to actual daily life situations, such as work, education, or relationships (Krawitz & Jackson, 2008), and also negotiate the process and meaning of leaving or completing therapy. This will have been a part of the care plan from the start but will become more of a focus as the service user moves into this last phase of therapy.

As an ex-service user reports, it is common that service users experience a range of affective states linked to separation and loss, such as anxiety, sadness, excitement, and pride (Krawitz & Jackson, 2008). The aim of the ending process is to ensure service users understand and reflect on their feelings and the meaning of completing SCM therapy (Bateman & Fonagy, 2016). Too little attention and consideration of this phase of SCM therapy can lead to the re-emergence of earlier ways of managing problems and a loss of this reflective or mentalizing capacity, leaving the service user feeling forgotten or abandoned.

The goals of this final phase of SCM, which need to be renegotiated with the service user, are to facilitate the service user taking greater responsibility for their own independent functioning, particularly with regard to applying skills that have been developed in therapy. It is also to consolidate further improvements in social stability and functioning, for example, in terms of education, employment and interpersonal relationships. There will be a collaborative process of agreeing a 'leaving or finishing therapy plan', including an agreement about follow-up appointments. Within this plan, it can be helpful to stimulate service users to take a lead role in how they would like their SCM therapy to end or complete, such as setting a date, what they will continue to work on and practice and what sort of follow-up appointments or further therapy might be useful. This is a matter of negotiation between the practitioner and service user. Some service users may find it difficult to end therapy, so may avoid the ending by seeking out frequent follow-up appointments. At the other extreme, there are service users often with severe difficulties who have had years of (not always helpful) contact with mental health services and so require a very gradual and longer period of support in adjusting to life without services, for example by incrementally increasing the time between follow-up/

> ### Box 11.5 Goals of Final Ending/Completion Phase of SCM
>
> - Not forgetting it! Keeping the sense of time, and progress/reviews in mind throughout the whole SCM pathway
> - Increased client responsibility for independent functioning
> - Consolidation of gains made in SCM already, especially in terms of social areas, such as work, education, and relationships
> - Collaborative negotiation of ending/completion phase, and agreement of follow-up appointments
> - Joint focus on the affective states and meanings of completing or ending SCM therapy

follow-along appointments over a period of a year. There may be a waiting time for some service users who seek further forms of therapy, as there are in most National Health Service (NHS) services across the United Kingdom. The goals for this phase are summarized in Box 11.5.

Unplanned Endings—Implementing Therapeutic Discharge

Occasionally, situations arise when a service user is transitioned out of the service at a non-transitional point or before completing the SCM programme. Sometimes this may be against their wishes. Examples of this include dealing drugs to group members despite previous warnings, assault, extreme passivity in the programme, persistently poor attendance, and/or bullying of others. Even during these times the discharge should still aim to follow as much as possible the PILP principles.

On some occasions, it may not be possible for the service user to engage in any therapeutic equivalent treatment programme offered by the service. At these times, the service or SCM team may need to take a carefully considered, clear therapeutic stance and review how to discharge the service user therapeutically as safely as possible from the service. This would be an alternative to the risk of being drawn into care and attachment patterns that are at best unhelpful and at worse can cause iatrogenic harm.

Therapeutic discharge can, if used appropriately be a way of shaping up active participation or shaping down therapy-interfering behaviours. Although seen as a last resort it can be helpful. The key to the success though is that the service should, whenever possible, be willing to accept the service user back and for the steps required for re-entry to the service be specified.

> ### Box 11.6 Steps to SCM Therapeutic Discharge
>
> - The decision should be a team decision, preferably an MDT
> - Rationale and aims of therapeutic discharge collaboratively discussed with the person and their supporters (e.g. family/friends, other agencies, GP)
> - Criteria for re-engagement/what would need to change for engagement/treatment to be more successful is clearly communicated to the service user and their support network (e.g. change in motivation, resolution or change to an external stressor, reduction in therapy-interfering behaviours)
> - Arrangements for rapid re-referral made and information shared with service user and support network on ways of re-accessing services (should the situation change/conditions for re-engagement be met).
> - Collaboratively review the safety plan and anticipate issues that may arise in primary care if discharged and information how to access out-of-hours services
> - Secondary care services remain available to GP for consultation (regarding risk, appropriateness of re-referral, relevance of third sector support).

The steps shown in Box 11.6 illustrate an implementing guidance for this type of therapeutic discharge. If not already done so, supporters/carers are referred/signposted for specific support related to their role.

Conclusion

There are multiple points of transition and ending for people undergoing SCM, all of which require careful consideration by the practitioner and clinical team. Such changes arouse considerable anxiety in service users who build strong attachments to their practitioners or services that support them.

Discussing in advance, at least 6 months before the ending of treatment, or before any planned change, the implications and meaning of the change will help ameliorate anxiety and increase a sense of choice and control. Collaboratively developing a phased and structured plan before changes occur provides some containment of anxiety and ensures epistemic trust is maintained throughout the service users SCM treatment pathway.

A transition plan should be the outcome of a process that has the elements of being planned, inclusive, linked, and personalized, as shown in Box 11.7.

Box 11.7 Transition Plan Elements

1. **Planned.** Careful consideration to the service user's attachment pattern and history that is paced, timed and ensures continuity of care
2. **Inclusive.** Involvement and co-production of the plan is demonstrated at every stage, supporting a strong collaborative therapeutic alliance. This includes key friends, family, and partners where applicable
3. **Linked.** Key practitioners from different services are identified and act as points of contact that are linked up. This may apply equally to MDT meetings and assessment clinics
4. **Personalized.** The plan should be personalized to the service user, based upon an understanding of their attachment pattern and clinical needs. This could include information from the service user that they feel is essential for all services to know, such as in a 'this is me' information sheet

---

In addition to planning for transitions, service users will need to know how they can access services at times of crisis following discharge, and some service users may require very gradual and phased withdrawal of care and support. Having integrated care pathways and systems supports such an approach.

References

Bateman, A. W., & Krawitz, R. (2013). *Borderline personality disorder: an evidence-based guide for generalist mental health professionals.* Oxford: Oxford University Press.

Bateman, A., & Fonagy, P. (2016). *Mentalization-based treatment for personality disorders.* Oxford: Oxford University Press.

Gonzalez, A., & Mosquera, D. (2012). *EMDR and dissociation: the progressive approach* (Rev.). Available from: Info@itradis.com.

Holmes, J. (2010). *Exploring in security: towards an attachment-informed psychoanalytic psychotherapy.* London: Routledge.

Kernberg, O. F. (2007). Countertransference: recent developments and technical implications for the treatment of patients with severe personality disorders. In B. Van Luyn, S. Akhtar, & W. J. Livesley (Eds.), *Severe personality disorders: everyday issues in clinical practice.* Cambridge: Cambridge University Press.

Krawitz, R., & Jackson, W. (2008). *Borderline personality disorder: the facts.* Oxford: Oxford University Press.

Mitchell, S., & Steele, K. (2020). Mentalising in complex trauma and dissociative disorders. *European Journal of Trauma and Dissociation,* https://doi.org/10.1016/j.ejtd.2020.100168

NICE. (2009). *Antisocial personality disorder, Clinical Guideline 77.* London: NICE.

NICE. (2009). *Borderline personality disorder, Clinical Guideline 78.* London: NICE.

NICE. (2015). *Personality disorders: Borderline and antisocial. NICE Quality Standard 88.* London: NICE.

NICE. (2015). *Transition between inpatient hospital settings and community or care home settings for adults with social care needs. Clinical Guideline 27.* London: NICE

NICE. (2016). *Transition from children's to adults' services for young people using health or social care services. Clinical Guideline 43.* London: NICE.

Steele, K. (2016). Attachment, dependency and collaboration in the psychotherapy of complex developmental trauma. *ESTD Conference*, Amsterdam, 15 April 2016.

Steele, K., Boon, S., & Van Der Hart, O. (2017). *Treating trauma-related dissociation: a practical integrative approach.* London: Norton & Co.

Winnicott, D. W. (1953). Transitional objects and transitional phenomena—a study of the first not-me possession. *International Journal of Psycho-analysis, 34,* 89–97.

12

Working with Families and Carers

John Chiocchi, Paula Slevin, Lisa Evans, Catriona Gray, Nicola Armstrong, and Kerry Anderson

Introduction

Like most mental health programmes, structured clinical management (SCM) programmes focus predominantly on the service user, helping them to learn skills and promote confidence in their own ability to cope with the challenges of daily life. However, any comprehensive SCM programme will also consider the system and family as essential parts of a pathway to recovery. It has long been argued that appropriate carer education programmes should be incorporated into the care and treatment offered to people engaging in mental health services in order to achieve better outcomes for both carers and service users (Gunderson & Hoffman, 2005). We know that families and friends are tremendously important in our lives. Because of the types of difficulties people diagnosed with personality disorder experience, interactions between them and their family members can be emotionally stormy and liable to misunderstandings, with mutual experiences of personal invalidation. This can lead to emotional exhaustion for family members who are doing the best they can with the knowledge and skills they have to support their loved one. They are often the first to notice when their loved one is becoming distressed and they play a crucial role in helping them to manage crises. They provide ongoing support which requires them to cope with their loved one's strong emotions or suicidal and self- harming behaviours, whilst also offering emotional validation and support in solving social problems. This is a role which requires skills many of us have not learned in the usual course of our lives (Hoffman, Fruzzetti, & Buteau, 2007). Families themselves report their need for better understanding and knowledge about the diagnosis and more support in their day-to-day caring roles (Giffin, 2008). Additionally, without an understanding of the intervention being offered, families may continue to react in habitual ways that inadvertently undermine the effort their loved one is making to put newly learned life skills into practice.

Carers and family members are not a homogenous group and might need different types of support at different times. Some people might find connecting with others and sharing their experience of caring for someone one who has a diagnosis of personality disorder both helpful and normalizing. Others may want to work with the person themselves to learn new skills and find ways of living better in relationship with one another. There are therefore two strands of carer and family work integrated into the overall SCM programme: a carer's education group and SCM family sessions.

This chapter starts by describing a personal journey from a carer perspective that led to the development of a co-produced Peer-Led Training Programme (a carer education approach). It then provides an overview of three different models of carer programmes and family intervention sessions for people diagnosed with personality disorder, as part of an SCM programme or pathway.

Co-production and the Peer-Led Carer's Training Education and Support Programme (TES)

Setting the context: a personal journey to developing a carers programme—John Chiocchi

For a number of years my wife and I found it a struggle to help and support our son. We had the typical experience of being 'bounced' around between primary care and secondary care mental health services because my son did not fit into the medical model of diagnoses at that time. When the impact of 'no longer a diagnosis for exclusion' (Department of Health, 2003) was changing the landscape for people diagnosed with personality disorder, my son was only then assessed by mental health services and finally given a diagnosis of emotionally unstable personality disorder (EUPD). This was at the time extremely difficult to understand and process, and we had many questions about the diagnosis: how did the disorder develop? How to help? Answers were not forthcoming and there was nothing in place for carers to access for support.

I felt so strongly about this that I raised this with a support worker allocated to us at that time. I was also disturbed by the lack of support and service provision not only for my son but also for others who had the same diagnosis and their families. The support worker signposted me to a monthly forum at a local mental health organization and also kindly encouraged me to attend the first few sessions due to my lack of confidence. This forum was the first time I was able to address my questions to the relevant people and could not only tell them about the lack of provision for those diagnosed with personality disorder but also their families and carers. Prior to that experience, it had become habitual to not be listened to.

At one of these meetings, a Trust director who chaired the meeting suggested I consider becoming a volunteer and help the organization make changes to service provision. This was to become life changing for me. Over the months and years, I became firmly established within the forum and I was then offered the opportunity to become one of two expert by experience (EBE) representatives, a service user

EBE and myself as a carer invited to sit on the Trust board. It made me extremely proud to be selected to represent the forum at this level. Again, it helped me gain confidence to talk directly to the board regarding my concerns about services within the Trust for people diagnosed with personality disorder. Eventually at one of the Board meetings, the operational director approached me about the proposed establishment of a personality disorder hub and asked if I would be interested in being involved. The answer to that invitation was a rapid 'yes'!

In 2010, Five Boroughs Partnership (Note: Five Boroughs changed to NWBH and then in 2021 NWBH split with Halton, Knowsley, St Helens and Warrington joining Mersey Care and Wigan joining Greater Manchester) in the United Kingdom established the Personality Disorder Hub (PD Hub). It comprised a number of practitioners: psychologists, psychiatrists, occupational therapists, community psychiatric nurses (CPNs), and, more importantly, EBEs who either had a diagnosis of personality disorder themselves or were caring for someone with that diagnosis. It took some time for the Hub to become embedded into the organization but it was clear that those who attended the business meetings had an absolute commitment to improve services for people with a diagnosis of personality disorder. The main remit of the Hub was to provide awareness training to enable staff to gain a greater understanding of the diagnosis and how to support people with personality disorder effectively.

This brings me to the essential question: how can we support carers and families? A co-produced working group developed a personality disorder awareness training for families. This was called CRISPS (Carers Require Information to Support Personality Symptoms). The 2 half-day sessions cover what a personality disorder is, how it develops, treatment and therapies, and coping strategies. Two carer videos were developed and participants reported they identified strongly with the themes and information the videos showed. Evaluation suggested positive outcomes: 'I have been given a greater knowledge of the illness; this will help me, my daughter, and family'; 'More courses please, with practical skills on dealing and coping'. The last quotation in particular drew my attention regarding what else could be developed.

In addition to these evaluations, the provision of psycho-education for carers of people diagnosed with personality disorder was highlighted in the National Institute for Health and Care Excellence (NICE) Quality Standard 88 (2015). Increased family involvement was also highlighted as predictive of better outcomes (Mottaghipour & Bickerton, 2005), providing additional strength to the proposal for the development of the training. In recent years, peer roles have been developed in mental health services and the rationale for the training education and support programmes being specifically peer led was emerging. Providers were seeing the benefit, having assisted the engagement of the carers in treatment and carers valued training with someone who had unique insight from personal experience and who was able to share their challenging experiences in a safe and supportive forum.

Community-based, free, peer-to-peer programmes complement services offered within the professional mental health system, and peers with lived experience may have a unique voice in delivering such programs (Day et al., 2011). From a peer perspective, family members feel understood by someone they see as the 'same as them'—that is, they experience that their concerns and emotional states have been accurately reflected from their perspective by another person whom they see as facing similar problems—this is uniquely powerful. This may allow family members to continue emotional involvement with loved ones in what can be at times very stressful circumstances.

The need to develop an extended support programme for carers as part of a treatment pathway led to the development of a formal proposal. A business case was developed and a CQUIN (commissioning for quality and innovation) payments framework was agreed to pay for the development of the service, with the proviso that carers' training should include all mental health diagnoses, not just personality disorder. A 12-month pilot project to deliver the carer's peer-led TES (Training, Education, Support) programme was commissioned. TES is a skills-based, peer-led programme of 20 × 2-hour training sessions. The first block of sessions cover invalidation, validation, improving relationships, coping with emotions, managing stressful situations, and it borrows ideas from family connection programmes (Hoffman et al., 2007), dialectical behaviour therapy (DBT), and mentalization-based treatment (MBT). The session content is provided via a PowerPoint presentation and participants complete exercises both in and outside sessions. This enables carers to consider a wider perspective of their experience; for example, how they feel if they are rejected or invalidated; can they reflect on how it might feel for the person they are caring for, thus enabling mutual understanding. This mentalizing approach can then alleviate some of the interpersonal misunderstandings between family members and the service user and how they impact on relationships.

The second part of the programme is teaching problem-solving with the aim of enabling the carer to support their loved ones to build resilience and to solve their own problems rather than trying to 'fix' the problem themselves, which can create dependency and importantly lead to burnout for the carer. Burnout and demoralization inevitably lead to withdrawal of support, which can reinforce a sense of abandonment in the person with borderline personality disorder (BPD). To measure effectiveness, carers completed a number of questionnaires as they progressed through the programme: WEMWEBS (Warwick Edinburgh Mental Wellbeing Scale; Tennant et al., 2007), BAS (Burden Assessment Scale; Reinhard, Gubman, Horwitz, & Minsky, 1994), and the FES (Family Empowerment Scale; Koren, Dechillo, & Friesen, 1992). These measures were administered at 3-monthly intervals to determine if the training programme improved mental well-being, reduced the emotional burden, and empowered carers in their role.

Evaluation also captures qualitative feedback. The following are quotations from families who have completed the programme:

'This programme has changed my approach to my daughter's illness. I can see a change in her as a result and she has commented how much better we communicate. It is an invaluable resource which will hopefully be on offer for all parents/ carers of family members with a mental illness.'

'I have thoroughly enjoyed the course. I have gained a tremendous amount of information to understand and continue support within future caring role. Also we have had time to express some of our feelings and concerns and received amazing support.'

'The course has been very well structured and delivered. I have gained knowledge and practical techniques to enable me to continue in my role and empower my son to be more independent.'

The success of the initial pilot study led to the carer consultant project obtaining a substantive role in the organization, that of specialist peer support worker, and the programme has now been extended across the entire organization. The data from the delivery of the programme have now been published (Chiocchi, Lamph, Slevin, Fisher-Smith, & Sampson, 2019).

Referral process and programme

Carers are referred to the programme via the mental health service in which they are working; for example, the community mental health home treatment team, assessing team, or in-patient ward. For service users on the personality disorder pathway, the referral is often made within the assessment process. To make a referral, practitioners complete a referral form which comprises the carer's details and the primary diagnosis of the service user. This then determines which awareness programme they will start (stage 1).

Once stage 1 is completed, they can progress to the family skills sessions (stage 2), and then finally to problem-solving techniques (stage 3). Figure 12.1 illustrates the programme overview.

Development of the CNTW Carers and Family Interventions—SCM Carer's Education Group (CEG)

The CNTW's Personality Disorder Hub Team's implementation of SCM also includes practitioners working directly with carers. In CNTW, the family programme was developed as in phase two of the pathway. Initially, the family programme was set up as a pilot. The proposal was for a seven to ten sessions and a psycho-education group for carers of clients being treated within the team was developed. The Carers Education Group (CEG) was developed by a team of practitioners from the

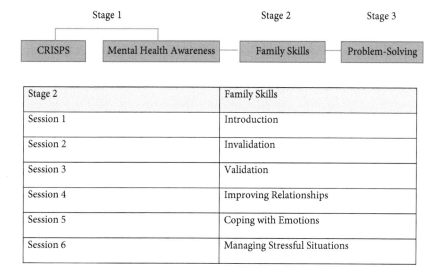

Stage 2	Family Skills
Session 1	Introduction
Session 2	Invalidation
Session 3	Validation
Session 4	Improving Relationships
Session 5	Coping with Emotions
Session 6	Managing Stressful Situations

Stage 3	Problem-Solving Techniques
Session 1	Introduction
Session 2	Supporting Recovery
Session 3	Relapse Prevention
Session 4	Managing Symptoms & Behaviours
Session 5	Communication & Problem-Solving Skills
Session 6	Barriers to Listening
Session 7	Conflict Situations
Session 8	Stages of Change in Behaviour
Session 9	Impact of Mental Illness on the Family
Session 10	Effect on Different Family Members
Session 11	Setting Boundaries & Limits
Session 12	Enhancing Relationships within the Family

Figure 12.1 Stages of Carer Training Programme

Hub, which included psychological therapists, specialist nurses, assistant psychologists, and specialist occupational therapists. The team met monthly to plan all aspects of the group as well as to allocate tasks and responsibilities. A needs analysis with six carers identified they needed further information on personality disorder and advice on how to respond best to the person for whom they care.

Referral process

Once teaching materials, psychometrics, and practical considerations were agreed, a presentation was delivered to the team to inform them of the CEG and referral process. Care coordinators within the team were required to identify suitable participants, approach their service users for consent for their carer to be invited to participate in the group, and provide their details to the CEG practitioners. Practitioners then invited potential participants to an individual information sharing session, where verbal and written information about the group was provided. This enabled participants' suitability for the group to be determined, their expectations to be agreed, their written consent given, and initial psychometrics to be completed.

Pilot group

The initial pilot group was taught over seven, weekly, hour-long sessions with an optional focus group in the eighth week seeking feedback from participants to inform improvements to the service. The modules taught each week were psychoeducation (e.g. personality disorder), DBT and mindfulness, validation and empathy, emotional regulation, problem-solving, mentalizing, and relationships. Ground rules were established at the initial session, which included issues of confidentiality and not talking over one another.

Evaluation—psychometrics

Pre- and post-group measures completed by participants were E-Kalm (measures empathy, knowledge and attitudes, learning, and management specific to the diagnosis of EUPD), BAS, WEMWBS, (measuring well-being), and the Caregiver Burden Scale. The Beck Depression Inventory (BDI) was also administered in order to enable practitioners to take into account depression as a confounding factor if required.

Outcomes

Post-group evaluations suggested that participants reported increased empathy, knowledge, management of symptoms specific to the diagnosis of EUPD, well-being and social function, and reductions in personal distress, feelings of guilt, and overall experienced burden. Subjective experiences identified from the focus group validated the psychometric results. During evaluation of the pilot participants also fed back their desire for less use of jargon, which was taken into account in planning the second group.

Developments

The second CEG was increased to 8 weekly, 1-hour sessions as well as a final focus group on week nine. The content of teaching materials was amended to include the updated ICD-11 (World Health Organization, 2018) and a widening of the referral criteria to include different types of personality difficulties. Topics covered in the weekly session included: psycho-education on aetiology of personality disorder (including attachment and biopsychosocial interactional causal model), DBT and mindfulness, empathy and validation, managing emotions (emotional regulation and distress tolerance skills), problem-solving, mentalizing, and the final session provided a recapitulation (which was flexible to the needs of the group). Understanding relationships was integrated into the content of all eight modules and carers were encouraged to consider how to balance their own needs with those of the person for whom they were caring. Results indicated that participant's knowledge of the diagnosis of BPD increased along with their awareness of options for treatment and support, and their ability to consider making positive changes in their own and other's lives developed. They experienced a reduced sense of burden, lower personal distress, less disruption to their activities, and a better perspective on their future with less upset and rumination about the past and lost hopes. Social functioning was also improved. Focus group feedback corroborated these psychometric results with qualitative feedback suggesting the main value was learning practical skills to cope with their role as a carer.

Evaluation

Overall feedback from participants suggested improvements in their style of communicating with the person they cared for and greater understanding of their difficulties and the processes underlying them. Feedback was not obtained from group dropouts, and this may have offered valuable feedback on how to improve the course. Responders also reported increased reflective awareness and new learning of applicable skills such as validation. At 3-month follow-up, results suggested the level of improvements was not likely to be sustained in the medium and longer-term. The results were similar to evaluation of personality disorder training programmes in that the helpful benefits of training diminish over time (Davies, Sampson, Beesley, Smith, & Baldwin, 2014). This suggests the need for ongoing access to a support system such as a regular meeting for sharing information, and ongoing learning for carers/families should be considered.

Group facilitators noted group cohesion was an important factor in participants' positive experience of the group along with the chance to vent or share their own personal experiences of their struggles in caring for their loved one. These needs were kept in mind by facilitators whose primary aim of the group was the provision of information.

SCM and Family Interventions

In this section, we describe how family interventions can be delivered by SCM practitioners within an SCM programme.

Although the terms 'family' and 'family meetings' are used throughout this section, the invitation to attend family meetings is extended to anyone with whom the service user has a significant relationship and who is identified as playing a part in their recovery. The aim in offering family work is to help families understand their own urges to variously rescue, withdraw, or confront their family member and to help them find ways of responding that avoids either reinforcing their loved one's difficulties or invalidating their experience.

Bateman and Krawitz (2013) advocate that family sessions cover a minimum of two topics: first, psycho-education around the diagnosis of personality disorder, and secondly, learning the specific skill of validation. Over 2 years, we invited families to meet together with us to explore 'understanding the diagnosis' and 'validation skills'. We explained that this was a new piece of work and that we were keen to learn from them in order to develop an intervention that would be most useful for families and carers.

Convening

While having a choice as to whether or not to engage in family work is fundamental, it was important that the offer of family work was available to all service users and their carers engaged in the SCM programme. Families are sometimes cautious about why they have been invited to a family meeting and can make assumptions that they are considered flawed or dysfunctional in some way and are blamed for their loved one's problems. People were assured that family meetings were an integral part of the whole SCM programme, open to everybody, and offered in response to needs that had been previously identified by families and service users.

In exploring the best place to meet with families, some people preferred to come into a clinic where the distinction between clinic and home allowed tricky conversations to happen more easily. Others, however, found the flexibility of being seen at home aided family involvement; for example, being able to offer appointments later in the day to accommodate family working patterns.

Conveners considered how to keep conversations safe for families and service users. Some families were able to continue to talk together constructively after the facilitators left; others began family work with a strict rule to not discuss anything outside the sessions. For these people, the facilitator's presence helped maintain safety. If a person has a co-occurring disorder for which they are actively being treated with another therapy, family work would not be offered as part of SCM.

Who should facilitate family sessions?

In SCM, the family work was developed to be structured in such a way so it could be easily delivered by generalist practitioners. Consequently, techniques common to most therapeutic modalities were used. However, over time it became clear that families with complex interactional, interfamilial, and social problems required practitioners who were experienced at managing multiple voices and perspectives. It therefore helps if at least one facilitator is experienced or has additional training in working with families, for example in systemic family therapy.

On occasion, a single facilitator can meet with families. This may be preferable to not meeting at all, although meeting with two facilitators opens up more possibilities for effective interventions. The second facilitator helps to ensure that each person has an opportunity to contribute and be listened to for example by attending specifically to anyone who seems withdrawn.

Facilitators are encouraged to talk with one another in front of the family to ensure thinking is transparent. Andersen's principles of reflecting team conversations (Andersen, 1995) are used which include remaining positive and curious, not offering direct advice but to offer knowledge or reflections tentatively, and not breaching confidences from conversations outside the family sessions. Although this was experienced as 'different' at first, service users and families found it validating and it was often a springboard for further conversations. As facilitators, it is a useful tool for putting a pause in a conversation which may be becoming less productive, allowing some thinking time, and giving the family some time to reflect. It also helps to establish trust when this may have been damaged through previous service or family experiences.

Facilitation by care coordinators

Service users had mixed views as to whether or not it was helpful to have their care coordinator as one of the facilitators. Some clients thought that having someone who knew them well helped them feel safe and allowed them to say what they needed, whereas others felt that not having their care coordinator present allowed them to speak more openly.

How often to meet and for how long?

Arrangements for family sessions are flexible and depend on the ability of families and practitioners to organize appointments. The time between meetings ranges from two to six weeks and the gap allows families to continue their conversations outside sessions if desired or to practise specific skills or homework tasks introduced in sessions. The length of each session depended on family preference. In principle, 1–1.5 hours was enough time to involve all family members in identifying problems and finding solutions without either them or the facilitators becoming exhausted.

Families were clear that they wanted to know how long sessions were to last and that the facilitator behaviour should guide families through the session with an outline of the topic, keep to time, and give a 15-minute warning before the end of the session.

Literacy

Many resources used in family meetings were printed and the language used, while familiar to practitioners, was not easily understood by all family members. Facilitators had to translate psychiatric language in to everyday, understandable concepts and terms. One or two family members also told us that the overuse of written resources felt like they were back at school. Facilitators therefore co-created resources using other forms of communication, for example videos, drawings, and games and role play.

The SCM family intervention

Table 12.1 summarizes the most up-to-date iteration of this work and we would like to thank each of the families who contributed to the development of the current version, which is always 'work in progress'.

Table 12.1 Six Session Outline of SCM Family Sessions

Session	Outline
1	Introduction to SCM family work, ground rules, and expectations
2	Goal session with individual family members
3	Understanding the diagnosis/diagnostic criteria and information sharing
4	Optional extra session—understanding diagnosis and information sharing
5	Validation, skills overview, and application to live problems or vignettes
6	Validation skills practice and endings

Next steps

Through a series of focus groups and individual interviews, families have reported that this intervention was helpful for them and that the themes explored were relevant.

> 'Understanding the diagnosis was crucial. Had been a grey area, no-one knew what it meant or how that conclusion had been made.' (Family member)
> 'Rather than feeling like they [parents] aren't listening, now feel like they are acknowledging and understanding.' (Service user)
> 'Use it [validation] all the time.' (Family member)
> 'Very beneficial to hear each person's view. Heart-warming to hear what they said to each other.' (Family member).

Having established the feasibility and acceptability of the sessions, the next step will be to evaluate the impact of the sessions formally for family members and service users.

Three Programmes Compared

All three carer's programmes were linked to or embedded within the SCM pathway, however routes into the programme differed. The TES was widely offered to carers, either via professional or self-referral, and did not rely on explicit consent from the service user. Service users may have been engaged in any one of the interventions offered across the pathway, alternatively they may have disengaged or never engaged at all. The programme was advertised via word of mouth and posters across different services within the pathway.

The CEG was exclusively offered to carers of service users care coordinated within the Personality Disorder Hub. Carers were approached following verbal consent from the client via their care coordinator. With regard to the SCM family sessions, service users engaged in the SCM programmes within both the secondary care community treatment teams and the Personality Disorder Hub were given the opportunity to invite their families to family sessions.

A number of similarities were evident across all three programmes; for example, all were delivered by two facilitators. This included the EBE in the TES whereas mental health professionals delivered the CEG and facilitated the family meetings. All three programmes included establishment of group rules (including confidentiality), psycho-education in relation to facilitating the carers' understanding of diagnosis as well as teaching the crucial skill of validation. Both the TES and CEG groups were structured, delivered weekly, didactic in style, held in a clinical setting, and with a focus on psycho-education in order to inform carers of optimal coping strategies. Both groups were invariably informed by DBT and MBT. They included explicit teaching of problem-solving, relationship skills, emotional modulation, as well as mentalizing.

The delivery of the family sessions was influenced by systemic family therapy and the sessions took place in both the clinical environment and home settings. A menu of activities was on offer, depending on the specific preferences of families, with the themes focusing on psycho-education and validation. Participants were encouraged to bring live relational problems to the sessions to practise validation skills. All three family and carer programmes encouraged reflective awareness in participants and all promoted the mentalization of both self and others. A message of blame was always avoided. It was deemed most beneficial when carers were able to engage in a process of understanding. All programmes were evaluated qualitatively with the group programmes also using quantitative measures. These included measures of well-being, burden, and knowledge. Feedback from all three programmes was overwhelmingly positive, however in all three there was a concern that facilitators could easily fall into the overuse of psychological jargon. Also, in relation to facilitation, in all three programmes participants mentioned that the attitudes of facilitators were key to enable trust and participation and that this wasn't just down facilitator knowledge or experience. The use of written materials was not deemed the most effective method of delivery. The implementation of role- play and videos as well as the active contribution of participants in trying out the techniques were deemed to be of most value. Ongoing delivery of the three programmes will take into account the feedback in considering the needs of carers in their role.

Conclusion

Whatever term is used, carer, family, friend, it is clear that people diagnosed with personality disorders live in community with others and that the term 'personality disorder' has not been well understood by service users or their loved ones and supporters. Providing programmes which help people to understand their experience and offer opportunities to develop practical skills for coping, including particularly the skill of validation, has been experienced by service users and those around them as helpful and supportive. In this chapter, all three programmes were co-created by service users and their supporters and it is likely that drawing on the knowledge of both EBE and Experts by Occupation will blend helpful interventions whatever the dominant therapeutic model. Attending to both the needs of the service user's wider support system and the resources they offer is integral to any SCM programme.

Having established that participants in all three programmes found the interventions acceptable, there is a need for further research into the immediate and longer-term impact of the programmes on service users' mental health and the well-being and resilience of those close to them and offering them support.

References

American Psychiatric Association. *Diagnostic and statistical manual of mental disorders (DSM)*. Arlington, VA: American Psychiatric Association. Retrieved from https://www.psychiatry.org/psychiatrists/practice/dsm

Andersen, T. (1995). Reflecting processes; acts of informing and forming: you can borrow my eyes, but you must not take them away from me! In S. Friedman (Ed.), *The reflecting team in action: collaborative practice in family therapy*. New York, NY: Guilford Press.

Bateman, A. W., & Krawitz, R. (2016). *Borderline personality disorder: an evidence based guide for mental health professionals*. Oxford: Oxford University Press.

Chiocchi, J., Lamph, G., Slevin, P., Fisher-Smith, & Sampson, M. J. (2019). Can a carer (peer) led psychoeducation programme improve mental health carers well-being, reduce burden and enrich empowerment: a service evaluation study. *The Journal of Mental Health Training, Education and Practice, 14*(2), 131–140

Davies, J., Sampson, M. J., Beesley, F., Smith, D., & Baldwin, V. (2014). An evaluation of knowledge and understanding framework personality disorder awareness training: can a co-production model be effective in a local NHS mental health Trust? *Personality and Mental Health, 8,* 161–168.

Day, C., Kowalenko, S., Ellis, M., Dawe, S., Harnett, P., & Scott, S. (2011). The Helping Families Programme: a new parenting intervention for children with severe and persistent conduct problems. *Child and Adolescent Mental Health, 16*(3), 167–171.

Department of Health. (2003). *Personality disorder: no longer a diagnosis of exclusion*. London: Department of Health.

Falloon, I., Fadden, G., Mueser, K., Gingerich, S., Rappaport, S., McGill, C., ... Gair, F. Meriden behavioural family therapy. Retrieved from https://www.meridenfamilyprogramme.com/.

Giffin, J. (2008). Family experience of borderline personality disorder. *Australian and New Zealand Journal of Family Therapy, 29*(3), 133–138.

Gunderson, J. G., & Hoffman, P. D. (2005). *Understanding and treating borderline personality disorder—a guide for professionals and families.* New York, NY: American Psychiatric Association Publishing.

Hoffman, P. D., Fruzzetti, A. E., & Buteau, E. (2007). Understanding and engaging families: an education, skills and support program for relatives impacted by borderline personality disorder. *Journal of Mental Health, 16*(1), 69–82

Hooley, J. M., & Hoffman, P. D. (1999) Expressed emotion and clinical outcome in borderline personality disorder. *American Journal of Psychiatry, 156,* 1557–1562.

Koren, P. E., Dechillo, N., & Friesen, B. J. (1992). Measuring empowerment in families whose children have emotional disabilities: a brief questionnaire. *Rehabilitation Psychology, 37*(4), 305–321.

Linehan, M. M. (2015). *DBT skills training: handouts and worksheets* (2nd Ed.). New York, NY: Guilford Press.

McGoldrick, M., Gerson, R., Petry, S., & McGoldrick, M. (2008). *Genograms: assessment and intervention* (3rd Ed.). New York, NY: W. W. Norton & Co.

MIND. (2018). *The consensus statement for people with complex mental health difficulties who are diagnosed with a personality disorder—shining lights in dark corners of people's lives'.* Retrieved from https://www.mind.org.uk/media/21163353/consensus-statement-final.pdf.

NICE. (2009). *Borderline personality disorder: recognition and management. Clinical guideline 78.* London: NICE.

Reinhard, S. C., Gubman, G. D., Horwitz, A. V., & Minsky, S. (1994). Burden assessment scale for families of the seriously mentally ill. *Evaluation and Program Planning, 17*(3), 261–269.

Siegel, D. J. (2011). *Mindsight: the new science of personal transformation.* New York, NY: Bantam Books.

Siegel, D. J. (2012). *Pocket guide to interpersonal neurobiology: an integrative handbook of the mind.* New York, NY: W. W. Norton & Co.

Tennant, R., Hiller, L., Fishwick, R., Platt, S., Joseph, S., Weich, S., ... Stewart-Brown, S. (2007). The Warwick-Edinburgh Mental Well-being Scale (WEMWBS): development and UK validation. *Health and Quality of Life Outcomes, 5,* 63.

World Health Organization. *The international classification of diseases (ICD) Version 11.* Geneva: World Health Organization. Retrieved from https://icd.who.int/browse10/2016/en#/F60-F69.

World Health Organization. (2018). *International classification of diseases for mortality and morbidity statistics.* Geneva: World Health Organization.

13

Adapting Structured Clinical Management for People with Intellectual Disabilities

Jill Everett, Mark Oliver, and Katie Cummings

Introduction

This chapter summarizes how structured clinical management (SCM) has been adapted as an intervention for people with intellectual disabilities (ID). There is no current guidance or qualitative or quantitative reports in the literature about SCM for people with ID. As such, this chapter combines definitional, philosophical, structural, political, cultural, and practical/clinical elements that can inform thinking about SCM in ID and provides a framework for adapting the available materials and piloting them with ID service users. The chapter is structured in two main parts: the first lays out these contextual elements, the second gives some examples of the adaptations made to the SCM workbooks to make them more accessible and acceptable to an ID population.

Beginning with some definitional elements, who are we talking about when we talk about people with ID? How is this diagnosis established? What is the prevalence of personality disorder within this population?

Definition of Intellectual Disability

Intellectual disability, learning disability, mental retardation, developmental disability, mental handicap, mental disability, mental deficiency, and mental sub-normality are terms used interchangeably around the world (World Health Organization, 2007). Yet these same terms can also refer to different populations which leads to 'disorder' in interpreting published literature as a term used in one country can refer to a different population when the same term is used in another. In this chapter we are applying the internationally preferred term 'intellectual disability' in order to be clear about the people we are working with, but at times the term learning disability will be used in the context of existing clinical and service descriptors, that is Learning Disability Community Treatment Teams. For the purposes of this chapter, when the term learning disability is used, it will be referring to ID.

Three elements need to be in place to make a diagnosis of ID (British Psychological Society, 2001).

1. Significant impairment of intellectual functioning. Generally operational-ized as a Full Scale IQ of below 70 on a standardized, norm-referenced test of cognitive ability (i.e. the most up-to-date version of the Wechsler Adult Intelligence Scale; currently the 4th UK edition (WAIS-IV UK) (Wechsler, 2008). This represents a population who score more than two standard devi-ations from the mean, equating to the lowest-scoring 2.5%.
2. Significant impairment of adaptive behaviour as measured by a standardized, norm-referenced test. The British Psychological Society (BPS) suggests the Adaptive Behaviour Assessment System, 3rd edition (ABAS-3) (Harrison & Oakland, 2015). and the Vineland Adaptive Behaviour Scales, 2nd edi-tion (Vineland-II) (Sparrow, Cicchetti & Balla, 2005) as being appropriate measures.
3. The deficits should have been lifelong—that is, before the age of 18.

Taken collectively, the diagnostic features of ID can be summarized as a lifelong presentation of comparatively poor functioning that is attributable to cognitive deficits. Note that this excludes features that can interfere with learning that are independent of cognition—attention deficit hyperactivity disorder (ADHD), dys-lexia, dyscalculia, and autistic spectrum conditions (ASC), although in the case of ASC the picture is somewhat muddied by historically established service commis-sioning, and this point will be explored later.

Intellectual Disability and Mental Health Needs

People with ID present with significantly higher risk of developing mental health problems than the general population. Challenging behaviour is also relatively common in people with learning disabilities, with estimated prevalence rates of between 5% and 15% across services (Emerson et al., 2001), often resulting in ex-clusion, adversity, trauma, and use of restrictive practices. The lives of people with intellectual disabilities can frequently be difficult, and can be further challenged by their vulnerability to exploitation and abuse (Franklin, Raws, & Smeaton, 2015). Improvement standards developed for National Health Service (NHS) Trusts fur-ther recognize that people with intellectual disabilities do not always receive treat-ment, care, and support that is safe and personalized and with the same access to services and outcomes as their non-disabled peers (NHS Improvement, 2018).

Intellectual Disability and Personality Disorder

As there is a high frequency of mental health issues within the ID population, it is expected that personality disorder would follow the same trend. Prevalence figures for people with diagnoses of both ID and personality disorders are rarely reported. What little research exists has been conducted within in-patient forensic settings, telling us relatively little about the ID population generally. Nevertheless, as an indicator, Lindsay et al. (2007) reported that the prevalence of any personality disorder within the forensic intellectual disability service was 39.3%, and with Borderline Personality Disorder (BPD) presenting with a rate of 10–13%. For comparison purposes, the prevalence of any personality disorder in the general population was found to be 9.1% in a US sample (Lenzenweger, Lane, Loranger, & Kessler, 2007), and the prevalence of BPD appears to be around 1.4% in the United States and 1.5% in the United Kingdom (González, Igoumenou, Kallis, & Coid, 2016). However, the greater prevalence of BPD in the forensic ID population compared to the general population may be explained by the tendency for people diagnosed with BPD and other personality disorders to be dealt with by criminal justice systems. Black et al. (2007) reported that 29.5% of male and female inmates in the Iowa prison system presented with BPD.

The situation is further complicated by some of the similarities in presentation between BPD and ID. Indeed, the list of problem areas of emotional regulation, impulse control, and interpersonal disorder defining BPD and targeted by SCM are found in many people with ID generally as these abilities rely largely on relatively sophisticated cognitive abilities and well-developed frontal lobe functioning (Muñoz-Ruata, Caro-Martínez, Martínez Pérez, & Borja-Tomé, 2013) which are not present in ID. Add to this behavioural presentations including deliberate self-harm, verbal and physical aggression to others and destruction of property, all of which would be frequently labelled as 'challenging behaviour' (Joint Commissioning Panel for Mental Health, 2013), it is not hard to see that the clinical overlaps between BPD and ID could make it difficult to separate the two (Cowen, 2018).

In short, the data currently do not exist to allow us to conclude the prevalence rate of BPD in the ID population with any confidence, but we can speculate that the lived experiences of many people with ID make them prime candidates for the emergence of significant levels of personality disorder. This lived experience is reviewed next, as the last decade has seen a significant shift in the expectations of how society supports people with ID. Unfortunately, the changes began with an abuse scandal.

Winterbourne View, Positive Behavioural
Support, and the Context of Care

Services do not exist in a social, political, or cultural vacuum. In the United Kingdom, the context in which people with ID are supported is in the long shadow cast by the Winterbourne View abuse scandal. When the BBC TV's Panorama programme sent an undercover reporter to work as a member of support staff in Winterbourne View care home, their hidden cameras revealed a shocking culture of abuse of the people with ID who were resident there (British Broadcasting Corporation, 2011). The staff, faced with the responsibility of supporting people with ID with challenging behaviour, had developed a culture of bullying and use of aversive practices to punish the residents for their behaviour and, worryingly, they used control and punishment for their own amusement.

The interpersonal and behavioural actions of people with ID and those of people diagnosed with BPD present similar emotional challenges to the care-giving workforce. In both groups the emotional responses of the caregivers fuel a destructive interaction: The challenging behaviour evokes fear and loss of control in the care giver who interprets the behaviour using emotionally loaded attributions and bases their understanding on the challenge the behaviour presents to them and their service, rather than on an understanding of the person themselves whose behaviour is an expression of underlying difficulties. Caregivers react to their own distress by trying to control the perceived threat, which fuels a culture in which the person in need of care is blamed and judged for their challenging reactions. This caregiver response leads to a cycle of strained and unhealthy relationships and increasingly socially unacceptable behaviours as the service user's needs remain unmet, when a suitable alternative approach is to look beyond the behaviour to understand the reasons why it is being displayed.

The outrage that followed the Panorama programme led to the closure of Winterbourne View, with 11 individuals subsequently pleading guilty to criminal offences of neglect or abuse, 6 of whom received prison sentences. An official government report into the scandal made a number of recommendations about the treatment of people with ID, foremost of which was that the recommended model of support for people with ID should be Positive Behavioural Support (PBS; Department of Health, 2012).

PBS is a framework for understanding challenging behaviour amongst people with ID, and a guiding set of principles to inform their support (Gore et al., 2013). PBS has a number of components but essentially advocates the understanding of challenging behaviour as functional, and that it represents an individual's response to dissatisfaction with the circumstances of their life. Aligned to this, PBS recommends the principal intervention strategy to be one of changing people's circumstances to prevent them from being exposed to such aversive experiences, and to teach them better and more adaptive ways to communicate their own needs.

In this context of delivery of care, if SCM is to be adapted and then adopted as a treatment for people with ID with emotional, impulsivity, and relational problems, it needs to be consistent with a PBS approach. PBS is fundamentally 'contextualist' in its philosophy (Singer & Wang, 2009) in that it assumes that behaviours can only be properly understood in the context in which they are shown. In other words, it is meaningless to separate the behaviour from the context and what is considered 'true' to a contextualist is defined as 'what works'. This underlying pragmatic, contextualist philosophy means that there is no *a priori* reason why interventions from other treatment models or approaches can't be applied (Hayes, Hayes, & Reese, 1988; Singer & Wang, 2009). So while SCM emerged from a different treatment tradition to PBS, the SCM techniques and approach can be used without conflict provided they are applied flexibly and with due consideration to the context in which the person lives their life (see Hayes, Hayes & Reese, 1988 for more details on integrating different philosophical world views). In conclusion, the general approach of SCM is not in philosophical conflict with PBS and may even be delivered in a way that can complement the PBS approach. So, just how best can SCM be delivered with PBS in a service context?

Configuring Services to Meet the Needs of People with Intellectual Disabilities

Recent equality legislation addresses the provision and availability of health services to people with disabilities (including intellectual disabilities). In practice, this legislation works in two directions: people with ID should, where possible, access mainstream services, and services that are available to mainstream populations should not be denied to people because they have a disability. Additionally, people with ID and mental health problems who are receiving psychological interventions should have them tailored to their preferences, level of understanding, strengths, and needs (NICE, 2016).

Public sector agencies have a statutory duty, under the Equality Act 2010 and the NHS and Social Care Act 2008, to make 'reasonable adjustments' to their services so that they are accessible and effective for people with intellectual disabilities. This legal duty is 'anticipatory', meaning that adjustments are required to be made in advance. People with ID consequently have an equal right to gain access to and benefit from mental health services, and all mental health services must presume that people with autism or ID will want to use their services and they must make arrangements in advance to accommodate them. The NHS Confederation, on behalf of the Department of Health, commissioned a report on the reasonable adjustments that were being made to mental health services to enable people with autism and ID to have access to effective treatment. Their report highlighted that 'few mental health services had comprehensively and systematically audited their practice and redesigned their delivery arrangements to ensure that people with autism or intellectual disabilities had fair access to effective interventions' (National Development Team for Inclusion, 2017, p.14). The Department of Health subsequently published a self-audit tool, the *Green Light Toolkit*, to support local efforts to benchmark and improve their mental health services for people with ID.

Subsequent guidance developed for commissioners of mental health services recommended that people with ID who have mental health problems may have needs that are better met within generic mental health services (Joint Commissioning Panel for Mental Health, 2013) and that secondary mental health services and ID services should be well-integrated so that individuals can receive coordinated care. The Commission on Acute Adult Psychiatric Care (2016) further identified the need for mental health services to be fully aware of the implications that it is 'likely to lead to more people with learning disability who may also have mental illness being treated in mainstream mental health services'.

Despite this decade-long direction of travel, tensions remain in enabling individuals with ID to access mainstream services due to both attitudinal and organizational problems. Mesa and Tsakanikos (2014) found that the majority of mainstream staff were unaware of the policy in relation to supporting people with learning disabilities in mainstream services and were significantly less confident about their training and experience and their perceived ability to communicate with, assess, and treat adults with learning disability when compared to those with mental illness. This position continues to be reflected in anecdotal reports from staff who report not feeling confident in meeting the needs of people with ID and not understanding why they should take on this additional responsibility when learning disability services exist within the Trust. The systemic pressure on practitioners to maintain a timely flow for service users along treatment pathways from receipt of referral to discharge can also be at odds with the need to make reasonable adjustments and to provide the extra time and planning that may be required to support people with ID. These tensions along with the integration of mainstream services with services for ID need to be taken into account when organizing treatment to address the needs of individuals with complex needs.

Practitioners working with people with ID and those working with individuals with personality disorder have considerable expertise in managing challenging behaviours and problems associated with emotional dysregulation and disorder with interpersonal relationships. Any treatment intervention for service users with ID and personality disorder is therefore likely to be effectively delivered at the interface of these services.

A case example for adapting the above into SCM is the Personality Disorder Hub team from Cumbria, Northumberland, Tyne & Wear. This service was established to work with people who experience severe and long-standing personality disorder and who engage in behaviours that place them at a high risk of harm. The

Personality Disorder Hub team works closely with sub-specialist practitioners and peer support workers with lived experience being embedded within community teams and facilitating the development of a tiered approach to assessment, intervention, training, and supervision. Initially, the developments of SCM as a treatment approach focused on mainstream services and did not extend to services for people with ID.

A key consideration therefore was how practitioners delivering SCM and other treatments for personality disorder in mainstream services could include people diagnosed with ID and personality disorder, consequently an additional pathway was created with appropriate adaptations for people with ID. To this end, practitioners were supported in making reasonable adjustments to their practice on a case-by-case basis, while acknowledging that there was going to be a sub-group of people with ID for whom this level of intervention would not be enough.

The Development of an SCM/ID Pathway

Within the UK NHS, geographically organized Mental Health Services have local service configurations that differ from their neighbours, and there may even be differences within the same organization. Here we present the implementation of an SCM/ID pathway in a Mental Health and Learning Disability Trust covering a large geographical area including the counties of Cumbria, Northumberland, Tyne & Wear and North Cumbria, an area of over 5,000 square miles. The geographical footprint is comparatively large for the population that it serves as it covers a substantial rural area as well as some larger population centres. The size of the organization and the different sources of funding across areas led to variations in levels of service provision and obvious differences in local custom and practice. There is an inherent tension between geography, funding source, urban/rural population, and an aspiration to provide consistent, equitable services to all the users of the Mental Health Service wherever they live.

The lack of appropriate provision for people diagnosed with ID and personality disorder is endemic in the NHS. There is reliance on specialist providers of care, often far away from service users' social support networks, for the most complex service users with ID and personality disorder who have persistent challenging behaviours. A Strategic Development Group, which included an intellectual disability clinician to represent ID and lead practitioners in Personality Disorder services was formed. This has since become the Personality Disorder and Complex Trauma Strategic Clinical Network (PACT) and ID services are a formal subgroup that reports to the network.

ID practitioners adapted the existing SCM group and individual materials and developed additional training materials for social care staff who are providing daily support to people with ID. All adaptations were checked for adherence to the

SCM model and changes ensured they were accessible for individuals with mild to moderate ID, as these are the individuals most likely to be able to engage in suitably adapted individual therapeutic work. 'Intellectual disability' covers a wide range of abilities, from people who score just below the clinical threshold ('mild') to people with increasing cognitive difficulties ('moderate'), to those who are severely and profoundly disabled. Training in the approach and use of the materials enhanced learning about ID and personality disorder increased the confidence of the practitioners to apply their developing skills in practice. Examples of this adapted material are presented later in the chapter. For those people with more significant ID and individuals either unable or unwilling to engage in individual therapeutic work, other appropriate interventions were considered using a tiered approach with the primary focus for the more impaired service users being on training for the staff providing community-based care and support.

In adapting SCM and the materials, the primary concerns were accessibility of individual and group work materials in terms of complexity and language, the emphasis on individual work, the issue of offering people a personality disorder diagnosis, and additional consideration around positive risk-taking in the context of the Mental Capacity Act (2005). There was a separate consideration around what the service response should be for people with a diagnosis of autistic spectrum disorder but without a diagnosis of ID.

In terms of personality disorder diagnosis, additional diagnostic labels may be unhelpful for individuals with ID, partly because they act as further barriers to accessing appropriate services and support. The National Institute for Mental Health in England guidance document 'Personality disorder: no longer a diagnosis of exclusion' (2003) highlights disparities in the availability of services for people with personality disorder and the reluctance of some practitioners and services to provide appropriate care and treatment. When this is combined with the barriers to appropriate healthcare already in place for people with ID, practitioners need to be circumspect about adding another diagnosis that adds stigma, stimulates a negative reaction in healthcare professionals, and leads to exclusion. A non-labelling approach is also more consistent with the PBS model, in which problems are considered to emerge as a result of a person's mismatch with their situation rather than as being something inherent within them.

Positive risk-taking enables individuals to have greater control over their lives and increased independence but necessarily involves an element of risk in terms of health and safety or potential for failure (Alaszewski & Alaszewski, 2002). Positive risk-taking focuses on managing risks because the potential benefits outweigh the potential harm, but this approach can be challenging for those who support people with ID. The UK strategy document, 'Valuing people now' referred to services getting the balance wrong between protecting vulnerable people and helping people have a meaningful life and argues that 'positive risk-taking should be a part of everyone's life' (Department of Health, 2007, p.77).

Positive risk-taking in the context of individuals with personality disorder can be particularly challenging for professionals, where the risks often include significant self-harm or suicide. Where it is unclear if an individual fully understands the risks and potential consequences of their actions, positive risk-taking has to be balanced against duty of care and the need to safeguard vulnerable people. An appropriate balance can be extremely difficult to achieve. The Mental Capacity Act (2005) applies to people with ID and requires consideration be given about whether they have the capacity to make decisions, including making unwise decisions. While capacity must be assumed unless assessed to be lacking, every decision opportunity faced by someone with ID is an opportunity for an MCA assessment. The assessor must establish whether the individual understands the nature of the decision and why they need to make it, can weigh up the pros and cons associated with the decision, and having demonstrated this, can communicate their decision. In such cases, even if someone makes a decision that appears to others to be unwise, they have the right in law to make it. If, however, the person is assessed as being unable to follow this process, they are deemed in law to incapable of making that decision, and a 'best interests' decision will have to be made. The responsibility for the decision-making at that point ceases to be that of the individual and becomes that of the person making the decision on their behalf. Provided this is done in the person's best interests, the decision-maker or carer will be protected from liability (Department for Constitutional Affairs, 2007). This makes positive risk-taking particularly difficult in this service user group because if the person lacks capacity, the responsibility for their actions lies with carers, support staff, or professionals. Allowing a service user to engage in self-destructive behaviours or failing to act when a service user makes decisions that could bring about their own death or lead to serious self-harm on the basis that they have mental capacity becomes clinically and professionally problematic; judgements around 'best interests' become especially challenging.

Autism Spectrum Condition

Studies suggest that approximately a third of people who have ID are also on the autism spectrum (Emerson & Baines, 2010). Similar prevalence figures of between 31% and 35.4% were reported as part of the adult psychiatric morbidity survey (Brugha et al., 2012). The needs of people with ID and those with autistic spectrum disorder are frequently assumed to overlap. Historically, services have been commissioned and given names such as 'learning disability and autism', even though our knowledge of autism now suggests that considering them in the same service makes less sense as their needs and the requirements around reasonable adjustments (and ultimately full-scale adaptations) for treatment and support tend to be very different.

Learning Disability Community Treatment Teams commonly focus on ID and services for people with autistic spectrum disorder are less clear. People with autism tend to be directed to mainstream services if they experience mental ill health and only to specialist learning disability services if they also have a significant ID and behaviours that challenge the ability of services to meet their needs. Adaptations of SCM for ID are unlikely to meet the needs of people with a diagnosis of ASD so efforts should initially focus on the needs of individuals with ID. The lessons learned from adaptation of SCM for ID can be shared with practitioners working more directly with people with autism with a view to more specific adaptation for the problems of their service users.

Materials Adapted for Individual SCM Work

An Individual Journey Booklet developed to support individual SCM sessions was adapted from the SCM individual service user workbook with key adjustments to the language and descriptors. For example, the original service user workbook describes four key problems in terms of; 'thinking, staying present and being yourself; acting quickly or in unsafe ways; managing and calming down feelings and relationship disorder'. Within the ID version, these have been amended slightly to 'thinking problems—it might be hard for you to know what you want or the sort of person you want to be; acting quickly without thinking—you might do things that end up hurting yourself or other people; difficulty understanding how you feel—you might find it difficult to know what you feel and what might help you feel better and problems with relationships—you might really like someone and then really hate them'.

Individual goals, once agreed with the service user, are scaled from 1 to 10 in terms of importance to the person and are further distinguished in terms of 'things I want to do more of' and 'things I want to do less of'. Problems, described as 'things that get in the way of reaching my goals' are RAG (traffic light system—Red/Amber/Green) rated for ease and rated both from the person's perspective and from the perspective of others, reflecting the key role of carers and family members, as shown in Figure 13.1.

A further adaptation, suggested by a group of self-advocates, was the inclusion of a formulation jigsaw, as shown in Figure 13.2, which they felt was more accessible for people with ID than the mainstream version.

Materials Adapted for SCM Group Work

The format and structure of SCM group sessions follows the general manual, which has an emphasis on practical problem-solving, making the approach particularly

My Problems
(Things that get in the way of reaching my goals)

Thinking Problems				Acting quickly without thinking			
How much of a problem is it?	Your rating	What others think		How much of a problem is it?	Your rating	What others think	

Difficulty understanding and coping with how you feel				Problems with relationships			
How much of a problem is it?	Your rating	What others think		How much of a problem is it?	Your rating	What others think	

• Red/Amber/Green

Figure 13.1 RAG*-rated Problems

helpful for people with ID, who can struggle to apply learned skills and generalize them to new situations. Adaptations to group work materials focused largely on the inclusion of more visual materials and learning aids; for example, each module begins with a visual session plan to aid the group's understanding of the content of each module. A summary of the adapted modules is shown in Figure 13.3.

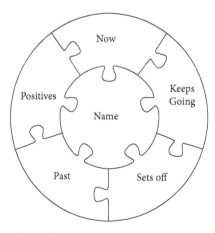

Figure 13.2 The Formulation Jigsaw

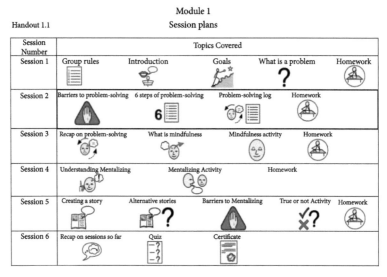

Figure 13.3 Adapted Module Summary

Problem-Solving Worksheets

The original problem-solving worksheets were also condensed into an accessible worksheet (Figure 13.4). The adapted worksheets are broken down into six simple steps to problem-solving, reducing the text and simplifying the structure of the worksheets allowing for a clearly defined message to be delivered to the group.

Accessible Learning Resources

Resources have been developed to teach the basic foundations of the SCM module. Individuals with an ID with co-occurring personality disorder may find it difficult to recognize emotions let alone distinguish between basic and social emotions. These basic skills related to recognizing and naming emotions are important to aid the understanding of body sensations and urges when these are discussed in subsequent sessions. Therefore, adaptations of SCM for ID may have to include more extensive psychoeducation with the use of visual resources and YouTube video clips.

Easy-to-Read Information

Adapting language and descriptors are key to aiding the understanding of each session's content; for example, 'Interpersonal Sensitivity' has become 'Relationship

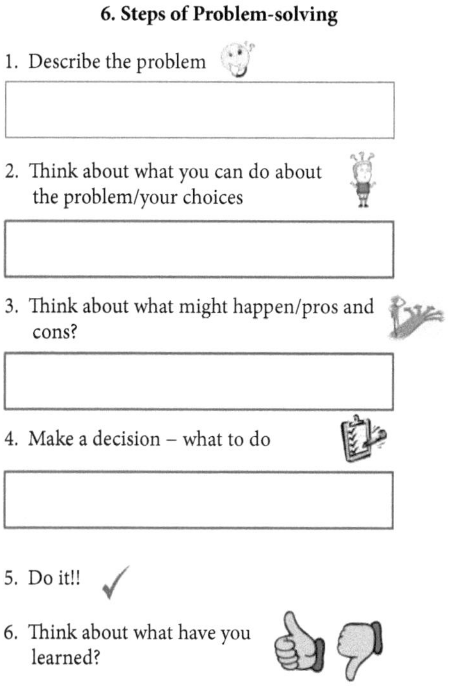

6. Steps of Problem-solving

1. Describe the problem

2. Think about what you can do about
   the problem/your choices

3. Think about what might happen/pros and
   cons?

4. Make a decision – what to do

5. Do it!!

6. Think about what have you
   learned?

Figure 13.4 Adapted Six-steps of Problem-solving worksheet

Sensitivity', 'Solving Insecure Attachment Problems' has been entitled 'Safety in Relationships' and 'Recognizing Unhealthy and Unsafe Relationships'. Further information has been simplified to meet the literacy needs of individuals with an ID and the content changed to provide easy-to-read information and increase engagement during group therapy sessions. Examples of easy-to-read resources are shown in Figure 13.5.

Practical Exercises

Practical exercises are integrated into each session to reinforce the core meaning of each session's teaching. Visual handouts have been developed to allow the group to easily follow step-by-step guidance on more mental based activities such as 'Surfing the Urge' and 'The Safe Box' (Figure 13.6). These resources allow the exercises to be accessed and practised easily at home or within the community setting in which the service user lives. More group-based exercises such as 'The Stop and Think Remote Control' and 'Card Sorting Exercises' have been developed to stimulate discussion and encourage the group to apply their knowledge to different social and personal narratives.

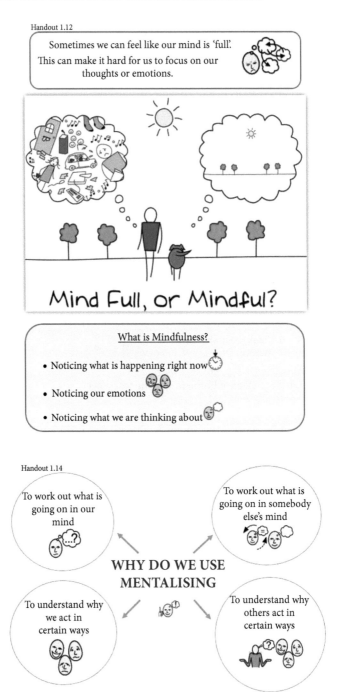

Figure 13.5 Example of Easy-to-Read Resources (© Henck van Bilsen, used with permission)

Handout 3.22

The Safe Box

1. Imagine a safe box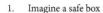

2. Are you going to leave your safe box in this room or put it somewhere else?

3. The safe box will be strong enough to hold all of your bad things (e.g. memories, thoughts, sounds, smells, and emotions)

4. What would your safe box have to be to hold all of your bad things? (e.g. a safe, lunch box, crate?

5. Can you describe the box to me? (Is it safe? What color? How big? What does it look life? What is it made of?)

6. Now imagine yourself putting all of your bad things inside your safe box

7. Now lock up your safe box

8. Is there anything that could make your box safer?

9. Are you happy that your box is safe?

10. If you have any bad things to to put into your box over the next week you can imagine locking them in your safe box

Figure 13.6 Adapted 'Safe Box' worksheet

Homework

The adapted homework sheets review previous session materials and require the group to apply this knowledge to themselves and encourage the use of newly learned skills at home or out in community settings.

Community Support Training Materials

A key additional component to the SCM-ID pathway is staff training for organizations that provide supported living and/or residential support to people with intellectual disabilities, reflecting the key role these staff frequently play in supporting people with intellectual disabilities and the potential for individual therapeutic work to fail without multi-agency understanding and cooperation. SCM has a problem-solving focus supporting the individual to develop an understanding of their own disorder and to recognize the problems that get in the way of addressing them whilst emphasizing a degree of self-advocacy in generating support from others to deal with them effectively. Provider staff can inadvertently undermine such efforts by problem-solving for the individual and acting in ways that support but potentially negate the need for the individual to manage their own disorder effectively. This dependence on others is often explicitly sought by the individual and it can be difficult for provider staff to know how best to respond.

Three levels of provider training have been developed, incorporating basic awareness raising about service pathways, personality function, and treatment (level 1), a more detailed understanding of personality disorder, SCM, and both the individual and group materials (level 2), and materials to support a more indirect approach (level 3). The rationale underpinning this approach was to ensure that where an individual is actively engaging in both individual and group SCM at level 2, provider staff have a more detailed understanding of the pathway and the work the individual is engaged in so they can not only support but also actively encourage and enable the person to implement and maintain their learning. At level 3, it is anticipated that the service user will either be unable or unwilling to engage in individual and group work but would still benefit from the SCM approach. In these circumstances, staff training would focus on the importance of validation, supportive problem-solving, and resilience work in an attempt to avoid staff burnout and placement breakdown.

Next Steps

The SCM approach for people diagnosed with ID and personality disorder incorporates the Individual Journey Book and focuses on developing service user understanding and application of problem-solving skills as the initial step. All materials for subsequent modules on emotions, impulsivity, and relationships are adapted to be within the reading and learning capacities of people with ID. Practitioners follow the SCM skills competency framework and integrate that with their specialist skills in working with people with learning disability. Peer discussion of cases and expert supervision is part of the programme. In keeping with good clinical practice there is continual review of the service development and the accessibility of the service pathway. There is a further need to evaluate the approach robustly and determine if it meets the needs of people diagnosed with ID and additional personality disorder, and whether it is effective in helping this complex and often marginalized group change.

Conclusion

In this chapter, we have presented the early development phases of a first attempt to adapt SCM for an ID population. People with ID are vulnerable to presenting with personality disorder and they have an ethical and legal right to have a service for their problems that takes account their particular needs. People with ID have a right to access mainstream services, but a group of people remain whose have enhanced needs which cannot be addressed in these services. It is suggested that for this group, SCM can be integrated with the dominant PBS approach satisfactorily, but that some adaptations to the model are required, with particular thought given to the use of diagnostic labels and how positive risk taking can be aligned with the Mental Capacity Act (2005). Examples of the adaptations have been shared in this chapter, including changes made to the materials and Individual Journey Books to illustrate the foundations of SCM for people with ID.

References

Alaszewski, A., & Alaszewski, H. (2002). Towards the creative management of risk: perceptions, practices and policies. *British Journal of Learning Disabilities, 30*, 56.

Black, D. W., Gunter, T., Allen, J., Blum, N., Arndt, S., Wenman, G., & Sieleni, B. (2007). Borderline personality disorder in male and female offenders newly committed to prison. *Comprehensive Psychiatry, 48*(5), 400–405.

British Broadcasting Corporation. (2011). *Panorama. undercover care: the abuse exposed.*

British Psychological Society. (2001). *Learning disability: definitions and contexts.* Leicester: British Psychological Society

Brugha, T, et al. (2009). *Autism spectrum disorders in adults living in households throughout England: report from the Adult Psychiatric Morbidity Survey, 2007.* Leeds: NHS Information Centre for Health and Social Care. Retrieved from http://www.hscic.gov.uk/catalogue/PUB01131.

Commission on Acute Adult Psychiatric Care. (2016). *Old problems, new solutions—improving acute psychiatric care for adults in England.* Retrieved from https://nhsproviders.org/media/2114/old-problems-new-solutions-report-lord-crisp-mhg-12-july-2016.pdf.

Cowan, A. (2018). Borderline personality disorder in individuals with intellectual disability. *Journal of Childhood & Developmental Disorders, 4*(2), 6. doi:10.4172/2472-1786.100069

Department of Health. (2007). *Valuing people now: from progress to transformation.* London: HMSO.

Department of Health. (2012). *Transforming care: a national response to Winterbourne View Hospital: Department of Health Review Final Report.* London: HMSO.

Department for Constitutional Affairs. (2007). *Mental Capacity Act Code of Practice.*

Emerson, E., & Baines, S. (2010). *The estimated prevalence of autism among adults with intellectual disabilities in England.* Stockton-on-Tees: Improving Health and Lives. Retrieved from http://www.improvinghealthandlives.org.uk/projects/autism.

Emerson, E., Kiernan, C., Alborz, A., Reeves, D. Mason, H., Swarbrick, R. et al. (2001). The prevalence of challenging behaviors: a total population study. *Research in Developmental Disabilities, 22,* 77–93.

Equality Act 2010. London: HMSO.

Franklin, A., Raws, P., & Smeaton, E. (2015). *Unprotected, overprotected: meeting the needs of young people with learning disabilities who experience, or are at risk of, sexual exploitation.* London: Barnado's.

González, R. A., Igoumenou, A., Kallis, C., & Coid, J. W. (2016). Borderline personality disorder and violence in the UK population: categorical and dimensional trait assessment. *BMC Psychiatry, 16*(1), 180.

Gore, N. J., McGill, P., Toogood, S., Allen, D., Hughes, C. J., Baker, P. A., . . . Denne, L. D. (2013). Definition and scope for positive behavioural support. *International Journal of Positive Behavioural Support, 3*(2).

Harrison, P., & Oakland, T. (2015). *Adaptive behavior assessment system* (3rd Ed.). Torrance, CA: Western Psychological Services.

Hayes, S. C., Hayes, L. J., & Reese, H. W. (1988). Finding the philosophical core: a review of Stephen C. Pepper's world hypotheses: a study in evidence. *Journal of the Experimental Analysis of Behavior, 50*(1), 97.

Joint Commissioning Panel for Mental Health. (2013). Guidance for commissioners of mental health services for people with learning disabilities. Retrieved from https://www.jcpmh.info/wp-content/uploads/jcpmh-learningdisabilities-guide.pdf.

Lenzenweger, M. F., Lane, M. C., Loranger, A. W., & Kessler, R. C. (2007). DSM-IV personality disorders in the National Comorbidity Survey Replication. *Biological Psychiatry, 62*(6), 553–564.

Lindsay, W. R., Hogue, T., Taylor, J. L., Mooney, P., Steptoe, L., Johnston, S., . . . Smith, A. H. W. (2007). Two studies on the prevalence and validity of personality disorder in three forensic learning disability samples. *The Journal of Forensic Psychiatry & Psychology, 17*(3), 485–506.

Mesa, S., & Tsakanikos, E. (2014). Attitudes and self-efficacy towards adults with mild intellectual disability among staff in acute psychiatric wards: an empirical investigation. *Journal of Mental Health Research in Intellectual Disabilities, 8*(2), 79–90.

Mental Capacity Act (2005). Retrieved from http://www.legislation.gov.uk/ukpga/2005/9/pdfs/ukpga_20050009_en.pdf.

Muñoz-Ruata, J., Caro-Martínez, E., Martínez Pérez, L., & Borja-Tomé, M. (2013). Frontal dysfunction in intellectual disability. In A. E. Cavanna (Ed.), *Frontal lobe: anatomy, functions and injuries* (pp. 1–66). Nova Science.

National Development Team for Inclusion. (2017). *Green Light Toolkit: a guide to auditing and improving your mental health service so that it is effective in supporting people with autism and people with learning disabilities. (Revised).* Retrieved from https://www.ndti.org.uk/uploads/files/Green_Light_Toolkit_2017.pdf.

NICE (2016). *Mental health problems in people with learning disabilities: prevention, assessment and management. NICE guideline 54.* Retrieved from https://www.nice.org.uk/guidance/ng54.

NHS Improvement. (2018). The learning disability improvement standards for NHS trusts. Retrieved from https://improvement.nhs.uk/documents/2926/v1.17_Improvement_Standards_added_note.pdf.

National Institute for Mental Health in England. (2003). *Personality disorder: no longer a diagnosis of exclusion*. Retrieved from http://personalitydisorder.org.uk/wp-content/uploads/2015/04/PD-No-longer-a-diagnosis-of-exclusion.pdf.

Singer, G. H., & Wang, M. (2009). The intellectual roots of positive behavior support and their implications for its development. In *Handbook of positive behavior support* (pp. 17–46). Boston, MA: Springer.

Social Care Act 2008. London: HMSO.

Sparrow, S. S., Cicchetti, D. V., & Balla, D. A. (2005). *Vineland adaptive behavior scales* (2nd Ed.). San Antonio, TX: Pearson.

Wechsler, D. (2008). *Wechsler adult intelligence scale* (4th Ed.). San Antonio, TX: Psychological Corporation.

World Health Organization. (2007). *World health statistics*. Retrieved from https://www.who.int/statistics.

14

Adaptations of SCM

A SCM Case Management Service and Personality Disorder Linkworker Role

Simon Graham, Jon Robinson, Rachael Juma-Smith, and Sharron Kayes

Introduction

In this chapter, we focus on adapting structured clinical management (SCM) in order to improve care pathways and treatment for people diagnosed with personality disorder. The National Health Service (NHS) system, which has historically often excluded service users diagnosed with personality disorder (Snowden & Kane, 2003), has, over the past 10 years, recognized their need for treatment and implemented evidence-based psychological therapies (Bateman & Fonagy, 1999; Dale et al., 2017; Linehan et al., 2006).

We describe and outline two adaptations to SCM as a treatment model for personality disorder. The first of these describes a specialist SCM Case Management Service based on SCM principles for service users who present with complex and severe personality disorder and who are assessed as being at high risk to themselves or others. The second adaptation focuses on the training of some mental health professionals as personality disorder linkworkers who provide individual SCM informed sessions in adapted form and apply SCM principles to the system of care surrounding the service user. Case management and linkwork are integrated in service provision when complexity, severity, and systemic risk are high.

An SCM Case Management Service

Our SCM Case Management Team comprises four psychiatric nurses with a reduced caseload of ten service users each, providing a 2-year pathway of treatment and support before service users are discharged back to generalist community mental health services. SCM case managers offer service users individual sessions, commonly once per week, using the principles and structure of SCM, and crisis meetings if necessary. The nurses are supported by weekly formulation sessions with a consultant psychiatrist and weekly clinical supervision by a senior clinical manager to support the maintenance and use of the SCM approach and skills.

Service users given priority for the intervention are those diagnosed with personality disorder who were deemed unmanageable in local services and had been sent to specialist in-patient units but are returning to community living, and those with the longest and most frequent local hospital admissions or regular attendances at emergency departments following high-risk events. The overarching aim of the SCM Case Management Team is to increase stability for service users through improved trust and self-regulation of distress, prior to service users moving on to the other social and psychological interventions within our wider service. Since the development of this service, no new service users have been sent to out-of-area placements, and all current service users are engaged in local services.

Service user profile and fit

Many service users were ambivalent about referral to the service and being asked to join an SCM skills group and work on their difficulties with the aim of developing greater independence. So initially, SCM case managers worked with service users using SCM principles focusing on the clinical stance, developing problem-solving skills, and enhancing motivation. Only when service users developed robust problem-solving skills and improved motivation were they referred to the SCM skills group. Data from the first 12 months (Graham, Sullivan, Briggs, Goodall, & Iraci Capucinello, 2019) showed that the new SCM Case Management Team had reduced hospital admissions by 80% compared to the previous year. It was also found that contacts with crisis teams and emergency departments had decreased during the same period of case management. Overall, there were cost savings made of approximately £2.5 million (Graham et al., 2019). These data support the view that service users diagnosed with severe and complex personality disorder with high risk can be supported and treated successfully in the community through a specialist SCM Case Management approach. This is a better alternative to hospital admission, which has been found to commonly be less helpful in the long term due to the risk of potentially stimulating iatrogenic dependency and regression (Bateman & Krawitz, 2013).

The work of the SCM Case Management Team in reducing hospital admissions for people diagnosed with personality disorder has resulted in more efficient use of the acute in-patient units and allowed the Trust to stop sending any person of any diagnosis out of area due to a local shortage of beds. Despite significant benefit for the majority, approximately 25% of service users were not stabilized by the SCM Case Management approach and continued to seek hospital admission. For this cohort there may need to be greater emphasis on supporting the wider system. This is covered in the Personality Disorder Linkworker section later in the chapter.

A related service development

In tandem with the developments of the SCM team, a specialist therapeutic Personality Disorder Day Service based on therapeutic community principles (Pearce & Haigh, 2017) was implemented. This provides an intensive intervention of social therapy groups, including creative, activity, psychological, and vocational groups during the week and a telephone and face-to-face crisis service. Service users are involved at the core of the Personality Day Service's work through regular meetings that support the running of the service, volunteering, co-facilitating the social therapy groups, and acting as senior members to help embed the ethos of the service by supporting new arrivals. The overarching aim of the Personality Disorder Day Service is to provide additional social support, with the shared service building acting as an attachment focus for service users (who might still be pre-contemplative for a formal therapy) becoming a therapeutic alternative to in-patient care.

This service is set up as a 4-year pathway and accepts any service users under SCM Case Management and direct referrals of service users diagnosed with personality disorder from generic community mental health services.

Staff within the service are trained in SCM principles alongside their therapeutic community skills and deliver SCM in individual sessions with service users. This ensures all clinical interactions are integrated, which is especially important within the crisis and day services to maintain a balance of empathic support alongside problem-solving and the development of personal autonomy and independence. As service users move through the Personality Disorder Day Service there are regular reviews intervals when people are assessed and encouraged to enter more formal psychological interventions (e.g. mentalization-based treatment (MBT), dialectical behaviour therapy (DBT), cognitive analytic therapy (CAT)) that are also on offer from our service.

Supervision is built into the programme with all staff attending formulation meetings and clinical supervision as well as participating in a reflective practice group.

By integrating three services—the SCM Case Management Team, the Personality Disorder Day Service, and the Psychotherapy Service—to work alongside each other within a single building, we have developed and maintain a clinical ethos as a specialist service. This supports our work with service users who were previously deemed to be too complex for community care and sometimes previously send out of area for care. The SCM Case Management Team focuses on providing clinical stability, ahead of the Personality Disorder Day Service promoting social engagement and inclusion, before service users engage with formal therapy.

Beyond our specialist service we have delivered training in SCM to the local community mental health teams as part of the plan that they implement this model for new service users as they move into their services from primary care. We support both community and in-patient services with offers of consultation and have also developed a policy, supported by the organization's executive team, to support clinically indicated risk taking. This is in recognition that prolonged in-patient care can exacerbate risks.

Adapting SCM in Job Roles: Personality Disorder Linkworkers

The role of the Personality Disorder Linkworker is slightly different from the case management service described previously. The linkworker role is to provide specialist case management, like that of the SCM Case Management Service, but with a greater emphasis on a consultancy ensuring safe 'patient' flow and engaging/supporting the wider system (multi-agencies). The linkworker provides both clinical work with the service user, ensuring the intervention components augment each other, and a systemic consultation and intervention to help with what can be the chaotic interaction between service users diagnosed with personality disorder and the services themselves. The greater focus on the systemic factors is to try and help, as illustrated earlier, a subset of service users diagnosed with a personality disorder who are frequently unable to engage in case management and/or structured evidence-based psychological treatments.

Referring to the personality disorder linkworker

Service user characteristics indicating referral to a Personality Disorder Linkworker are identified in Box 14.1. Traditionally, if there is no enhanced case management team these service users would have been offered a nominated mental health professional such as a coordinator of care (care coordinator) to stabilize

---

Box 14.1 Indicators for Referral to Personality Disorder Linkworker

- High usage of services within the community such as police, Accident and Emergency, and ambulance services.
- Previous involvement with mental health services but has frequently disengaged from services or struggles to participate in treatment programmes.
- Repeated or lengthy hospital admissions.
- May not have an awareness of SCM or other evidence-based therapies and the potential advantages of engaging in this approach.
- Presenting with a number of high-risk behaviours.
- Service user in frequent contact with several care/service agencies.

their interactions with services. However, rarely has the coordinator been trained in the special needs of people diagnosed with personality disorder. Consequently, service users with the highest level of complexity and need are put with a practitioner who has not had specialist training and frequently with a job plan and case load that does not allow them to accommodate the needs of the service user. The result of this can be twofold. First, service users and coordinator may feel stuck in a relationship that fails to engender change and can increase dependency on services. Second, this may engender frustration and disappointment for both parties due to the lack of a clear systematic focus towards self-agency and time to do the job properly.

The Personality Disorder Linkworker role is a hybrid of an SCM practitioner and a care coordinator. The role is similar to the SCM Case Manager described previously but with some minor differences. The role has a system-wide focus working with the service user and the wider system of care provision such as primary care, probation, social care, housing, in order to encourage more integrated support and wider understanding and knowledge about working not only with an individual service user but also with service users diagnosed with personality disorder generally. The recommended case load of a specialist Personality Disorder Linkworker, like the SCM Case Manager, is ten service users presenting with complex and severe personality-related problems and high risk.

Beyond core professional training, the Personality Disorder Linkworker requires additional specialist training in personality disorder, including both personality disorder awareness and a therapy-based training. A key difference of the Personality Disorder Linkworker from the SCM practitioner role is that they can work more intensively with service users in crisis offering additional flexible sessions, as well as supporting other professionals from the wider system who are involved in providing support. The Personality Disorder Linkworker, like that of the SCM case manager, would take the SCM clinical stance as described in Chapter 3 and thus is always looking to self-agency where possible. They would also ideally have specialist skills and experience in delivering evidence-based interventions for personality disorder for instance SCM, MBT, or DBT. Box 14.2 describes the SCM-informed clinical stance of the linkworker and case manager described earlier.

Therapeutic agreements

The Personality Disorder Linkworker, like the SCM practitioner, has explicit discussion about the role and expectations for both the service user and themselves. Despite often high levels of chaotic engagement, the linkworker keeps the core SCM principles and there would still be the expectation of active participation from the service user. They would continue to focus on change and building self-agency although there may be an increased awareness of realistic expectations (compared to service users in the SCM programme). A key difference between

Box 14.2 Clinical Stance of Personality Disorder Linkworker

- Basic interviewing skills: these are used by practitioners in their everyday practice and are based around open questions which will lead to an elaboration of the topic. The clinician's goal is to elicit a conversation where the service user feels that they are able to talk about themselves and work on their own solutions. The linkworker actively listens to what is being said and will feed back to the service user so that the service user can recognize that they are being understood.

- Authentic and open: reacting as a person and showing natural responsiveness. The practitioner needs to show the service user that that they are open in their thoughts and attempting to understand what the service user is talking about by asking curious questions.

- Not knowing stance: this stance is used in MBT, SCM, and is also part of the adaptive model of SCM stance. This stance means that the clinician does not have to have the solutions, rather different experiences to that of the service user that can provide an opportunity to explore each other's perspectives.

- Openness and acknowledgment of mistakes: all clinicians make mistakes, whether this be a misunderstanding of the service user's situation or by saying something in the wrong context. The clinician should be aware of the mistakes that they make, accept responsibility for any perceived errors and reflect back that they are trying to understand the service user's perspective.

- Empathic approach: empathy is an approach that allows the linkworker to be able to comprehend the service user's emotions so that person feels understood. By being understood a therapeutic alliance is built, which is part of the core treatment strategy.

- Awareness of possible trauma: by using a trauma-informed approach there is an awareness that people may have traumatic and adverse experiences and that this may consequently impact on them developing trusting relationships and feeling safe within services. This trauma-informed approach ensures the service user is culturally, emotionally, and physically safe, as well as the clinician having some comprehension of the service user's anxiety, which might be focused on to ameliorate it during the intervention. The linkworker's goal is to build trust with the service user by being consistent and non-judgemental (i.e. not evaluating something as good or bad, instead sticking to the observable facts of the situation).

- Providing choice: the linkworker aims to ensure that the service user has a choice about what they do and the practitioner has an appreciation of the needs for an approach that honours the service user's dignity.

- Collaboration: the service user and practitioner work in a collaborative fashion, understanding that improvement happens in relationships with shared decision-making.

- Focus on strengths: the linkworker attempts to gain an understanding of the service's strengths which helps in the development of a safety plan, and the service users' strengths are built on and validated.

the linkworker and SCM practitioner is that the linkworker also provides consultancy on service users who do not agree to work with or are not working with the linkworker directly. The linkworker may then support staff from other teams and agencies who are also supporting the service user by attending professional meetings to support care planning.

As described above, whenever possible it is important to encourage service users' active participation and where possible they would look to see them in clinics or be as active in their interactions as possible, perhaps using Internet-based meetings rather than telephone if they are not able to get to clinics. Despite this, there is an acknowledgement of realistic expectations and sometimes as part of the engagement process a more assertive engagement approach may be required. This may involve initial case conferences and multi-professional meetings with home visits or sessions at General Practice (GP) clinics. Note that home visits are kept to a minimum wherever possible (e.g. assessment process), and meeting in GP clinics is preferred over seeing service users at home.

The components of the adapted SCM role for Personality Disorder Linkworkers are shown in Box 14.3.

As such, the adapted role of the linkworker is different from that of an SCM practitioner who is delivering the SCM psychological intervention. The flexibility of the Personality Disorder Linkworker role enables them to work more adaptively in addressing the barriers preventing the service user from engaging in SCM or

---

Box 14.3 Components of Adapted SCM for Personality Disorder Linkworker

1. Duration of Personality Disorder Linkworker involvement is 3–6 months, ending with a review to formulate a person's suitability for evidence-based therapies.
2. Joining up the fragmented parts of the system through liaison with other services, to ensure the provision of coordinated multi-agency care, so there is consistency in the care provided to the service user.
3. Speaking to carers and family members to support and signpost them to any educational materials or support groups.
4. Supporting generic care coordinators through provision of supervision to them about service users on their case loads.
5. Developing collaborative care plans with service users and other professionals.
6. Formulation of risks and risk assessments.
7. Supporting the transitions from in-patient care to the community.
8. Supporting the education to the wider system through sharing expert knowledge around the diagnosis of personality disorder.
9. Undertaking a regular 3-month review, if required.

another specialist therapy. They can be more assertive in follow-up and engagement than practitioners in SCM or other specialist therapies as the role is to work with the service user and the system to address barriers to engaging in a potential therapy option.

Development of a care plan

A personalized care plan (Walker & Rogers, 2011) is a way of engaging and collaborating with a service user with long-standing difficulties. It is an effective approach that prioritizes the service user's decisions and personal goals. The care plan should take a person-centred approach and be collaboratively developed with the service user. The care plan identifies the service user's difficulties and potential goals and sets out an action plan. The care plan should provide clear and concise guidance for the service user themselves, the linkworker, practitioner, and other services involved in the system of care.

The care plan should identify the duration of the practitioner's involvement with the service user as this ensures that service user is aware of a timescale for the intervention including a mid-point review date. This provides the service user with a clear trajectory of the practitioner's involvement right from the start.

The care plan mirrors that of an SCM contract in that it clearly defines roles and expectations for both the practitioner and the service user. It differs from a care coordination plan as there is a clear identified end point to the involvement of the role at the outset.

Safety planning

A personalized safety plan is a separate safety/contingency plan, which is a working document that is developed during the initial assessment process (see Chapter 4 for an example). This is an important part of the care of people diagnosed with BPD as it focuses on how to manage life-threatening risks. Developing a safety plan can reduce risk and make it less likely that the service user will employ maladaptive coping strategies when in distress.

The Personality Disorder Linkworker should focus on devising a safety plan with the service user from the first appointment to help the service user develop autonomy and generate choice about actions. The safety plan is regularly reviewed in a way that encourages the service user to use adaptive strategies to manage distress. It is a step-by-step plan that includes what the service user can do to improve things, and what they should not do. The plan should also extend to provide guidance on how family, friends, carers, and services might best respond, including responses that can lead to an increase in emotional distress and are not helpful and so should be avoided. Significant effort and focus in ensuring the safety plan is personalized is necessary to make certain it is 'owned' by the service user. There should be a focus on the service user's strengths and positive strategies that have helped previously.

The final part of the safety plan focuses on what interventions mental health services can provide that reduce the service user's distress, and what service users have experienced as invalidating. With the consent of the service user, the safety plan is shared and discussed with all those working alongside the service user across the wider system. This ensures a whole system approach to care, thus increasing consistency of application and continuity across different services. The safety care plan will often include what to do if the person presents in crisis including expectations and goals around admission to hospital. The plan should be developed as collaboratively as possible acknowledging sometimes this can be difficult when service users have a poor relationship with services. The safety plan should try to avoid being too restrictive, for example never admit or alternatively treating the service user as fragile and having unrealistic expectations for what inpatient care can do for them.

Whole systems approach to care

The linkworker works across the whole system, including other mental health teams (in-patient, community, liaison) as well as organizations across the wider system (e.g. police, primary care, probation, housing, social care, etc.). This ensures consistency of treatment offered to service users and coordination of interventions provided by all those working with them. Of particular importance in this role is managing the transition of the service user into and out of psychiatric in-patient units. The linkworker facilitates both admissions and discharges to ensure a safe transition of the service user through the psychiatric and wider system. Another important role of the linkworker is to support all professionals involved in the care of the service user in developing a positive therapeutic risk-taking approach in discharge planning. As such, the Personality Disorder Linkworker's role supports and enables the wider system to improve its care for people with BPD, seeking to overcome barriers within the system, for example from overly cautious risk management which can trap a service user in in-service user facilities for longer than necessary.

Supervision

Personality Disorder Linkworkers have regular protected time for weekly supervision to support effective functioning of their role. If weekly sessions are not viable, the time interval should not be longer than once every 2 weeks. Supervisors should have expertise in working with people with complex relational and emotional needs, be SCM trained, and have knowledge of both the personality disorder pathway and role. The structure and topics for discussion in supervision are shown in Boxes 14.4 and 14.5 respectively.

Box 14.4 Supervision Structure for Personality Disorder Linkworker

1. Service user risks/presenting difficulties
2. Review of progress made by service users and end of care date
3. Reflecting on the health and wellbeing of linkworker
4. Reviewing the relational dynamics with the service user for example: exploring dynamics around withholding versus treating them as too fragile/special; relationship/idealization
5. Monitoring additional roles/case capacity
6. Skills development
7. Personal development plan

Box 14.5 Supervision Topics for Personality Disorder Linkworker

1. Service user risks/presenting difficulties
2. Review of progress made by service users and end of care date
3. Reflecting on the health and wellbeing of linkworker
4. Reviewing the relational dynamics with the service user for example: exploring dynamics around withholding versus treating them as too fragile—special relationship/idealization
5. Monitoring additional roles/case capacity
6. Skills development
7. Personal development plan

Conclusion

This chapter outlines how the principles of SCM are extended to areas beyond direct psychological intervention. SCM brings a unifying philosophy that allows different teams within a service to work together in an integrated way as long as this is coordinated using trained SCM Case Managers. In an extended version of this role, a Personality Disorder Linkworker goes beyond face-to-face direct therapeutic work to support the internal and also wider system in delivering treatment and support for people diagnosed with personality disorder but still following the principles of SCM.

The development of the Personality Disorder Linkworker role and the Personality Disorder Case Management Team in services shows how healthcare organizations can extend their service availability to people diagnosed with personality disorder and coordinate all services involved in treatment. What is common to the roles is extending the ethos of SCM to engage and motivate those service users who are unable to participate initially in direct psychological intervention. Instead, the psychological philosophy of SCM is used to inform either service provision within the whole of the health and social care system or the care plan organized around the individual service user.

References

Bateman, A., & Fonagy, P. (1999). Effectiveness of partial hospitalisation in the treatment of borderline personality disorder: a randomised control trial. *American Journal of Psychiatry, 156*(10), 1563–1569

Bateman, A. W., & Krawitz, R. (2013). *Borderline personality disorder: an evidence-based guide for generalist mental health professionals.* Oxford: Oxford University Press.

Castillo, H. (2015). *The reality of recovery in personality disorder.* London: Jessica Kingsley Publishers.

Clark, D., & Layard, R. et al. (2009). Improving access to psychological therapy: initial evaluation of two UK demonstration sites. *Behavioral Research Therapies, 47*(11), 910–920.

Dale, O., Sethi, F., Stanton, C., Evans, S., Barnicot, K., Sedgewick, R., et al. (2017). Personality disorder services in England: findings from a national survey. *British Journal of Psychiatry Bulletin, 41*, 247–253.

Graham, S., Sullivan, K., Briggs, L., Goodall, M., & Iraci Capucinello, R. (2019). Preliminary service evaluation of a personality disorder case management service. *Personality and Mental Health, 13*(2), 65–74.

Haigh, R. (2013). The quintessence of the therapeutic environment. *Therapeutic Communities, 34*(1), 6–15.

Kane, E., Reeder, N., Keane, K., & Prince, S. (2016). A cost and economic evaluation of the Leeds personality disorder managed clinical network—a service and commissioning development initiative. *Personality and Mental Health, 10*(3), 169–180.

Linehan, M. M., Contois, K., Murray, A. M., Brown, M. Z., Gallop, R. J., et al. (2006). Two-year randomised controlled trial and follow-up of dialectical behaviour therapy vs therapy by experts for suicidal behaviours and borderline personality disorder. *Archives of General Psychiatry, 63*(7), 757–766.

MacKeith, J., & Burns, S. (2011). *Mental health recovery star: user guide.* London: Mental Health Provider Forum and Triangle Consulting.

NICE. (2009). *Borderline personality disorder: treatment and management. Clinical Guidance 78*. London: NICE.

Pearce, S., & Haigh, R. (2017). *The theory and practice of democratic therapeutic community treatment*. London: Jessica Kingsley Publishers.

Snowden, P., & Kane, E. (2003). Personality disorder: no longer a diagnosis of exclusion. *Psychiatric Bulletin, 27*(11), 401–403.

Walker, R., & Rodgers, J. (2011). *Implementing personalised care planning for long term conditions*. SD Publications.

15

Adapting SCM for Complex Trauma and Dissociation

Stuart Mitchell and Kerry Anderson

Introduction

Studies show rates of 37–68% comorbidity of post-traumatic stress disorder (PTSD) with borderline (emotionally unstable) personality disorder (BPD) (Harned, Korslund, Foa, & Linehan, 2012; Hefferman & Cloitre, 2000). Up to 70% of service users diagnosed with personality disorder have reported childhood experiences of sexual abuse (Bateman & Krawitz, 2013; Gunderson, 2008; Zanarini, Frankenburg, Reich, Hennen, & Silk, 2005) and neglectful caregiving (Putnam & Silk, 2005; Zanarini et al., 2000), whilst others do not report such histories (Zlotnick et al., 2003). The relationship of personality disorder to complex trauma is complicated (Gunderson, 2008; Herman, 1997), and there is considerable overlap, as well as distinct differences, in the differential symptom criteria (Cloitre, Garvert, Weiss, Carlson, & Bryant, 2014; Ford & Courtois, 2014).

Current diagnostic criteria for PTSD (American Psychiatric Association, 2013) potentially overlap with most of the DSM-IV criteria for BPD (Ford & Cortois, 2014), and these in turn are remarkably similar to complex PTSD symptoms, according to ICD-11 (World Health Organization, 2018). Complex PTSD involves the core symptoms of PTSD (intrusions, avoidance, and physiological hyperarousal) 'plus three additional features that reflect the impact that trauma can have on systems of self-organization, specifically problems in affective, self-concept, and relational domains' (Ford & Cortois, 2014; p.3). Whilst these core features of complex PTSD closely mirror the central difficulties in BPD, namely abandonment anxiety and alternating idealization and denigration, they are also quite distinct (Cloitre et al., 2014; Ford & Courtois, 2014). It seems that personality disorder has multifactorial aetiology, with trauma and neglect being just two of the many potential risk factors, alongside genetics and social and developmental experiences (Bateman & Krawitz, 2013; Laporte, Paris, Guttman, & Russell, 2011). Adverse and traumatic experiences place a person at risk of many psychiatric sequelae, including major depression, anxiety, bipolar affective disorder, obsessive compulsive, eating, dissociative, psychotic, somatoform, and personality disorders (Bateman & Fonagy, 2016; Steele, Boon, & Van Der Hart, 2017). Cloitre et al. (2014) have attempted to distinguish PTSD from Complex PTSD and BPD in their latent class analysis. They found that Complex PTSD could be distinguished from BPD in four key areas: abandonment anxiety, unstable sense of self, unstable and intense interpersonal relationships, and impulsiveness (p.1). Similarly, Ford and Courtois (2014, p.1) in their review argue that it is 'unwarranted to conceptualise complex PTSD either as a replacement for BPD, or simply as a sub-type of BPD'.

In terms of the impact of complex PTSD on the service user who has comorbid personality disorder, it leads to heightened affect dysregulation, intrusions, dissociation, history of suicide attempts and self-harm compared to service users without complex PTSD (Cacowski, Neubauer, & Kleindienst, 2016). In relation to dissociation and suicide attempts, the effects of complex PTSD seem closely related to early childhood sexual abuse (Cacowski et al., 2016). Dissociation is often a key feature of BPD (Ford & Courtois, 2014), but this is usually seen as a transient state during episodes of extreme stress, especially relational abandonment anxiety (Bateman & Fonagy, 2016; Ford & Courtois, 2014). Whilst depersonalization and derealization are common in BPD, up to around one-third are found to have chronic or severe states of dissociation or a 'cluster' of dissociative symptoms (Zanarini, Frankenburg, Jager-Hyman, Reich, & Fitzmaurice, 2008; Steele et al., 2017). This evidence has been used to suggest that there may be a dissociative sub-type of BPD (Ford & Courtois, 2014; Gonzalez & Mosquera, 2012), which is related to severe early childhood trauma (Steele et al., 2017). Dissociation could be one of several (e.g. affect regulation) common factors which link BPD with complex PTSD (Ford & Courtois, 2014).

When service users diagnosed with PTSD and BPD have Dialectical Behaviour Therapy (DBT), they have a worse outcome than when they do not have comorbid PTSD due to their unaddressed trauma (Barnicot & Crawford, 2018; Barnicot & Priebe, 2013). When such therapies are adapted to take into account the post-traumatic symptoms, prognosis and progress in treatment are improved (Barnicot, 2014). Since we found considerable comorbidity of complex trauma and dissociation during implementation of SCM in a specialist personality disorder team, adaptations of the model were considered about how to address trauma-related problems. An SCM Trauma Stabilization (SCM-TS) programme was developed. In line with extant research and international experts in trauma (Mosquera, 2019; Ogden and Fisher, 2015; Steele et al., 2017), a phase-oriented treatment model of working with trauma, focusing on stabilization, processing, and re-integration was used (Herman, 1997). Since SCM is a stabilizing generalist treatment, we focused on how to enhance the trauma stabilization aspects of the standard SCM approach, hence SCM-TS.

Whilst generalist practitioners may be more able and experienced at recognizing the problems related to different aspects of personality disorder, they are frequently less able to recognize aspects of complex trauma and dissociation (Steele et al., 2017). It has been recognized that these difficulties are often more difficult to assess due to their hiddenness, the different meanings attached to the symptom of dissociation in routine practice, the different diagnostic classification systems, and the lack of training on working with complex trauma and dissociative disorders (Steele et al., 2017). The initial challenge is to help practitioners improve their assessment of complex PTSD and dissociation.

This chapter will outline what SCM-TS is and how it was developed so that it can be used by generalist practitioners to address complex PTSD and trauma-related dissociation alongside personality disorder problems. This involved a focus in three areas: clinical intervention methods and materials, training, and supervision. Some qualitative data will be presented on how generalist practitioners have found implementing this adapted form of SCM-TS. Finally, we will suggest areas of future research and areas for further clinical development.

SCM-TS Clinical Interventions

SCM-TS is an individual intervention (one session of up to an hour weekly) based on the principles of SCM but adapted to the presenting trauma-related problems brought by the service user. An SCM-TS client workbook (Mitchell, 2019) was developed to supplement the individual sessions and to provide a focus for the work. The work may take up to 1–2 years, depending on the severity of the presenting problems and severity of the personality disorder present. Group work has been provided successfully for service users with complex trauma-related dissociation (Boon, Steele, & Van Der Hart, 2011), but this was not the format we began with. The approach used was based on knowledge of what is effective when treating service users in the stabilization phase of complex trauma according to expert consensus and recent research (Boon et al., 2011; Steele et al., 2017).

Individual SCM-TS Sessions

In SCM-TS sessions, the practitioner is working with the service user to help them improve stability in emotional, psychological, and behavioural functioning because this is affected by adversity and traumatic experiences, both in the distant past and present. The aims of this are to improve daily life functioning and coping with the effects of adversity and trauma. This covers the effects of trauma on the personality functioning of the service user, managing emotions, especially being either hyper-aroused or detached and shut down, self-harm and suicidal behaviour, dissociated voices or parts of the person, amnesia and memory problems, triggers, and relationship sensitivity especially where current safety in compromised. It does not cover processing traumatic material and memories or integrating traumatic parts of the personality into daily life post-processing or in-depth trauma-focused therapy such as eye-movement desensitization and reprocessing (EMDR) or trauma-focused cognitive behaviour therapy (TF-CBT). Core skills are taught to service users as applied specifically to their current trauma-related difficulty, such as grounding, mindfulness, self-compassion, mentalizing, coping with voices, self-harm, and PTSD symptoms. After much alliance building and psycho-education about trauma, dissociation, the nervous system, and the concept of the 'window of tolerance' (Ogden & Fisher, 2015; Siegel, 1999), the intervention is carefully paced so it is within the service user's window of tolerance and focused on the current presenting issues.

For example, John presented with personality problems (impulsivity, emotional detachment, and relationship sensitivity), voice hearing and flashbacks, and some amnesia in his daily life. He would approach each session with rapid talking about his latest crisis in his living situation or with his partner and his fears of being attacked (partly unrealistic) which would make it difficult to focus on the problem areas agreed with him at the outset. With careful use of validation, and exploration of what was happening in his mind using the clinical stance, it became clear that he was hearing voices towards which he was highly phobic and avoidant. With psycho-education about how his voices might be trying to help him, it was possible to get some understanding of when they appeared and what functions they served. This enabled John to become more curious towards the voices and less avoidant. Further psycho-education about the window of tolerance and how different parts of him felt (some were hyper-aroused, whilst others were detached) at different times about the same subject, with sensitive exploration carefully managed by the practitioner he was then able to begin further dialogue with his voices/parts and use different stabilization strategies with each of them. This was then linked to his safety plan, so that different parts of him could be helped by him in different ways to become safe when they were triggered by current situations, or internal triggers, such as a critical and hostile voice. Gradually the SCM-TS sessions focused on what worked best for his parts and voices so that all of him felt more in control and responsibility for his daily life functioning. This is entirely in keeping with the aim of SCM: to learn problem-solving and safety planning skills whilst improving daily functioning.

The Problem Areas Addressed in SCM-TS

To help structure the sessions in SCM-TS, the problems are clearly defined in core domains or areas of functioning that are linked to the most common effects of traumatic experiences. As yet, there is no group SCM-TS so the sessions are individually tailored round the core areas, in line with the problems identified and formulated with the service user. The problem areas can be focused on flexibly with the service user, much as they are in the standard SCM approach in individual sessions. The only difference is that there is no group in which to develop inter-personal skills and learn problem-solving and other skills alongside other service users. We anticipate that this element of the SCM-TS programme will be developed shortly and will complement the individual sessions.

The main problem domain categories and skills developed in SCM-TS to manage them are developing knowledge, basic, intermediate, and advanced skills in managing the effects of trauma. These are detailed in Boxes 15.1–15.3.

Box 15.1 Knowledge and Basic Skills in SCM-Trauma Stabilization

- Knowledge:
  - o Psycho-education (trauma, adversity, complex trauma, dissociation, the nervous system, and window of tolerance)
- Basic skills:
  - o mindfully recognizing how different parts of the self are affected (the idea of 'parts and gifts', linked to dissociation and motivational systems)
  - o coping with trauma-related triggers and memories (identifying, planning and rehearsing strategies; containing memories)
  - o improving daily life functioning (sleep, eating, relaxation, daily structure)
  - o building resources and strengths for daily life (mentalizing, greater relationship understanding, improved cooperation ,and ability to maintain present awareness and manage emotional triggers).

Box 15.2 Intermediate Skills in SCM Trauma Stabilization

- Containing and regulating emotions in all parts of the self, including fear, anger, and shame (different strategies for different parts)
- Managing PTSD-type symptoms, but not treating traumatic memories (containing these until a later time)
- Coping with detachment, shut down, and numbing (through sensorimotor and trauma-sensitive yoga exercises)

Box 15.3 Advanced Skills in SCM Trauma Stabilization

- Building relational communication, connection, and cooperation with different parts of the self (building adult self, connecting and soothing younger parts, containing and negotiating with more critical and hostile parts); and reducing internal and external fears and phobias towards parts, thinking, feeling, and attaching
- Managing present safety and stabilizing parts (internally and externally)

Psycho-education

In individual sessions, the SCM-TS practitioner will provide some information using the SCM clinical stance to help the service begin to make sense of their trauma-related problems. For example, here is an extract from the workbook, which can be discussed sensitively with the service user:

When we are facing a trauma, or threat of some kind, our instinctive response is to feel overwhelmed with fear or terror. We then tend to do something to help us cope and survive these dangers. The most *common ways of coping* that we all tend to engage in, and have learned over thousands of years, are as follows:
- **Fight**—our bodies try to fight to survive, through shouting, hitting out, or acting in an aggressive sort of way to deal with the threat to us or others. We may do this when there appears to be no escape possible from the threat.
- **Flight**—this is the tendency to feel fear and anxiety, and to run away or escape from a dangerous situation. Later on, using drugs, medication, or alcohol may serve the same purpose.
- **Freeze**—this is the initial response when faced with threat, to stand very still and motionless, and assess the danger present. You may have heard of this as the 'rabbit in headlights', and it is something animals do too.
- **Submit**—this is the response of trying to please or appease the other person so they cause us less harm, or to appear as small as possible by hiding away.
- **Play dead**—this is the response when we cannot escape or fight and is a way to shut down the body so as to appear dead. This can lead to fainting or a loss of speech and numbness.
- **Dissociate/shut down**—if any of the above do not appear to work sufficiently then the response may be to shut down inwardly, and detach from the experience so that it becomes an 'it's not happening to me' experience.

We may have different conflicting emotions and urges at the same time. For example, we may have an urge to run away but also an urge to hit the person who is threatening us. This can leave us feeling very confused, and unsure of ourselves and our motives. This is simply how our brain is trying its best to cope with the threat.

Soothing, calming, and grounding—basic skills

In SCM-TS, the practitioner will be helping the service user develop basic skills for soothing, calming, and grounding the body and the mental states of different parts of them that feel currently affected by trauma. It can be useful to do this at the start of each session to ensure the service user is 'fully present' and not dissociated, or to calm a hyper-aroused part in mind and body. Taking a subjective unit of distress (SUDS) rating of 1 to 10 before and after the brief exercises can immediately show how effective the intervention has been. Just seeing an improvement of one or more points in the direction of being present is effective.

Again, here is some of the material from the workbook, which can be used in bite-sized pieces as necessary to focus the work, or for the practitioner to learn from memory and implement when needed. The worksheets can be then given to the service users as a reminder to practice between sessions to reinforce learning and reduce dissociation.

> Being able to calm and soothe the mind and the body is important whenever we feel overwhelmed with emotions, so that we quickly feel safer and more in control. We may have been triggered by upsetting things in the present, which remind us of traumatic things from the past. If we grew up in an environment where we were not soothed or reassured by parents or other adults, then we might struggle with knowing how to do this to ourselves as adults. Your body may easily get into a state of high arousal or terror, so you then need to learn how to calm and soothe your mind and your body. In this way, you will be providing yourself with the care and nurturing you may not have had enough of as a child, or by becoming your own best friend. This helps you cope at most times, but especially when you are in a crisis. The sections on **Mindfulness and Compassion are very closely linked** to the exercises in this section.
>
> The exercises here are useful at any time, but especially when you are approaching a crisis, or finding it really difficult to cope. There are several ideas here. Try and finds out what works best for you, practice them regularly, even when you aren't in a crisis so they become familiar to you. **Incorporate the most useful ones into your 'safety plan'**. It takes lots of effort and determination to change our usual response, so be kind and encourage yourself to use them as best you can. Here are some ideas to try.
> - **Providing reassurance to yourself**, and all parts of you, that you are here together and you will do your best to get through the current crisis. You may

imagine you are all in a circle, providing each part of you with what it needs to feel safe and secure in the present.

- **Using your compassionate self.** Using your compassionate self to provide you with what you need right now, to have wisdom, warmth, and courage to face what is difficult, and to know that it is painful, but you have survived it before and can do so again. To meet your needs with compassion, kindness and care.
- **Using the 5 senses.** Using all 5 senses, to reduce your distress to calm the body and your mind.
  - **Vision**: look at a beautiful painting, photos of people you love, flowers, a candle flame, children playing, animals, scenes of nature, a sunset or sunrise, the stars at night, people dancing etc. Child parts of you may like to watch a children's film or TV programme.
  - **Taste**: have a cup of your favourite hot drink, eat some of your favourite foods, treat yourself to a desert, chew a piece of gum, realty taste the food you eat slowly and mindfully.
  - **Sound**: Listen to soothing or invigorating music, the sounds of nature, the sound of laughter, children playing, the voice of someone you love, sing or play your favourite song or instrument. Do it mindfully, focusing on the sounds going in the ear and out.
  - **Touch**: Take a long hot bath or shower, wear silky soft fabrics, snuggle under the covers of your bed, brush your hair, rub lotion on your hands or massage part of your body, stroke a cat or dog, hug someone, wrap up in a blanket, feel the breeze on your skin, hold a safe object. Some people like to hold a 'grounding object' like a stone or pebble or to squeeze a soft ball, or place a cold compress on your head or neck. There is more on this under 'grounding' later in the workbook. Do these things one at a time mindfully and slowly.
  - **Smell**: Use your favourite soap, shampoo or lotion, light a scented candle, wear your favourite perfume or aftershave, light a wood fire on a cold day, bake a cake and enjoy the aroma, smell pleasant aromatherapy oils. Do these things mindfully, one at a time.
- **Using activities.** It may help to do some activity, like reading your favourite book story or poem, drawing their thoughts or feelings, releasing feelings by crying, shouting or hitting pillows, writing things down and then tearing them up, or by exercising (e.g. walking, running, gym, yoga, tai chi, mediation), walking the dog, playing with other pets, doing other creative activities.
- **Bilateral stimulation.** Some people find that just by gently **rocking** from one foot to another, or **tapping** their knees alternately, and saying something soothing, like 'this will pass', 'let it go', 'I am safe now' allows the brain and body calm down and feel safer and stronger in the present moment. Giving yourself alternate **butterfly hugs** can also help, whilst saying similar soothing words, until you are calmer. It is important not to do this too quickly so that your

brain doesn't process traumatic material from your past, and to do it briefly and slowly for a short time (say 10–15 seconds, 2–3 times, or as long as it still feels calming).

- **Safe place imagery**. When feeling unsafe, it can help to make a comforting place at home, using some of the ideas above, or to create a safe imaginary place where you can go to in your mind to feel calm, safe and secure, such as a beach or a wood. This may be real place you know of, or an imaginary place you have created. Here, you can use all your 5 senses to really get a picture of it in your mind, and perhaps also give it a cue word, so it comes to mind easily, such as 'calm' or 'peace'. This can be a helpful technique to use also when parts of you need to be somewhere else while you are at work or undergoing some adult activity (e.g. medical procedure).

Advanced skills—parts work and managing dissociation

In SCM-TS, the practitioner will aim to build more advanced skills and awareness at the pace the service user can bear within their window of tolerance. These skills will include parts work, pacing, and regulating and managing phobias of internal and external triggers (e.g. a critical voice telling them to kill themselves or harm someone).

Below is some of the material that is discussed with the service user as it applies to them in any session. The parts work is complex and requires careful pacing and mentalizing on the part of the practitioner so it does not overwhelm the service user or be outside of their window of tolerance.

> **Feeling made up of parts**. Here, the person may feel that they are made of different 'parts' or aspects that do not feel like them, but nonetheless influence them from within. The person does not feel whole, but in parts that are to varying degrees separate to the adult person who lives their life. These parts are not 'things' or 'people' but are ways of mentally organizing what experiences we have been through in a way that makes sense. They are enduring patterns of thinking, feeling, perceiving, predicting, sensing and behaving, often organized into different and sometimes contradictory senses of being one person. Such parts may intrude into daily life experiences, and sometimes even 'take over' control of the person's body for a period of time, that the person themselves cannot later remember. Such parts may take on more of separateness to the person, with their own feelings, sensations, memories, and may have been given a name too, which explains something about their purpose or meaning in the person's life.
>
> **Intrusive symptoms, like voices**. The person may hear voices or see visions which are often linked to their traumatic experiences, and are not usually psychotic, as in a diagnosable psychotic disorder. The quality and nature of the voices

are usually different when linked to trauma and adverse experiences, than in psychosis.

Beginning to stabilize parts. All parts of the person are parts of the person as a whole, so they should be given equal attention. No part can be 'got rid of', as they are all important in the person's recovery, and no one part should be blamed, as it is the whole person who is responsible for their life. Try and be curious about the positive purpose of each part in your life as a whole. To stabilize parts, it helps if the person can learn to:

- **Acknowledge and accept** the existence of the part(s) **non-judgmentally.** The part has had a difficult 'job' to play in your life up to this point. Can you wonder what job they have had to play to help you?
- **Do not begin with sharing traumatic memories.** Stop parts with the message, that 'I hear you, but we cannot do this right now'.
- **Begin with education about dissociation, grounding, orientation, containment and helping the person accept and care for parts inside.** For example, can you check inside and see what that part of you is worried about? What can you do right here, right now to help this part feel less worried/scared etc.?' 'Does this part know that you an adult now, it is 2021, and you are safe here in this office?' 'Could you ask that part and any other part who shares those feelings, sensations etc. to send all that to the container we described earlier for safe keeping?' Aim to build inner compassion, care, collaboration, communication, curiosity and control—the '6 C's'.

Pacing and regulating. Severe childhood and adult trauma and adverse experiences can lead the service user to have great difficulties with regulating their emotions and relationships. As you begin SCM Trauma Stabilization therapy, you will be learning to use a balance of various skills:

- **Pacing yourself:** only go at the speed you can comfortably manage, not too fast and not too slow. Start with inner experiences related to the present, not the past. Your practitioner will 'check-in' frequently with you to see how the pace of therapy is going, and to reduce the intensity or speed of it going too fast to manage. This may include you **'doing a little bit at a time'**, so the skill is broken down into smaller steps that are easier to manage (e.g. 'would you be able to notice what you are feeing right now for 10 seconds?').
- **Self-regulation.** Using various emotion regulation strategies to calm, reassure and support ourselves when we are alone (e.g. describing and accepting emotions, accepting, 'acting opposite' to change emotions, radical acceptance, mindful distraction and distancing techniques, such as imagining a small TV screen far away, using a remote control, fast forward, stop or turn off the

recording etc). It is important to try to learn when to use self-regulation (e.g. coping with chronic crises) and when to use relational regulation (e.g. when feeling very alone and in pain or scared).

- **Relational regulation.** This is when the relational presence or mind of another is felt as a safe and calming influence on us. It helps us restore our own sense of safety and connection. This builds trust and hope in recovery. However, it is important that for some people too much warmth and care from the practitioner can evoke some parts of people to cry out for further contact and support, increasing conflict and difficulty with learning and separation. Here, the best approach is for the therapist to work with you in a **collaborative way** so that you can feel supported, but you can also learn to remain independent and build you own sense of being in control of yourself and your life.

Content of Training in SCM Trauma Stabilization

A 2-day training programme for SCM-TS was developed, based around the service user workbook and the key domains and skills that would be taught. This was delivered initially to practitioners who were members of a specialist personality disorder team and therefore already experienced in providing SCM, DBT, or MBT therapies for personality disorder. In the SCM pathway, the phasic framework for treatment of personality disorder (Livesley & Larstone, 2018) was used, adapting phases 1 to 3 of the pathway to the service user's needs and current degree of stability. Adapted SCM-TS in this context refers to strengthening the service users existing psychological and somatic resources, both internal and external (Ogden & Fisher, 2015) whilst recognizing trauma-related signs, and teaching strategies for coping with these as they arise. The basic content of the 2-day workshop is shown in Box 15.4.

The aims of the workshops are to provide practitioners with an overview of the effects of trauma and adversity, including basic neurobiology, teach skills in basic stabilization tasks, such as grounding, containment, and distancing, and to practise using the SCM-TS client workbook.

Practitioners' Experiences of Implementing SCM Trauma Stabilization

A focus group was formed to discuss practitioners' experience of treating complex trauma and comorbid Personality Disorder using an SCM-TS approach. Most practitioners found the workshops helpful alongside clinical supervision. Some practitioners inevitably found implementing SCM-TS stressful due to the effects of listening to harrowing material related to trauma and the feelings and reactions

---

Box 15.4 SCM Trauma Stabilization (SCM-TS) Workshop—Programme Outline

---

- Assessment and recognition of trauma-related effects, including dissociation
- Basic neurobiology of trauma
- Pacing and regulation strategies
- Treatment planning, psycho-education, resource development, and safety planning
- Containment, distancing, flashback/nightmare protocols, and managing dissociation
- Use of SCM Trauma Stabilization client workbook
- Vicarious traumatization and clinician well-being strategies
- Phase 2 readiness and phase 3 integration work

---

this evoked in them. Clinical supervision was therefore useful not only as a guide to following the model but also as a source of containment and support for the practitioner. The same was true of informal peer support, particularly in the use of the service user workbook.

Using the SCM-TS workbook

The SCM-TS service user workbook helps to provide a focus for individual sessions so that the clinical work does not drift or become unfocused and ineffective. The content sections of the workbook are shown in Box 15.5.

The workbook is intended to be used as a guide rather than a prescription, or a set of tasks to be completed, and used flexibly when needed as a reminder of the problem area to be worked on or as a reminder about what to practise outside the clinic office between sessions. Despite this, practitioner anxiety may result in it being delivered in a too directive way which can overwhelm both the service user and the practitioner. It is important therefore to provide ongoing support and supervision to the practitioner to ensure they do not rush through the exercises in a prescriptive or linear way. This may include providing individual handouts and worksheets separately as the focus of topic is discussed rather than in one large document or workbook.

A related issue is pacing, timing, and sequence of the different SCM-TS tasks and knowing what to do and when with service users. In early SCM-TS sessions, the practitioner should aim to assess the service user's window of tolerance (for emotion, thinking, being present, and attaching). The clinical work can then focus

---

Box 15.5 SCM Trauma Stabilization Client Workbook—Content

General introduction

- How to use this workbook
- What is trauma and adversity and the steps to recovery?
- How does trauma and adversity affect the brain, mind, and body?
- What is my 'window of tolerance'?

General skills

- Mindfulness
- Reflection and mentalizing
- Compassion and self-care
- Soothing/calming
- Safety planning
- Distraction, containment, and distancing
- Grounding
- Resourcing

Specific problem areas

- Self-harm and suicidal thoughts and behaviours
- Shame and self-forgiveness
- Dissociation and shutting down
- Flashbacks and nightmares
- Hearing voices and visions
- Mood swings
- Unusual beliefs

Sources of further resources and support

---

on topics relevant to the service user's current situation and formulated problem areas at the pace that they can manage without being under- or over-challenging. Often, it is well known by trauma experts that 'the slower you go, the faster you get there' (Steele et al., 2017).

It may help with some servicer users to adapt the written materials to a format that suits them or matches their particular learning style. For example, some service users may prefer the use of colour, artwork, puzzles, or grounding objects in order to stay present in the moment. This may include making laminated posters of how the brain works, or the traffic light system of recognizing emotional arousal. Others find words too difficult to think about so may prefer gentle movement, gestures, and body exercises in order to re-establish present connection and safety.

It is worth considering that for a generalist practitioner the SCM-TS intervention may feel like a 'new' intervention, despite it being an adaptation of a model they may already know as standard SCM. For this reason, there needs to be clear limits on what is expected of the SCM-TS practitioner. It is a stabilization type of generalist treatment and not a trauma specialist type of treatment.

Conclusion

Adapting SCM for trauma stabilization means fully considering the trauma-related difficulties, listening and formulating these collaboratively, and supporting service users in learning new skills to address these difficulties. It is possible with good training and ongoing supervised practice to embed this adapted form of SCM within a specialist personality disorder community team. We also think this can be implemented within generalist mental health services as an adapted and stabilizing form of SCM with a relatively short training programme, ongoing clinical supervision, and access to the clinical workbook materials to supplement the clinical work. Research into evaluating the effectiveness of this intervention in clinical services is needed to ensure outcomes are in line with other evidence based approaches to personality disorder and comorbid trauma-related problems.

References

American Psychiatric Association. (2013). *The diagnostic and statistical manual of mental disorders* (5th Ed.). Washington, DC: American Psychiatric Association.

Barnicot, K., & Crawford, M. (2018). Posttraumatic stress disorder in patients with borderline personality disorder: treatment outcomes and mediators. *Journal of Traumatic Stress, 31*, 899–908.

Barnicot, K., & Priebe, S. (2013). Posttraumatic stress disorder and the outcome of dialectical behavior therapy for borderline personality disorder. *Personality and Mental Health, 7*, 181–190. https://doi.org/10.1002/pmh.1227

Bateman, A., & Fonagy, P. (2016). *Mentalization-based treatment for personality disorders.* Oxford: Oxford University Press.

Bateman, A., & Krawitz, R. (2013). *Borderline personality disorder. an evidence-based guide for generalist mental health professionals.* Oxford: Oxford University Press.

Boon, S., Steele, K. , & Van Der Hart, O. (2011). *Coping with trauma-related dissociation: skills training for patients and therapists.* New York, NY: Norton & Co.

Cacowski, S., Neubauer, T., & Kleindienst, N. (2016). The impact of posttraumatic stress disorder on the symptomatology of borderline personality disorder. *Borderline Personality Disorder and Emotion Dysregulation, 3*, 7.

Cloitre, M., Garvert, D. W., Weiss, B., Carlson, E. B., & Bryant, R. A. (2014). Distinguishing PTSD, complex PTSD, and borderline personality disorder: a latent class analysis. *European Journal of Psychotraumatology, 5*, 25097.

Ford, J. D., & Courtois, C. A. (2014). Complex PTSD, affect dysregulation, and borderline personality disorder. *Borderline Personality Disorder and Emotion Dysregulation, 1*, 9.

Gonzalez, A., & Mosquera, D. (2012). *EMDR and dissociation: the progressive approach.* http://www.Intra-tp-com

Gunderson, J. G. (2008). *Borderline personality disorder: a clinical guide* (2nd Ed.). Washington, DC: American Psychiatric Publishing Inc.

Harned, M. S. (2014). The combined treatment of PTSD with borderline personality disorder. *Current Treatment Options in Psychiatry, 1*, 335–344.

Harned, M. S., Korslund, K. E., Foa, E. B., & Linehan, M. M. (2012). Treating PTSD in suicidal and self-injuring women with borderline personality disorder: development and
preliminary evaluation of a dialectical behavior therapy prolonged exposure protocol.
Behaviour Research and Therapy, 50(6), 381–386.

Heffernan, K., & Cloitre, M. A., (2000). Comparison of posttraumatic stress disorder with
and without borderline personality disorder among women with a history of childhood
sexual abuse: etiological and clinical characteristics. *Journal of Nervous & Mental Disease,
188*, 589–595. https://doi.org/10.1097/00005053-200009000-00005

Herman, J. (1997). *Trauma and recovery*. New York, NY: Basic Books.

Laporte, L., Paris, J., Guttman, H., & Russell, J. (2011). Psychopathology, childhood trauma,
and personality traits in patients with borderline personality disorder and their sisters.
Journal of Personality Disorders, 25(4), 448–462. doi:10.1521/pedi.2011.25.4.448

Livesley, W. J., & Larstone, R. (Eds.). (2018). *Handbook of personality disorders: theory, research and treatment* (2nd Ed.). London: Guilford Press.

Mitchell, S. (2019). *Individual SCM trauma stabilisation: client workbook* (2019 Ed.).
Unpublished: CNTW NHS Foundation Trust, UK.

Mosquera, D. (2019). *Working with voices and dissociative parts: a trauma-informed approach*. Institute for the Treatment of Trauma and Personality Disorder (INTRA-TP).

Ogden, P., & Fisher, J. (2015). *Sensorimotor psychotherapy: interventions for trauma and attachment*. New York, NY: Norton & Co.

Putnam, K. M., & Silk, K. R. (2005). Emotion dysregulation and the development of borderline personality disorder. *Developmental Psychopathology, 17*(4), 899–925.

Siegel, D. (1999). *The developing mind*. New York, NY: Guilford Press.

Steele, K., Boon, S., & Van Der Hart, O. (2017). *Treating trauma-related dissociation: a practical integrative approach*. New York, NY: Norton & Co.

World Health Organization. (2018). *International classification of diseases and related health
problems* (11th Ed.). Geneva: WHO.

Zanarini, M. C., Frankenburg, F. R., Jager-Hyman, S., Reich, D. B., & Fitzmaurice, G. M.
(2008). The course of dissociation for patients with borderline personality disorder and
axis II comparison subjects: a 10 year follow-up study. *Acta Psychiatrica Scandinavia, 119*,
291–296.

Zanarini, M. C., Frankenburg, F. R., Reich, D. B., Hennen, J., & Silk, K. R. (2005).
Psychosocial functioning of borderline patients and axis II comparison subjects followed
prospectively for six years. *Journal of Personality Disorders, 19*, 19–29.

Zanarini, M. C., Skodol, A. E., Bender, D., Dolan, R., Sanislow, C., Schaefer, E., & Gunderson,
J. G. (2000). The collaborative longitudinal personality disorders study: reliability of axis
I and II diagnoses. *Journal of Personality Disorders, 14*, 291–299. https://doi.org/10.1521/
pedi.2000

Zlotnick, C., Johnson, D., Yen, S., Battle, C. L., Sainslow, C. A., Skodol, A. E., & Tracie Shea,
M. (2003). Clinical features and impairment in women with borderline personality disorder (BPD) with posttraumatic stress disorder (PTSD), BPD without PTSD, and other
personality disorders with PTSD. *The Journal of Nervous and Mental Disease, 191*, 706–
713. https://doi.org/10.1097/01.nmd.

PART 4
SYNTHESIS AND FUTURE DIRECTIONS

16

Service User Experiences of SCM

Robert Watts, Amy Maher, Lisa Weaving, and Donna Potts

Introduction

The emphasis on service user and carer involvement in the design and delivery of health services has become increasingly prominent in government policies over the past 30 years in England. This began with the National Health Service and Community Care Act (1990), which recommended that local authorities consult with service users on their community care plans, and was followed by the National Service Framework for Mental Health (1999), which identified user involvement as one of its core principles. User involvement continued to expand, with a new emphasis on patient experience in the document 'High quality care for all' (Britain & Darzi, 2008), and so the principles of contemporary mental health policy endorse service user and care involvement in care planning through to national guideline development (Department of Health, 2011; Harding, Pettinari, Brown, Hayward, & Taylor, 2010; Healthcare Commission, 2008). The aims of this approach are to improve the culture and responsiveness of services, to improve the quality of care, and to improve facilitation of peoples' recovery. Such policies are supported by evidence demonstrating that service users want to be involved in care planning (Bee, Price, Baker, & Lovell, 2015). Despite this increasing emphasis on service user involvement in national and local mental health policy, there is evidence to suggest that shared decision-making needs to be enhanced in practice (Storm & Edwards, 2013), so local care planning and development of interventions and care pathways should consider service user involvement as integral to good-quality care. Service user involvement can be described as a continuum depending on how much power is held by the service user. Different levels of participation can be identified (Peck, Gulliver, & Towel, 2002; Storm, Hausken, & Mikkelsen, 2010); this should involve, on a primary level, interactions between service users and healthcare professionals but there may be local service management opportunities and then finally service planning opportunities. Therefore, involvement may take place both on an individual level, participating in decisions made about one's care and treatment, through to participating in decisions concerning mental health service design.

Service user involvement has been regarded as an important part of the development of personality disorder and SCM programmes, on an organizational, individual, and treatment development level, as described in earlier chapters of this book. From the earliest level of service planning through to implementation, services for people diagnosed with personality disorders are recommended to be co-developed between experts by experience (EBE) of living with personality disorder, people with expertise in caring for somebody diagnosed with a personality disorder, and experts by occupation (EBO). EBEs form part of the ongoing structure of services, meeting at regular intervals as a governing body to consider the services on offer and their quality, organization, and responsiveness to the needs of the service user. This is commensurate with the Royal College of Psychiatrists' (Department of Health, 2020) recent recommendations for service design for people diagnosable with personality disorder, which suggests involvement in decision-making as a democratic process with EBEs to avoid marginalization and isolation.

With the expansion of SCM to a greater number of mental healthcare providers across the United Kingdom and in Europe, it is imperative that service users who have received SCM programmes are involved in developing the intervention in order to continue to improve the quality of care and recovery focus within this approach. There are a number of commonalities of generalist mental health treatments for people with emotion regulation and interpersonal difficulties that have been identified by Bateman and Krawitz (2013) as important in the delivery of SCM. These include the practitioners' therapeutic stance, the therapeutic relationship, practitioner monitoring, and skill development. It is therefore helpful to explore whether service users identify such themes as important to them in their SCM treatment and whether other themes emerge as significant in service users' views of their treatment. The study described in this chapter was undertaken in two NHS mental healthcare providers in the United Kingdom. The aim of the study was to gather service users' experiences of SCM to inform the continued development of SCM and to inform the implementation of SCM in the future.

Method

Due to the exploratory nature of the study, a qualitative research design was selected in order to capture a diversity of participant views on the SCM programme.

Participants

A convenience sampling approach was employed, whereby current service users of community mental health services who had completed at least 10 months of SCM, were approached by practitioners and asked if they would be interested in taking part in a focus group about the programme. In Cumbria, Northumberland, Tyne & Wear NHS Foundation Trust (CNTW), two focus groups were arranged in localities where SCM has been running for at least one cycle (six months). Focus groups were arranged in different areas of the North-East. SCM had been offered for 12 months for one focus group and SCM had been offered for around 24 months for another. Of three eligible participants in one area, two elected to take part in the focus group. Of the 16 eligible service users in the other, six elected to take part in the focus group. In North West Boroughs Healthcare Foundation Trust (NWBH Note: in 2021 NWBH split with Halton, Knowsley, St Helens and Warrington joining Mersey Care and Wigan joining Greater Manchester), SCM had been offered in some areas for 5 years. In order to get a wide sample of views, practitioners from across the whole Trust were asked to invite individuals who had completed at least 10 months of the programme and who were still open to NWBH as current service users. Of 16 identified eligible participants, 11 attended the arranged focus groups; six attended one focus group and five attended another focus group.

Procedure

One to two weeks prior to the focus groups, prospective participants were sent or given an information sheet about the focus group and a copy of the questions that would be asked. The information sheet outlined the aim of the group, who would be facilitating it, how it would be recorded, and how data would be stored. All focus group participants completed a consent form prior to commencement of recording. Focus groups lasted up to 1.5 hours, depending on group size. Each group was recorded using a digital dictation device and the conversations were transcribed. Data coding and analysis were undertaken within a constructivist framework and employed thematic coding following the guidance of Braun and Clarke (2006). All data were analysed by one of the authors (AM). A credibility check of the analysis was undertaken by another author (RW) at step 2 of the six-part analysis and emerging themes were agreed by the two authors. A member check of the final themes was undertaken with a small sample of focus group participants from CNTW (Doyle, 2007); changes were made to the results section following their feedback.

Ethical considerations

Both organizations' Research and Development panels granted approval that this study met ethical guidelines. Participants were informed at the outset that taking part was voluntary and non-participation would not impact their care and treatment. Informed consent was gained from all participants for the use of data for the purposes of the study and this chapter. Participants understood they were able to withdraw consent at any point, including during the focus group. Participant confidentiality was prioritized and service user-identifiable information was withheld from the final report.

Results

Responses were gathered from participants' discussion regarding six key questions about their experiences of SCM.

1. How do you think being involved in SCM has impacted on your well-being/daily living?
2. What do you think about the individual SCM work and support?
3. What do you think about the SCM group work?
4. What do you think about the different modules?
5. What do you think about the accessibility of the group?
6. What do you think about the length of time of the SCM intervention?

As the themes emerged, it became clear that they could be categorized into three overarching themes: development through SCM, enabling factors for effective SCM, and barriers to effective SCM.

Development through SCM Self-understanding and awareness

Across both Trusts service users' feedback suggests personal development and recovery through the SCM process. This includes an increase in confidence:

'It [SCM] changed me, it's made me more confident'. (CNTW)

'Seeing new people come in [SCM group] and see a completely different person in a couple of months they've got their confidence and able to share what they're feeling'. (NWBH)

Increased awareness and understanding of emotions were also noted:

'Because I am more aware of my emotions I now feel I can see things that are wrong in that relationship'. (NWBH)

'I think I've got a better understanding of what's wrong with me and why I react the way I do ... having that knowledge I guess has helped in other environments in terms of things like at work'. (CNTW)

Examples of pre- and post-behaviour changes

Service users also shared poignant examples of their behaviour and thoughts pre- and post-SCM to illustrate how SCM had changed them:

'It's really helping me get my life back on track, I've managed to get a job, maybe I will have a job with the NHS. All these things have happened, and I never dreamt it. If someone would have said to me a year ago this would have happened, I would have said Nah.' (NWBH)

'The best part of it is when they [parents/friends/social services] tell you that you've changed and it's not a bad thing, you're a lot calmer, a lot more focused, you're able to do stuff, you don't get as angry'. (NWBH)

'And even spending because at one point my spending was getting really reckless and a lot of impulse buys and I think having been through the whole module on impulsivity. I'm a lot more conscious now about what I'm buying, you know so if I want to buy something online for example I'll put it in the basket and leave it for a day.' (CNTW)

Enabling Factors for Effective SCM Attachment and therapeutic relationship

Throughout the discussions, it became clear that another important theme to emerge is the development of therapeutic relationship, and the fit of the attachment style between the service user and practitioner. Service users stated that being well matched is important:

'I think he listens, understands but even if he sometimes doesn't understand he can sort of empathize if that makes sense. I think I've probably got on his nerves a little bit if I'm honest but, but yeah, I think it has to be, I think if you're not well matched to the person who, who you're with, in the group, and you go to one on one I can imagine that being quite difficult. But I think me and my individual talking therapist are quite well matched.' (CNTW)

It was also highlighted that feeling listened to and checking in with the service user is a key aspect:

'I like how my CPN is now, how every session she'll ask how, what self-harm's been like and how at risk I am like suicidal feelings and stuff and she'll always check that kind of at the beginning and I like how she does that.' (CNTW)

It suggests that curiosity and genuine interest in the service user's well-being helps develop the relationship, which influences service user's experience of SCM and how well they engage. Service users also acknowledged how hard it could be to develop a therapeutic relationship at the start:

'You get failed by a hell of a lot of services.' (CNTW)

'One of my main issues is trust and it's taken a long time to be able to trust her. It doesn't just happen. You can't just assume you walk in a room and I'm going to trust you. So it has taken time to build that therapeutic relationship you know.' (CNTW)

Psychological approach

Another aspect service users felt made a difference to them was that SCM was a psychological approach, focused on relationships and skills building rather than medication. They offered examples of the different experiences they had with the medical model, versus their experiences in SCM:

'I've spoken to a consultant or my GP about some of the issues that I've had, and I feel like sometimes they don't listen, or there is a time pressure. Whereas with [SCM practitioner] I know that like I have an hour with him once a week.' (CNTW)

'Half the time people don't listen to you because they just think, oh well, you're doing it for attention where in Structured Clinical Management people listen to you, they understand you.' (NWBH)

Service users went further and suggested that had they received SCM earlier, they could have avoided unsuccessful medical intervention:

'People think that hospitals and drugs and medication is the answer to everything. It's not, its therapy. If this is what we'd have had years ago it would have helped us.' (NWBH)

Peer support

One theme that emerged across the focus groups was the key role that peer support plays in the effectiveness of SCM. Discussion suggests that peer support in the group setting is crucial given that it means the service users feel less alone:

'I think sometimes it's feeling like you're not alone, because in the SCM group it's like you're a family. The people in the group know what it feels like to be you and they're not going to say, "oh you're doing it for attention or this or that", so it's easier. I could cope with life better than dealing with the challenges I was dealing with at the time.' (CNTW)

Working alongside people who have shared experiences is felt to be validating and understanding:

> 'Being around other people with similar illness massively helps, don't feel it's just you with the weight on your shoulders. There's a lot of other people like that. It helps a lot.' (NWBH)

Peers suggesting solutions to problems was considered to be a valuable asset:

> 'I think as well for me coming to the group lets me know that I'm not on my own … As a group collaboratively we can sometimes help each other which is obviously where the problem-solving thing comes in. However, I think that having the group instead of just having one person perspective from your care coordinator, you are then actually getting input from other professionals and other service users and sometimes that can be quite valuable.' (CNTW)

As important was developing a relationship and sense of camaraderie with peers:

> 'I liked talking about homework in the group because you heard others thinking and their ideas, lots to learn from. Especially with the problem-solving aspect, that really worked well with the group hearing other solve problems together and sharing ideas.' (NWBH)

Responsibility and empowerment

This theme depicts service users' feedback around the SCM approach, which helped them develop greater responsibility and self-agency in their own recovery; this was seen as an important part of how they were able to flourish and improve. Feedback suggested this was different from other therapies they had undertaken:

> 'In all the other (therapies) I was never challenged on my behaviour. If you get challenged you have to hold your own and say I accept that. I need to do XYZ to change it. The other ones felt like bubble wrapping and drip feeding. You need to put the action in for you to get there.' (NWBH)

Service users reiterated the need for them to engage fully in the process and take responsibility for their own recovery:

> 'It just changes your life, but you've got to put a lot into it to get a lot out of it.' (CNTW)

'I'm 46 years old and I'm suddenly feeling like an adult, I've been molly-coddled my whole life, and now I've got to take responsibility.' (NWBH)

Individual and group combination

This theme highlighted the service user's feedback that doing individual sessions alongside group was important in terms of the effectiveness of the therapy:

'I don't think it would be as successful if it wasn't running alongside one on one (sessions) because if it was just a group and then I wasn't able to discuss what happened in the group with, with [my SCM practitioner] actually I would probably find it quite difficult.' (CNTW)

Group and individual sessions complement each other as individual sessions help with understanding of the skills learned in group:

'I found the one to one's beneficial, I know the groups where more like the skills based but the one to ones were more like personalized so you could think about what you learned and what was going on for you.' (NWBH)

As well as this, individual sessions allow a more personalized depth of conversation that can't happen during the group session:

'I found the one to one's very helpful—similar to what [another service user] was just saying, personalized and going at your own pace and helping with your specific issue. In the groups you feel like you can hide a bit behind other people but in the one to one you are faced to think about yourself, which is nice because it's helpful.' (NWBH)

Longer time frame

Another key theme that emerged was the importance of a longer time frame. This theme had two threads. First, service users reported they felt a positive aspect that made SCM stand out and be effective compared to other therapies was the 12–18-month time frame:

' I think one of the main things for me is that the fact that the programme is not just 8–10 weeks as in some therapies. To get to the root of the problem is a bit like trying to put a sticky plaster on a cut when you know you need stitches. Having done eight sessions of CBT you skim surface whereas this is tackling the problems that nobody really has ever seen or got to the bottom of.' (CNTW)

It was suggested throughout that the longer time spent in SCM compared to previous therapy and repetition of modules helped to increase understanding:

'Well, we went over everything twice in the group didn't we? I felt like it was just right at 18 months.' (NWBH)

'I really need a second round of group, everything's so not going into my head.' (CNTW)

Second, there was a strong theme that emerged regarding the programme needed to be longer still:

'Our process was 18 months with check in sessions – bank sessions – I had some extra one to one because I still needed that support but I felt like the group could have gone on longer. There were loads to take in a short time, I think if it was longer it would be easier.' (NWBH)

'This is my second time doing it and what if I'm still not fixed, what happens after the third time?' (CNTW)

Service users expressed a desire for them to be able to decide how many rounds (6-month blocks or cycles) of SCM they could do and that it should be decided on an individual basis:

'It should be up to you because if you don't feel right in yourself and not ready to go, that should be like right well you need extra time. I get told all the time by my CPN that once group is over then we're going to have to start pushing you to do things.' (CNTW)

However, this did appear to be influenced by the very nature of their attachment difficulties, as further themes emerged suggesting a fear of abandonment contributing to their wanting SCM to continue without limit:

'What happens at the end of 18 months if you are not fixed? Do they just kick you out in the cold?' (CNTW)

Suggestions were made that a way to overcome this would be with a good transition:

'There's something about the ending being gradual. You just sort of got dropped. I had become dependent on it really.' (CNTW)

'I don't think we should have been discharged so quick after the 18 months. I felt like I still needed something and didn't have anything then.' (NWBH)

Module length

In CNTW, individual and group workbooks have been created, and the group work divided into four discrete modules which are 6–7 weeks' duration. Service user's feedback suggested module length should increase to help with understanding:

> 'It wasn't until the second time round I started to understand that. There is too much put into the short amount of time, like learning about different types of relationships and like I think there's just too much pressure.' (CNTW)

> 'I thought more time should have been spent on self-harm, suicidality and enhancing relationships. That's something that I really, really struggle with.' (CNTW)

Problem-solving

Problem-solving was also a theme that emerged, as service users discussed how problem-solving was beneficial:

> 'I've learned from that problem and I do think the problem-solving module one is beneficial. I do think that the problem-solving should stay and that was the best bit of module one.' (CNTW)

> 'I think it's good to know problem-solving straight away because it's essential and it's good to learn mindfulness and mentalizing.' (CNTW)

> 'I liked talking about homework in the group because you heard others thinking and their ideas, lots to learn from. Especially with the problem-solving aspect, that really worked well with the group hearing other solve problems together and sharing ideas.' (NWBH)

However, there were barriers to completing the problem-solving part of the session; that is, if people didn't have a problem to bring:

> 'I think some weeks are difficult because some people don't necessarily have a problem to bring so that's been difficult and there's been weeks where we've been so engrossed in what we've been doing that actually we've decided that we didn't want to do the problem-solving.' (CNTW)

Another barrier was that there wasn't always the time at the end of the session to attend to problem-solving:

'The length of the session was fine but when there was so much in one session, we ended up not being able to do the problem-solving.' (CNTW)

Barriers to Effective SCM Difficult modules

Service users in CNTW stated that some of the group-delivered modules were difficult to complete, and they experienced some of the modules as triggering, which they felt made their mental health worse. Modules people experienced as difficult were the Enhancing Relationships and Mentalizing Attachment modules:

'I found that was one of my worst modules because of the relationship you have with people, you've got to think about it and my relationship with my mam was crap, really was.' (CNTW)

In addition, the Impulsivity, Self-Harm and Suicidality module was found to be challenging:

'I really struggled with the self-harm and suicidality module because it was getting to the point of being nearly unmanageable. I think it is particularly difficult in a group environment because it's very personal.' (CNTW)

Indeed, feedback suggested that sometimes topics in the group could trigger abrupt shifts in thinking about problems and the effectiveness of existing coping strategies:

'[attended hospital] begging them to section me ... the reason that I mention that here is because that stemmed from the problem-solving exercise that we did in group so that's how triggering it was.' (CNTW)

Topics could also facilitate discovery of unhelpful coping strategies:

'It was giving you ideas of self-harm, I can still remember it now, thinking oh so that's another way.' (CNTW)

Service users suggested the need for a cool down or grounding period at the end of sessions, to help combat this:

'When it was about suicide and self-harm there should be something at the end that helps you wind back down. When I used to leave, I had awful thoughts in my head.' (CNTW)

It was also suggested that mindfulness should be increased and be run throughout the modules:

'Mindfulness should go throughout the whole thing, it shouldn't stop, like it and obviously problem-solving doesn't stop so mindfulness shouldn't stop.' (CNTW)

Inconsistent SCM practitioner

Inconsistencies with SCM practitioners emerged as a theme that disrupted therapy, impacted upon engagement, and triggered fears of abandonment:

'I've connected really well with someone and then they've had to leave and I've already got a fear of abandonment so I was really resentful to my next worker because I couldn't be bothered to make this relationship again.' (CNTW)

A service user highlighted that short and abrupt transitions can be interfere with therapy:

'I nearly got kicked out of group because I got told she was leaving and then I didn't go to any of my sessions for about 3 weeks because that was me saying no, that's the relationship over for me.' (CNTW)

This depicts the impact that poorly executed transitions can have and further illustrates an importance for the need to develop a good therapeutic relationship. It was suggested that a slower transition, with joint sessions, where the service users could be prepared, would be preferred:

'Maybe having sessions with that worker and your new worker so you can all do some work together.' (CNTW)

Group dynamics and commitment

Group dynamics (interpersonal habitual patterns that are fixed or rigid) emerged as a key feature to how well SCM worked. However, there were also situations in which group dynamics were a barrier to effective engagement:

'When one of them [other service users] doesn't speak and the other one sits and brags about doing drugs every week, every day, multiple times a day, it's so, so hard and I feel quite disappointed because the first time we did it we all gelled.' (CNTW)

'People in and out all the time is more destructive than a new solid person joining.' (NWBH)

'I feel that I would get used to new people joining as long as they are committed to the group.' (NWBH)

To aid this, group rules should be created collaboratively, and boundaries respected:

'We have group rules like no oversharing, one voice at a time. And the other therapies never adhere to those group rules. We have been the ones to come up with them, before it's been the staff writing it down.' (NWBH)

There was also some discussion around group being closed to foster a sense of commitment, trust and safety. Another group dynamic was about gender. There were different opinions on this, with both positives and negatives regarding the mixed gender groups:

'I was anxious when we did have that lad in our second group and especially when he sat next to me because I've had abusive relationships, I've been assaulted by a bloke before so it was difficult.' (CNTW)

'I don't mind about girls and boys mixing together, that really does not bother me.' (CNTW)

'I think it's good to have a mixture; it gives you different perspectives. Different genders might not have different sorts of problems.' (NWBH)

Environment

Another emerging theme was the impact environment can have. Service users stated:

'It's all about the environment, if you feel comfortable and the room is one of the most important things, because if you don't feel comfortable you're not going to talk are you.' (CNTW)

'A comfy room would be a better place for the room to help me feel relaxed. The way they have done the family I feels like that might be a cosy place and more relaxed and homely.' (NWBH)

'I preferred [a hospital-based environment] over this one. I don't know, maybe it just the placebo effect or the fact that you go to a hospital to talk about your mental health as opposed to in a room like this environment.' (CNTW)

Resoundingly, it would appear that the suitability of the environment should be considered when organizing a place to facilitate SCM as service users made it clear that having somewhere comfortable was important to them.

Discussion

Previous research into the effectiveness of SCM has demonstrated measurable behaviour changes, such as in reduced suicidality, self-harm, and hospitalization, and improved social functioning (Bateman & Fonagy, 2009; Bateman & Krawitz, 2013). However, the current study sought to explore the meaning of emotional and behavioural changes and the process of the therapy from the service users' perspective. As demonstrated through the first of the two overarching themes emerging from the data, there is a generally shared view that participation in SCM brought about a reduction in what participants viewed as previously problematic behaviour and increased effective ways of dealing with life's challenges, enabling service users to experience a life worth living.

A number of factors emerged that appeared meaningful in contributing to the effectiveness of SCM: the quality of the relationship with the individual practitioner and the nature of the approach the practitioner took were spoken about in positive terms and appeared to be enabling factors in effective treatment. As demonstrated in a review by Levy (2005), service users diagnosed with BPD are highly likely to have an insecure attachment style (Bowlby, 1977), which is likely to create a significant barrier to effective engagement in close relationships. An SCM practitioner who is positive about the treatment and therefore able to instill hope, who is empathic and validating, as well as being attentive to the therapy relationship, is critical in the success of SCM as a treatment. In this study, the empathy displayed by practitioners, the curiosity and the time taken to build a trusting relationship were regarded as important by service users in the SCM focus groups. This demonstrated the importance of prioritizing development of these skills both in SCM training and in ongoing supervision of practitioners.

It may also be suggested that the emotional safety and containment offered by the individual practitioner and the group framework could create a secure base that could enable increased ability of service users to take responsibility for their emotional stability and behaviour. As such, the structure of the therapy and the attunement of the therapist to the service user empowers the user to start being less reliant on services and others to manage their emotional distress outside planned appointment times.

SCM follows other evidence-based therapies developed for treating people diagnosed with personality disorders, such as dialectical behaviour therapy (DBT) (Linehan, 2014) and mentalization-based therapy (MBT) (Bateman and Fonagy, 2016), in offering a group therapy component as part of the overall treatment. In DBT the group tends to focus on building skills, whilst in MBT the mentalizing group component utilizes the group as a training ground for service users to develop their interpersonal mentalizing.

The group work in SCM seeks to offer elements of both these therapies, with the learning of skills such as problem-solving, mindfulness, mentalizing, distress tolerance, and interpersonal effectiveness, as well as giving space to focus on individual problems whilst fostering supportive and constructive group processes. It was clear from service user feedback that the group work was often a positive component in treatment due to the influence of other people. Others were seen as a yardstick with which to compare oneself, normalizing socially unacceptable behaviours such as self-harm and suicidality, as well as being able to appreciate that other people have had adverse life experiences. In addition, others became a source of skills and ideas when problem-solving, which expanded the availability of useful skills and was helpful in empowering service users to take responsibility for their treatment seeing others doing just this. What we emphasized and is a key finding from this study was just how important the peer support and sense of belonging that a group gives the service users.

Similarly to DBT and MBT, SCM treatment is recommended to be 12–18 months, although this does vary from service to service and can often be up to 2 years in duration. The relatively long duration of these therapies reflects the recognition among experts on personality disorder that robust and lasting change in emotion regulation and interpersonal difficulties requires a long-term therapeutic frame, both with individual practitioners and the service as a whole. This longer duration was captured as a positive aspect of SCM treatment, with it being viewed as important to take longer in order to fix underlying issues rather than offer a 'quick fix'. It was also noted that service users shared anxieties about the ending of treatment even after this longer duration, demonstrating that for some service users 18 months may not be long enough to facilitate meaningful changes in long-standing personality difficulties.

It is useful to acknowledge the difficulties that service users find with SCM to facilitate service development where possible, in order to meet their needs in better ways. It was observed that some service users found topics such as suicidality and interpersonal sensitivities extremely difficult to discuss in a group setting. This fits with the experience of authors of this chapter who facilitate SCM groups. With reference to the earlier differentiation between DBT and MBT it may be helpful for

Trusts that are developing group work modules to focus on a skills-based approach to such difficulties; offering distress tolerance and interpersonal effectiveness modules as found in DBT group work (Linehan, 2014).

It was also recognized that the relationship with one's individual SCM practitioner is an extremely important aspect of care, so regular supervision for that practitioner is vital. This ensures there is sufficient reflective time for that practitioner to consider the effectiveness of their therapeutic alliance and guard against counter-relational enactments and therapeutic ruptures which are likely to be harmful to the service user. Similarly, unhelpful group dynamics were discussed and regarded as interfering with the treatment. Managing a group of service users, all with their own sensitivities, and keeping the therapeutic environment challenging enough to create positive change but not so challenging that people become anxious or angry, is a difficult balance for group facilitators to achieve. Sometimes they may get it wrong or become drawn into unhelpful dynamics within the group. It is therefore important that supervision for group facilitators is weekly (if the groups are weekly) to enable reflective space for looking at group dynamics and their role in them, as well as time to problem-solve difficulties in the group.

Finally, the physical environment emerged as a relevant theme, with observations regarding the importance of the meeting rooms feeling like a comfortable and safe environment in which to meet.

Conclusion

As demonstrated through four focus groups across two UK NHS Trusts that are delivering SCM in community settings, there is much to celebrate from the views of service users of this treatment. From those who attended these focus groups there was a general sense of optimism and affirmation regarding the role of SCM in their care and treatment, and the specific foci on key elements of the treatment is helpful in assuring practitioners that this approach is generally well received and can lead to meaningful change. It is, however, important to recognize that there are significant barriers that can impede service user recovery in this treatment, notably difficulties in relationships with individual practitioners, unclear or sudden transitions, and difficulties in groups. Such challenges can be avoided by careful planning of how SCM is offered, ensuring once up and running it can be consistently resourced, and that both individual and group practitioners receive sufficient regular supervision. The planning of such resources at initial set-up will ensure a high-quality SCM treatment package that will be benefit service users with emotion regulation and interpersonal difficulties.

Limitations

This study focused on service users who had been in SCM for a minimum of 10 months and as a result were views of service users who stayed in the programme. These may be views from service users who liked this approach and for whom the programme had worked. For any future study, it would be useful to talk with service users who dropped out of SCM or did not like this approach.

Acknowledgements

The authors wish to thank Nicola Armstrong, Patient and Carer Involvement facilitator at CNTW, for her involvement in the Haughton CNTW focus group, along with Jade Bamford, Psychology Assistant, and Charlotte Davidson, SCM Practitioner, at NWBH, as they also gave up their time to facilitate other NWBH focus groups. The authors also wish to thank the service users from both Trusts who freely gave up their time to participate in these groups and offer their thoughts on this intervention. Without their input this study would not have been possible.

References

Bateman, A., & Fonagy, P. (2009). Randomised controlled trial of outpatient mentalization-based treatment versus structured clinical management for borderline personality disorder. *American Journal of Psychiatry, 1666*, 1355–1364.

Bateman, A., & Fonagy, P. (2016). *Mentalization-based treatment for personality disorders: a practical guide*. Oxford: Oxford University Press.

Bateman, A., & Krawitz, R. (2013). *Borderline personality disorder: an evidence-based guide for generalist mental health professionals*. Oxford: Oxford University Press.

Bee, P., Price, O., Baker, J., & Lovell, K. (2015). Systematic synthesis of barriers and facilitators to service user-led care planning. *The British Journal of Psychiatry, 207*, 104–114.

Bowlby, J. (1977). The making and breaking of affectional bonds: I. aetiology and psychopathology in the light of attachment theory. *British Journal of Psychiatry, 130*, 201–210.

Braun, V., & Clarke, V. (2006). Using thematic analysis in psychology, *Qualitative Research in Psychology, 3*(2), 77–101.

Britain, G., & Darzi, A. (2008). *High quality care for all: NHS next stage review final report*. London: The Stationery Office.

Community Care Act. (1990). http://www.legislation.gov.uk/ukpga/1990/19/contents

Department of Health. (2011). *No health without mental health: a cross-government mental health outcomes strategy for people of all ages*. London: Department of Health.

Department of Health. (2020). *Royal College of Psychiatrists PS01/20. Services for people diagnosable with personality disorder*. London: Department of Health.

Doyle, S. (2007). Member checking with older women: a framework for negotiating meaning. *Healthcare for Women International, 28*, 888–908.

Harding, E., Pettinari, C. J., Brown, D., Hayward, M., & Taylor, C. (2011). Service user involvement in clinical guideline development and implementation: learning from mental health service users in the UK. *International Review of Psychiatry, 23*(4), 352–357.

Healthcare Commission. (2008). *The pathway to recovery: a review of NHS acute inpatient mental health services.* London: Healthcare Commission.

Levy, K. A. (2005). The implications of attachment theory and research for understanding borderline personality disorder. *Development and Psychopathology, 17,* 959–986.

Linehan, M. (2014). *DBT skills training manual* (2nd Ed.). London: Guilford Press.

Peck, E. Gulliver, P., & Towel, D. (2002). Information, consultation, or control: user involvement in mental health services in England at the turn of the century. *Journal of Mental Health, 11*(4), 441–451.

Storm, M., & Edwards, A. (2013). Models of user involvement in the mental health context: intentions and implementation challenges. *Psychiatric Quarterly, 84,* 313–327.

Storm, M., Hausken, K., & Mikkelsen, A. (2010). User involvement in in-patient mental health services: operationalisation, empirical testing, and validation. *Journal of Clinical Nursing, 19,* 1897–1907.

17

Practitioners' Experiences of SCM

*Sarah Hanmer, Donna Potts, Robert Watts, Amy Maher, Isaac McCann,
Darren Ellis, John Ludden, Karen Finch, Melanie Jones,
Lisa Weaving, and Kristine Allam*

Introduction

The principles of structured clinical management (SCM) have been outlined in earlier chapters of this book. This chapter focuses on the experiences of SCM practitioners in UK National Health Service (NHS). To date, there have been no published explorations of the experiences of mental health professionals providing SCM to service users with a diagnosis of borderline personality disorder (BPD). When considering the implementation and future development of an intervention, the qualitative experiences of both practitioners and service users can be useful to review in terms of quality improvement (Kitzinger, 1995). The aim of this chapter, therefore, is to provide a reflective account and summary of the experiences of practitioners delivering SCM in two NHS Trusts in the United Kingdom. It is hoped that this will help inform and shape the implementation of SCM in any type of mental health service. Key themes emerging from discussion with practitioners at two focus groups that took place in late 2019 will be discussed. Some elements of the chapter will overlap with, and refer to, Chapter 16 and Chapter 18 of this book.

Context

The authors of this chapter work in two NHS Trusts in the United Kingdom—North West Boroughs Healthcare NHS Foundation Trust (NWBH Note: in 2021 NWBH split with Halton, Knowsley, St Helens and Warrington joining Mersey Care and Wigan joining Greater Manchester) and Cumbria, Northumberland, Tyne & Wear NHS Foundation Trust (CNTW)—where SCM has been offered as an intervention to those with a diagnosis of BPD since 2014 and 2017 respectively. As expected, there are some differences as to how SCM has been developed and implemented in these areas and even within the same Trust. Therefore, this has understandably impacted on and influenced the experiences of practitioners delivering SCM, along with the success and challenges they may have faced.

North West Boroughs Healthcare NHS Foundation Trust

In NWBH, SCM has been part of a standard offer of care to those with a diagnosis of BPD since 2014. Initially, it was offered within Borough Recovery Teams (equivalent to community mental health teams) as an addition to the care coordinator's normal role as an identified practitioner overseeing a patient's overall care. A number of care coordinators trained across the Trust and managers of teams enabled them to hold a small case load of service users being treated with SCM (two to three) with supervision from a Clinical Psychologist. SCM training was (and still is) provided in-house by suitably qualified practitioners and refresher dates are offered at regular intervals to ensure model adherence and support with any barriers to implementing locally.

Over time, NWBH has recognized that those with a diagnosis of BPD were not always able to access the most appropriate support, nor was the National Institute for Health and Care Excellence (NICE) guidance being followed efficiently and equitably. Therefore, a co-produced Borderline Personality Disorder Pathway was developed, that went live in 2017. The pathway allowed increased access to effective and collaborative assessment, intervention, and family/carer support. As a result of the pathway, it also meant that most boroughs created SCM practitioner job roles, whose primary job was to provide SCM to service users with a diagnosis of BPD, whilst other boroughs kept the original model of offering SCM alongside care coordination roles.

Cumbria, Northumberland, Tyne & Wear NHS Foundation Trust

In CNTW, Bateman and Krawitz's (2013) treatment guide for generalist mental health professionals working with people with diagnoses of BPD was used to guide individual practitioners working within the Personality Disorder (PD) hub since its inception in 2014. The full SCM programme (individual and group) has subsequently been offered in Sunderland and South Tyneside Community Treatment Teams in partnership with the PD hub since 2017 for service users with either diagnoses of BPD or high traits of BPD. Northumberland in 2018 and North Tyneside later followed this in 2019 as more community teams received training in SCM. SCM training is provided in-house by a PD expert in a train-the-trainers model, which was then delivered locally by suitably qualified practitioners, and the work has been further enhanced by the development of an SCM manual (Mitchell, 2017), service user workbooks, and local and Trust-wide implementation groups. SCM is currently delivered across most areas of CNTW by trained community treatment practitioners and PD Hub workers. In the community teams, this is alongside their generalist roles (i.e. care coordinator).

Box 17.1 Focus Group Questions

1. What are your thoughts on SCM?

2. What was your experience of starting SCM (individual/group)?

3. What has been your experience of using supervision alongside SCM?

4. What have been some of the challenges of implementing SCM where you work?

5. What have been some of the benefits of implementing SCM where you work?

6. Is there anything else you would like to add about your experiences of SCM?

The Focus Groups

In order to gather the data on the experiences of practitioners delivering SCM in the United Kingdom, the authors arranged two focus groups, one in each region, of 19 SCM practitioners. Two senior practitioners facilitated the groups, focusing on a series of semi-structured questions (see Box 17.1). The design of the questions was to allow open and flexible discussions in order to gather information about practitioner experience.

Analysis of the Data

A total of 19 practitioners delivering SCM took part in the focus groups, ten CNTW staff and nine NWBH staff. The focus groups lasted from 90 to 120 minutes and were audio-taped and subsequently transcribed verbatim. Data were analysed using thematic analysis (Braun & Clarke, 2006). Thematic analysis was chosen for its applicability across an array of epistemological and theoretical positions. Thematic analysis is done, generally, in six steps:

1. Familiarizing oneself with the data
2. Assigning preliminary codes to the data in order to describe the content
3. Searching for patterns or themes in the codes across the different interviews
4. Reviewing themes
5. Defining and naming themes
6. Producing a report

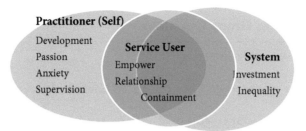

Figure 17.1 Thematic Map of Primary Themes

Identified Themes

Three key overarching themes were identified from the data: Practitioner (self), Service User, and the System. Within these three overarching themes were nine sub-themes (Development, Passion, Anxiety, Supervision, Investment, Inequality, Empower, Relationship, Containment), some of which applied across each of the main themes. Figure 17.1 demonstrates a thematic map showing how the identified themes related to each other. Figure 17.1 also, significantly, applies the Service User theme as central to the experiences. Interestingly, the themes identified were shared across both NHS Trusts and therefore, the data are not differentiated by Trust.

The main themes identified related to the general findings in the data in relation to how the practitioners started their responses. For example, there was a high use of 'I' (self), 'they' (service users), and 'team' (system). It felt pertinent that these also seem to fit with how many of us make sense of our experiences: self, other, the world (Beck, 1976). Each theme and sub-theme are discussed in more detail below, with extracts to demonstrate them.

Practitioner (self)

During both focus groups, this theme was identified throughout in relation to the focus on the self in the data. This was named as a key theme due to the use of 'I' in much of the feedback but also because of the importance of the practitioner in how they have experienced SCM.

'I found it quite useful' (female, CNTW)

Within the key theme of 'self' there were four main sub-themes identified that did not overlap with other themes: Development, Passion, Anxiety, and Supervision.

Development

Many of the discussions highlighted the shift in confidence, knowledge, and skills as an SCM practitioner.

> 'I think when you first start you're always afraid of saying the wrong thing … When I first started I thought "I'm not a psychologist so I can't really speak in that way" and was afraid of making it worse … and the penny drops that I can't say much worse than they are already feeling. So it's all right to talk about those things even though you are not a psychologist.' (male, NWBH)

> 'I reflect on my work when I first started to then what my clinical practice is like being group facilitator has been brilliant.' (female, CNTW)

Some practitioners also identified that it meant that they had developed further than their traditional roles (i.e. no longer felt like just a nurse), and that this gave them confidence in understanding service users more, along with feeling that they themselves (as staff) had benefitted.

> 'I would say I've lost touch with my nursing qualification really … but that gives me then the ability to … understand more deeply what's going on for the clients … it was learning in action.' (female, NWBH)

> 'I'm learning for the first time ever, and I think that the benefits for me have been huge.' (male, NWBH)

> '… a very bare skeleton actually and we have added lots to ours.' (female, CNTW)

> '… for me this whole year has been a complete learning curve.' (female, NWBH)

Passion

This sub-theme was by far one of the clearest themes relating to the practitioner. Both focus groups identified how passionate practitioners are in relation to providing and being involved in SCM. Practitioners spoke with enthusiasm throughout and this demonstrated how rewarding SCM can be to the staff delivering it. The authors have selected just a few quotations to demonstrate this theme; however, it could have been an entire chapter in itself.

> 'You go into work quite passionate and it's quite rewarding.' (male, NWBH)

> 'The benefits to us as practitioners are amazingly invaluable … for the past 5 years of that (my job) I have enjoyed my job immensely more than I had for the time before that. I feel passionate, I'm engaged.' (male, NWBH)

> 'I'm ahead of the game with this, this is a system that works … I know exactly what to do … I like going to work.' (male, NWBH)

'SCM and that has just changed my whole career and when I am now, where I am today.' (male, NWBH)

'... it's a common theme in the room, to do this properly ... you need passion, you need to believe ... I think everybody here does. It's got to be the right people delivering it ... That passion, that belief, must be there first.' (male, NWBH)

'... if you're passionate and you believe in the pathway and you bring that across to your clients and they buy into it and they then have hope.' (female, NWBH)

'... it's really kind of motivating.' (female, CNTW)

'... it's that job satisfaction ... you're actually seeing people through a full actual process.' (female, CNTW)

Anxiety

Practitioners identified that anxiety about their work with people diagnosed with PD was important. They focused on two aspects: anxiety provoked by the work and reducing anxiety. What was understood from the data was that one implementing SCM with the client group evoked for some practitioners considerable anxiety. This, in part, related to delivering new interventions (e.g. SCM techniques or organizing groups):

'Starting SCM with individuals I found really nerve wracking, it was really anxiety provoking and is totally different to anything that I have done.' (female, CNTW)

Along with wanting the treatment to succeed:

'I'm quite anxious about the group. I want it to succeed.' (male, NWBH)

On the other hand, SCM was seen as a model that contained and reduced anxiety. Some of this, in part, was due to the supervision, structure, and framework it provides which will be discussed in more detail later in the chapter, but SCM also helped staff feel more able to manage risk and know how to work more effectively. They described feeling more able to go home and not worry about their service users, which historically they may have done when they were not working within a structured model:

'I think reducing my anxiety is also about how to manage risk ... it helps me out with my personal anxieties which is quite nice and quite refreshing.' (male, NWBH)

Supervision

Supervision was highlighted by the authors as a sub-theme. Whilst the authors recognize that there are overlaps with many of the other themes identified, the emphasis on supervision by practitioners, even outside of the specific question on supervision, left the authors feeling that this needed specific attention. Within the sub-theme of 'Supervision' three other mini themes were identified (see Figure 17.2). This section can be read in conjunction with Chapter 18 of this book. Practitioners discussed supervision as necessary for their own well-being:

'... supervision is good for offloading... it actually helps me with my mental health.' (male, NWBH)

'It prevents burning out.' (male, NWBH)

They also identified supervision as allowing them to feel part of a mutually supportive team and to share in clinical decisions:

'It's shared ownership of the kind of risks as well as the positives ... you don't feel like you are just on your own ... it's a shared thing.' (female, CNTW)

'... you had to become a team unit.' (female, CNTW)

'... just shared a lot, it just meant it worked so well.' (female, CNTW)

'Shared experience isn't it. So even if the psychologist isn't there you still feel confident to meet and work things out between yourselves.' (male, NWBH)

'It's nice to make decisions ... clinical decisions within supervision about what you're doing with the client ... you feel validated.' (male, NWBH)

'It makes it like a team decision within the SCM team rather than it feel like ... it's your responsibility, it gives the whole team a sense of shared responsibility ... with obviously the client at the forefront.' (female, NWBH)

In addition, supervision allowed the time and space for reflection. This was not just to reflect on the process of SCM but also on what the service user or practitioner was bringing to the individual and group sessions:

'SCM supervision ... got us all to bring it together and really think about each other's experiences and challenge them.' (female, CNTW)

'I think having the time to reflect fully... '. (female, CNTW)

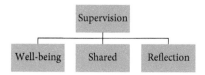

Figure 17.2 Supervision Themes

'I think the supervisions help kind of, shape that as well ... in terms of anxieties around groups and how to improve.' (female, NWBH)

'Fundamental really ... it gave me the safe space to say "I've messed up" ... just time to think really.' (male, NWBH)

'It's a bit reflective of what the group's like almost because you have to make a commitment to go every week, you have people that have more experience and people that are coming in new ... you have a commitment to being open and honest.' (male, NWBH)

'We have had issues amongst even the staff ... our relationship is facilitated (in supervision)' (female, CNTW)

'... that self-reflection is ... the stuff that I have grown the most from.' (female, NWBH)

The focus groups and themes pulled from them clearly demonstrate that supervision is a key aspect in successfully and safely implementing SCM, not just because of the monitoring of the clinical work but also the benefits it provides to practitioners and service users.

System

This theme was identified in both datasets. The premise of this theme was the place of SCM as a service in relation to wider system challenges. In particular, three themes were identified that were independent from the other themes: Resources, Funding, and Inequality.

All three themes were felt to be particularly important for senior managers and commissioners to consider when planning implementation of SCM locally. They were seen predominantly as challenges and obstacles that got in the way of and otherwise positive picture about implementing SCM.

The two sub-themes were: Investment and Inequality.

Investment
This was identified from the focus group data and particularly emphasized areas such as resources, funding, and respect from the whole system for the model of SCM.

In relation to resources, this focused primarily on challenges with staffing, such as staff retention, their time as SCM practitioners being agreed by the management as an important part of their clinical role and being allocated accommodation to run SCM groups safely.

'... our lack of resources is a big factor, to the very basics of - we haven't got a room to facilitate it ... it's all good will (staff and third sector agencies).' (male, NWBH)

'... we have had a little bit of an issue with venues and just being able to secure a suitable venue ... you have to have an environment conducive to running a group.' (female, CNTW)

'... people not respecting our time to do SCM.' (male, NWBH)

'... some of the challenges, I think it's like the staffing of it ... having the staff to run it ... but that's more of a kind of system issue than an actual problem with the intervention.' (female, CNTW)

'... staffing is definitely an issue and the pressure of being in the community treatment team.' (female, CNTW)

Focus group feedback highlighted that these challenges placed pressure on SCM practitioners as they attempted to maintain the programme, even when their own motivation to implement the programme was high. Appropriate facilities and practical and psychological support for SCM were often seen as something that did not get priority from managers and the wider system. These factors added to the efforts required to maintain an effective service and endangered the goodwill of SCM practitioners.

'It impacts on the staff, staff that were willing to implement SCM are no longer working within the teams ... I guess if management aren't on board with then then that's the message that's being cascaded across the team.' (female, NWBH)

'... it was quite grass roots led as well, I didn't feel we particularly had a great deal of support from our kind of clinical pathways leads ... they had many things that were taking priority.' (female, CNTW)

However, there were times when managers were on board and all parts of the system could see the benefit:

'I think you're right there I think that ... the manager recognizes that the crisis stuff is getting managed more effectively, and there's not as much pressure on the team.' (male, NWBH)

The focus group data also identified challenges related to the attitudes and investment in a positive culture surrounding SCM as an important service for people with complex relational and emotional needs and/or whose problems are consistent with BPD. This concern was not based on whether funding was available of not but was related to whether people across the managerial system valued what SCM brings to services, service users, and staff.

'You need investment in it ... they're (Services) not investing in people (staff) and they're not investing in the service users.' (male, NWBH)

'The challenge is, it's about a cultural shift, so there is stuff about operational management being on board and whether they see it as a priority.' (female, NWBH)

'... they are concerned that there may be a financial cost ... so that's an extra pressure on us facilitators to try and find solutions for.' (female, CNTW)

Inequality

Inequality was identified from the data with two areas of inequality being identified: (i) inequality in what services within the same Trusts were offering, and (ii) external wider system opportunities

In relation to the inequality within Trusts, both focus groups identified differences across their own services:

'... it's a postcode lottery.' (male, NWBH)

'You wouldn't think that we actually work for the same Trust would you?' (male, NWBH)

'... inequality in terms of the provision of SCM.' (female, CNTW)

In relation to external inequality, the focus groups identified the current political climate as something that may limit the progress outside of services that our service users can make:

'... it's about actually what services are actually in for them to link in to, I think the government cutbacks and all the rest, and there has been a lot of constriction on what is actually available so, I think that potentially holds some of our people back.' (female, CNTW)

'... people need to build a life as well as manage symptoms ... the challenges out there for just a lack of other places to belong.' (female, CNTW)

Service users

Involvement and interaction with service users were identified as key themes due to the importance they play in the experiences of practitioners delivering SCM, along with the system in which the practitioners work. All sub-themes identified overlapped with other key themes (e.g. Self and System). The sub-themes identified were:

1. Empower (Self and Service Users)
2. Relationship (Self and Service Users)
3. Containment (Self, Service Users, and System)

It was interesting for the authors to see such an overlap between the different the components of SCM, and it clearly highlighted the triangle of care that practitioners and services often seek.

Empowerment

The theme of 'empowerment' was identified throughout the focus group data and was linked to not only empowering the service user but also the SCM practitioner themselves. In relation to both it was very much around confidence building and personal development, but less of a focus on skills.

> 'There's something about empowerment for all of us as human beings isn't there? If you're "othered" in society "oh this is a difficult person" you'll use your power in that system in maybe a negative way to get hear ... and then you're not "othered" anymore (in SCM) ... those people are empowered ... changing the system ... retraining us as staff ... it's inclusive and they are using their power in a positive way.' (female, NWBH)

> '... it feels collaborative and empowers the patient to kind of work on what, in a more holistic way it feels, to work on what they want to work on.' (female, NWBH)

Relationship

Relationships were referred to throughout the data. This theme was highlighted across self and service users. Practitioners identified that experience of reciprocal relationships between themselves as practitioners and others involved in the same work gave them confidence:

> 'I feel like I am part of this niche circle of SCM friends.' (female, CNTW)

In addition, they identified the reciprocal relationship between practitioners and service users as essential:

> 'It's about helping people understand their difficulties and their triggers so it gives them a vocabulary that they can talk to us ... doing some of the work around attachment.' (female, CNTW)

> '... getting to really know somebody.' (female, CNTW)

> '... there's a lot more than what the skills are, it's about the relationships between people.' (female, CNTW)

> 'I think predominantly for me it's about the relational element of structured clinical management.' (female, NWBH)

> '... it is about you both in a room, every single week, same time, same place and it is about the relationship that you have.' (female, CNTW)

Reciprocal relationships between the service users themselves was also vital:

> '... they are building the trust in that room as well with other people....they can actually overcome that (lack of trust) and have those meaningful relationships with other people.' (female, CNTW)

Containment

Finally, the theme of containment was highlighted across all of the data. This transcended the component parts of self, service user, and systems, relating to the structure of SCM and what it provided across the three levels in terms of consistency, containment, and a general framework. Much of the data highlighted that these were key to the success of SCM and impacted on many of the other themes identified.

Practitioners highlighted the emotional and mental containment for themselves, which also aided the reduction in anxiety that was identified as an earlier theme:

> 'We have got a framework to go from start to finish with something which I think is really useful.' (female, CNTW)

> 'I know where it starts, I know where it finishes and I know exactly what people are doing in the middle. That organizes me.' (male, NWBH)

> '... I suppose I like the structure of it as well ... I kind of enjoyed using that structure.' (female, CNTW)

> '... a more boundaried approach.' (female, NWBH)

> '... it feels easier doesn't it as well?' (male, NWBH)

> 'I have containment, consistency and a framework ... a lot safer ... I go home without worrying.' (female, NWBH)

> 'I don't understand why more people don't want to do it (SCM) ... why don't they want to feel contained?' (male, NWBH)

> '... compared to care coordination, because I do both, ... it does feel a lot clearer what I'm doing with someone ... yeah it feels a lot more contained.' (female, NWBH).

> '... now we have a framework to understand it, and a structure for us to offer up, something that's going to be really consistent.' (female, NWBH)

> 'For me it's nice to have a framework which you know is for experience for the first time rather than medication.' (female, NWBH)

In addition, service users seemed to feed back to practitioners that they found the containment helpful and important:

'It makes people feel like we are all reading from the same book if you like, it helps to kind of contain a lot.' (female, CNTW)

'I know that they (service users) are going to be contained by that (length of SCM).' (female, CNTW)

'... a framework for him (service user) to maybe think about his relationships.' (female, NWBH)

'... transparent conversation ... right from the very beginning.' (female, NWBH)

Practitioners also identified the containment provided to the other services and the system as a whole from the clear plans for service users and staff. Services saw real value in a coordinated, organized, and focused treatment outline for service users that had been challenging to them:

'... they (services and service users) are seeing the benefit in multiple areas.' (female, CNTW)

'... they (system) feel quite relieved when they know somebody who is accessing their services is even known to the PD hub or is having SCM ... they know their care plans will be robust.' (female, CNTW)

'... the impact on the wards, ward feedback is that this is great, this is somewhere now for these people that we really struggled with that we may be had to put out of area that we maybe feel like we're doing something with ... there's many bits of the system that feedback how good it is.' (male, NWBH)

'... it's allowed me to umbrella into services in the Borough to develop whole systems approaches to people's care.' (female, NWBH)

'... it benefits duty ... it benefits staff, it benefits other staff that are not doing SCM, you've got GPs it benefits A&E. I think like you say it's the whole, it's everything, the service.' (male, NWBH)

Conclusion

Despite the data being gathered across two different NHS mental health providers, both covering large and differing geographical areas, the key themes elicited showed remarkable similarity with regards to the implementation of SCM. Each theme clearly demonstrates that SCM not only benefits the service user (clinical evidence) but also the practitioner and the wider system.

Overall, it was found that practitioners reported SCM offers them a framework which strengthens their skills and confidence, combining a balance of learning, enhancing their general role in services, and increasing job satisfaction. Whilst anxiety may have been high at the start of utilizing SCM or working with this client group, practitioners reported that over time, SCM provided a feeling of containment which left them trusting the model and feeling empowered in the work they were delivering.

The focus groups also identified that practitioners found that SCM strengthened their relationships with service users in that it provided them with a collaborative structure in which change felt realistic and achievable. As has been found in other areas, supervision also played a key role in promoting well-being, confidence, and containment, and demonstrates the importance of having this support in place.

One of the most heartening findings was a general sense of enhanced job satisfaction whereby practitioners felt they 'enjoyed' their work, were more engaged in their roles, and believed they were truly able to make a positive difference.

However, the data also highlight key challenges that need to be considered when planning to implement SCM locally. Critically, SCM is more likely to be successfully implemented when there is involvement of service leads and these service leads can see the benefit of this approach. It is then more likely that resources will be made available for the programme. The main resource issues identified during these focus groups were practitioner time and the availability of appropriate venues for group work. SCM is therefore best implemented at a service level, with training in this approach being offered to service leads and practitioners. In this way, the need for frequent and structured appointments, supervision, and suitable rooms is appreciated by those responsible for the allocation of resources.

Acknowledgement

With thanks to SCM Practitioners in CNTW and NWBH for taking the time to participate in the focus groups.

References

Bateman, A., & Krawitz, R. (2013). *Borderline personality disorder: an evidence-based guide for generalist mental health professionals*. Oxford: Oxford University Press.

Beck, A. T. (1976). *Cognitive therapy and the emotional disorders*. New York, NY: Penguin.

Braun, V., & Clarke, V. (2006). Using thematic analysis in psychology. *Qualitative Research in Psychology, 3*, 77–101.

Kitzinger, J. (1995). Qualitative research: introducing focus groups. *British Medical Journal, 311*, 299.

Mitchell, S. (2017). *Structured clinical management (SCM): a therapist's manual*. Northumberland, Tyne & Wear NHS Foundation Trust.

18

SCM Supervision in the United Kingdom

Julia Harrison, Robert Watts, Genevieve Quayle, Sarah Hanmer,
Rachael Line, Darren Ellis, Amy Maher, and Louise MacDonald

Introduction

In this chapter, the key principles of clinical supervision for structured clinical management (SCM) will be outlined. The experiences of SCM supervisors, supervisees, and team managers from two contributing National Health Service Trusts in the United Kingdom (Cumbria, Northumberland, Tyne & Wear NHS Foundation Trust (CNTW) and North West Boroughs Healthcare NHS Foundation Trust (NWBH Note: in 2021 NWBH split – Hatlon, Knowsley, St Helens and Warrington Boroughs going to Mersey Care NHS Foundation Trust and Wigan going to Greater Manchester) will be used to illustrate how supervisory arrangements have been implemented and to give an overview of how SCM can be delivered and supervised according to the skill mix and resources of services.

Supervision Models and Their Application to SCM

The Care Quality Commission (2013) advises that supervision is essential for all registered professionals and support staff within health and social care. This helps ensure that service users and their carers receive high-quality care at all times from staff who are able to manage the personal and emotional impact of the work. SCM is an evidence-based approach that enables generalist mental health practitioners to work effectively with people diagnosed with borderline personality disorder (BPD). It is therefore important that supervision structures are considered as part of the implementation of this approach and that experienced supervisors with adequate understanding of the model are identified at an early stage.

Given there are likely to be differing supervisory functions and roles involved in the implementation of SCM, clarifying their differing purposes can be useful. Proctor's (1986) model of supervision suggests different foci exist: formative, normative, and restorative. The formative approach focuses on the skills development of the supervisee; normative upon the managerial and quality control aspect of the supervisee's practice, and a restorative approach on the well-being of the supervisee.

Managerial supervision commonly has a normative focus, with the supervisor having accountability for, and authority over, the work of the supervisee, and it balances a service-level focus with the development and well-being (restorative) needs of the supervisee. Clinical supervision has more of a formative focus, providing the opportunity for skills learning and practice, reflection on the therapeutic work, and the supervisee's personal and professional responses to it, with the aim of self-development in the context of application of the SCM programme. Both managerial and clinical supervisors are instrumental in the embedding of SCM within a service and so consideration of the functions of both roles should be considered when negotiating the resources needed for implementation of SCM.

When considering implementation of SCM supervision, it is helpful to review existing approaches to supporting people who implement treatments for people with personality difficulties. Both dialectical behaviour therapy (DBT; Linehan, 2014) and mentalization-based therapy (MBT; Bateman & Fonagy, 2016) are specialist evidence-based therapies for people diagnosed with BPD (NICE, 2009). SCM shares some similarities with both these approaches and all are long-term and highly structured psychological interventions. The learning embedded within DBT and MBT can be used to inform both the frequency and structure of supervision sessions for SCM.

DBT and MBT recommend weekly supervision meetings for all staff members involved in the delivery of full therapy programmes (Anna Freud Centre, 2018; Swales, 2010). This ensures good communication between group and individual practitioners, frequent reflective space to consider the emotional impact of the work, and a space to maintain knowledge of the models used. There is also close attention to monitoring model adherence and competence of the therapist and team. Within MBT supervision, an adherence and competence scale is used to provide a focus for the training and supervision of practitioners (Anna Freud Centre, 2017). DBT similarly utilises an adherence scale (Linehan & Korslund, 2003). SCM draws on the supervisory frameworks of these psychological models to allow successful implementation of treatment within community care teams.

SCM Supervision Delivery—General Principles

Some of the general principles informing delivery of SCM supervision discussed in this chapter were developed from information collated from staff questionnaires and interviews. Relevant healthcare staff including clinical team leads and managers, SCM supervisors, and SCM supervisees were invited to participate in online surveys specifically tailored to their role.

SCM is an integrated treatment approach that incorporates all aspects of good clinical care coordination with an active intervention phase focusing on core modules of problem-solving, emotional regulation, impulsivity and other risky behaviours, and mentalizing attachments and relationships. It is also helpful to plan an ending or 'next steps' phase in which the service user both consolidates learning and thinks about how to maintain skills and progress.

The SCM practitioner is often, but not always, in the position of delivering psychological interventions whilst simultaneously in some cases carrying out a care coordination and liaison/advocacy role. This dual role can give consistency to the service user, thereby having a sound clinical rationale. Although there are clear benefits to this, the dual role of the SCM practitioner can present challenges to the practitioner and the wider mental health and social system, and these problems will consequently present in supervision.

Within the SCM model there is clear guidance regarding the provision of supervision with the recommendation that all SCM practitioners receive monthly group expert-led clinical supervision as a minimum, alongside peer-led team supervision (Mitchell, 2018). This is in line with typical NHS supervision policies. Where a service user's group therapy and individual SCM sessions are provided by different practitioners, both practitioners should preferably attend the group supervision. Where this is not possible, arrangements need to be put in place to ensure good communication, information sharing, and reflection across the team. Feedback from both Trusts on the delivery of SCM supervision is shown in Box 18.1.

SCM Supervision Resources

The supervisee's training needs in becoming a proficient and competent SCM practitioner cannot be met solely by individual or group clinical supervision. It is unrealistic to expect one type of supervision to be an adequate format to meet the multiple functions of supervision effectively as described previously. Feedback from both Trusts about how their learning was developed over time is shown in Box 18.2.

Just as SCM delivery requires a team approach and integration of multiple clinical perspectives, SCM supervision draws on a variety of resources and processes. In order to provide a high-quality treatment programme that has effective governance and supervision, there has to be ongoing development of supervisee skills using a range of supervisory techniques and processes targeting all aspects of an SCM programme. These are described in Box 18.3.

SCM supervision requirements place time and resource demands on services. In busy secondary care community teams, these requirements may be concerning to service leads and managers, and the time allocated for supervision becomes eroded over time. A balance needs to be struck between what is recommended as a 'gold standard' for service provision and what is pragmatic and feasible within current local resources and service constraints.

It is important to keep in mind however, that the time and resources invested in supporting SCM delivery through supervision is invaluable in equipping staff

Box 18.1 In Practice: Delivery of SCM Supervision in CNTW and NWBH

Within the contributing NHS trusts, the clinical supervision of SCM was found to be primarily provided by clinical psychologists (67%), with a smaller number of supervisors from occupational therapy and nursing disciplines. There is a requirement that supervisors are adequately trained in SCM, and it is desirable that they have experience in delivery of SCM, whether group or individual, as well as experience of clinical supervision. Survey respondents reported an average of 16 years post-professional qualification experience and an average of 4 years post-SCM training.

As staff have become more experienced in delivery of the model, SCM practitioners have themselves begun to develop additional peer supervision groups, such as leading on 'Share, Learn, and Do' forums where staff can become familiar with skills, strategies, and components of the model, and share their experiences of delivery.

The contributing Trusts are endeavouring to maintain the recommended frequency of supervision; in some services weekly supervision is scheduled for group facilitators with an invitation to individual practitioners to join. Local guidelines have been developed regarding acceptable attendance levels, with a minimum of fortnightly participation required. There are likely to be differences in how much supervision is prioritized depending on the type of service offering SCM. Within CNTW, the Personality Disorder Hub seeks to maintain fortnightly individual supervision of SCM clinicians, and this is important given that all service users on staff caseloads have complex needs and high risk difficulties. Within CNTW Community Treatment Teams, in which a service user's presenting difficulties are less complex and clinicians maintain high case loads of service users with other mental health difficulties, there is less time available to maintain frequent supervision:

'Within our Community Treatment Team the current arrangement is a monthly peer supervision session ... there is occasionally individual scaffolding outside of this but I do not offer formal individual supervision.'

An alternative arrangement has been separate supervision forums for staff providing individual and group SCM, with a monthly 90-minute forum provided for practitioners delivering one-to-one SCM. This is in addition to their monthly individual clinical supervision.

It was found that although modes of delivery and frequency may vary slightly, there was a consistent investment in provision of good-quality supervisory and support systems.

The majority of supervisees surveyed indicated that SCM supervision supported their practice with 61% reporting that this was *always* the case, and another 33% reporting that supervision *often* (11%) or *sometimes* (22%) supported their SCM practice.

Frequency of supervision was highlighted as helpful:

'I find the frequency and quality of supervision I receive extremely beneficial. I feel it is an integral part of enabling me to deliver the model in an effective way. I feel very well supported.'

The complex demands of providing both care coordination and psychological interventions was raised with survey respondents. The majority of supervisees (68%) had previous experience of care coordination and 66% of supervisors also reported having care-coordination experience. Supervisors surveyed indicated that this experience was useful in helping them fully understand the pressures and demands of the role, particularly the difficulties of integrating the varied aspects.

to meet the needs of their service users more effectively and in supporting staff welfare and clinical confidence and resilience. A more resilient and clinically effective workforce can lead to lower levels of staff sickness and burnout, improved outcomes for service users, and more focused and shorter treatment pathways. As Boorman (2009) noted in a review of UK NHS staff well-being, improved resilience in staff can help the NHS achieve its four key targets of improved quality, innovation, productivity, and prevention. Feedback from SCM staff, clinical managers, and team leads on how they have collaborated effectively is shown in Box 18.4.

SCM Supervision—Specific Demands

For effective clinical implementation, individual and group SCM practitioners face a number of demands and require a variety of skills. Supervision focuses synergistically on a number of related issues. First is the practitioner–service user relationship and SCM Clinical Stance. Second is fostering the development of techniques, generic clinical skills and SCM strategies and intervention. Third is closely attending to issues of safety assessment and management. Finally is regularly monitoring adherence to the model and any relational dynamics that may

Box 18.2 In Practice: Facilitating Staff Learning within CNTW and NWBH

Within the contributing NHS trusts, despite SCM training eliciting positive feedback, it was evident that training alone was not enough for staff to go on and confidently deliver treatment. Perceptions were that although SCM training provided a good foundation and awareness of the underpinning principles and treatment targets, staff often felt daunted by the demands of ongoing treatment provision.

Both supervisors and supervisees referred to this in their survey responses. 'A steep learning curve' was described, with 67% of supervisors suggesting that SCM training alone prepared practitioners only moderately (50%) or a little (17%). Respondents emphasized the need for 'ongoing supervision and support getting clinicians up and running', and highlighted '(one) can only be confident by doing, not just the theoretical underpinnings'.

Respondents also highlighted that SCM training may at times assume an existing knowledge base of skills or theory that in reality individual staff lack, and therefore again supervisory processes are vital to identify and address gaps in competencies and confidence.

Issues were also raised about how to monitor the quality of resources that were often gathered on an individual basis from a variety of sources in order to deliver SCM skills-based interventions

Within NWBH this issue was addressed by the development of quarterly refresher days where practitioners meet to network, share practice, consider barriers, and further develop skills.

In CNTW there are now a number of therapist manuals and service user workbooks to aid the delivery of both individual and group SCM. This has been of significant help to clinicians; however, the drawback to this positive development is that as with any model, considerable preparation and planning time is required to become familiar with the materials and competent in the delivery of skills and strategies. The trust also developed the 'Structured Clinical Management Implementation Checklist' (Harrison & Mitchell, 2019) which is described further in this chapter.

In addition to the methods above, both Trusts reported the provision of local SCM implementation meetings where issues, including model adherence, drift, and supervision needs can be fed back and discussed. As an aid to this, one of the participating Trusts has also developed a database to record outcomes and highlight issues such as model drift, attrition, etc.

Box 18.3 In Practice: SCM Supervision Resources within CNTW and NWBH

Within the NHS Trusts implementing SCM and contributing to this book, a number of supervision resources have been developed:
- Individual supervision using the 'SCM Implementation Checklist'
- Supervision of group facilitators and group programme
- Monthly group supervision to familiarize staff with the model and its components, using manuals and workbooks.
- Monthly 'Share, Learn, and Do' groups to practise specific skills and strategies
- Monthly supplementary groups to discuss complexity factors such as complex trauma and dissociation that may present obstacles to engagement
- Complex case discussion groups using SCM principles to formulate
- Scaffolding of other services and staff
- SCM refresher and networking days to ensure adherence to the model and address barriers or challenges within local teams
- Supervision checklist/tasks
- Extra training on group delivery

---

arise between the practitioner, service user, and the wider mental health system (Bateman & Krawitz, 2013).

Attachment and therapeutic alliance

Regarding the common difficulties that the supervisee may encounter, it is important to remember that at its core, SCM is an attachment-based model. As such, there is an emphasis on the development of a secure therapeutic attachment between practitioner and service user in order to foster safety, which supports therapeutic progress. Without a strong therapeutic alliance, practitioner and service user may experience drift, relational rupture, or avoidance of treatment (Horvath & Symonds, 1991). In SCM, the role of the therapeutic alliance is a vital component in problem identification, agreeing collaborative goals, increasing task engagement, and improving overall outcomes.

Individuals referred for SCM treatment present with a number of features that may make achieving a therapeutic relationship more difficult to achieve. Service users diagnosed with BPD show considerable mistrust in the world and are wary of talking openly to new practitioners, most have experienced childhood trauma and encountered continuing adverse interpersonal relationships. The attachment

Box 18.4 In Practice: Collaborating with Managers and Team Leads

The contributing services noted the resource demands involved and that at times, careful negotiation with team managers and leads has been needed to secure the time needed for training and supervisory activities. Team managers were also surveyed to gather their perspectives about the resourcing and supervision of the model.

Of the 13 respondents, all of whom worked in community settings, a majority of managers (92%) reported that they believed SCM to be 'very much' or 'moderately' of benefit to service delivery, service users, and clinician skillset.

Despite this largely positive response, the majority of managers (77%) indicated that they were not trained in SCM, and only a small number (12%) felt that they had a good overall understanding of the SCM model and its components. This is perhaps an issue due to the time demands of full SCM training.

Additionally, whilst they had suggested valuing the model, issues were also highlighted about the resource demands placed on teams due to the high number of service users who could benefit, and the resulting need for training, delivery, and effective supervision:

'there is already effective supervision in the team, which means there is little need for separate';

'we have practitioners trained in SCM but no capacity to deliver';

'As far as I am aware there is currently no access to SCM supervision.'

Comments suggested a disparity between geographical areas in which there are SCM-trained clinicians but no supervisors or group facilitators who can embed the whole treatment package, and areas in which this has been possible. Areas in which SCM has become embedded as a treatment have tended to be well supported by team leads who have attended the training or have some knowledge of treatments offered to service users with emotion regulation and interpersonal difficulties.

In response to the issues presented by managers, within one of the contributing Trusts a 1-day training package has been designed specifically for managers, with the aim of providing an opportunity to communicate the benefits of allocating resources and also problem-solving together the obstacles that arise.

styles activated in any interaction are insecure and often disorganized, anxious, or dismissive, which can evoke strong counter-relational responses in the practitioner leading to reciprocal interaction that can at times either enhance or hinder progress. Additionally, the complexity and pervasiveness of presenting problems may make agreeing and maintaining a shared therapy focus difficult at times. Maintaining a balance between validation of distress, effort, and intentions, and supporting commitment to change can be a challenge for the practitioner also.

Not only should attachment and therapeutic alliance between the SCM practitioner and service user be considered but also the alliance and attachment styles of the supervisor and supervisee. Effective supervision requires the right balance between support and challenge. If this balance is not achieved, and the supervisor leans towards constant validation and support, this can inhibit the development of skills. Conversely, too high a level of challenge can result in a supervisee feeling overly criticized, with the potential for a relational rupture to occur if the supervisee reacts by becoming dismissive of any challenge or guidance or feels inadequacy or even shame arising from feelings of failure or humiliation. Lastly, the supervisory relationship may at times mirror the relational dynamics or patterns that are occurring in SCM treatment and therefore provide a useful reflective tool if both supervisor and supervisee can maintain awareness of this phenomenon. How the working alliance mirrors the supervisory process is illustrated in Figure 18.1.

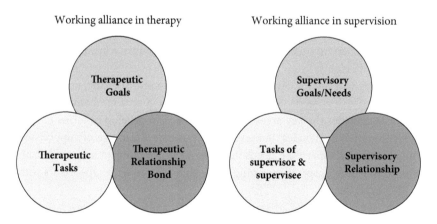

Figure 18.1 Mapping the Working Alliance onto Supervisory Processes

Assessment, formulation, safety management, safety planning, and goal-setting

If the supervisee is engaged in the initial phase of SCM work, supervision will focus on more practical tasks such as developing a clear understanding of formulation of the service user's presenting difficulties, including understanding and management of risk behaviour in the context of the formulation. Where service users are referred from children and young people's services, supervision might need to focus on a transfer of care and be used to assist the practitioner in ensuring the service user's transition is planned, linked and collaborative (see Chapter 11). Supervision of practitioners delivering these early stages of treatment can be used as a reflective space for development of the service user's care plan and prospective treatment. It can be used to assist the practitioner to develop a hierarchy of treatment goals, to set a time frame and trajectory of therapy, and negotiate contracts between service user and practitioner. It is likely that the levels of risk with which the service user presents will change over the course of treatment and supervision is a useful context for the practitioner to 'step back' from the situation and reflect with others on what is effective or not effective in managing risk.

Skills development

In the intervention phase, the practitioner is asked to teach and model skills that help the service user problem-solve, reduce impulsive and risky behaviours, increase emotional regulation, and develop robust skills in mentalizing and improving the quality and safety of relationships. This requires familiarity and competence in delivering psychoeducation and skills-based psychological intervention strategies. The practitioner may be delivering sessions on an individual basis or in a group setting, and additionally may have to adapt the intervention programme for service users who display significant trauma-related problems or cognitive impairments.

Supervisees will have varied levels of experience and training, resulting in different supervision needs. Supervision is therefore a setting in which practitioners can consider the key areas which they need to develop in terms of specific skills and competencies. Supervisors in turn need a range of supervision resources to meet supervisee needs and the service requires a system that allows supervisees with specific training needs to be placed with supervisors with matching expertise.

Clearly, the role of the SCM supervisor can be challenging. However, there is great reward and fulfilment professionally and personally from seeing practitioners become more resourced and skilled over time. Supervisees sometimes refer to a point at which 'the penny drops' and they start to feel intrinsically more confident about positive risk management, making decisions about whether to 'do' or 'not do' something, and delivering specific skills or modular interventions. Such supervision needs are detailed in Box 18.5.

Box 18.5 In Practice: Meeting Multi-factorial Needs in Supervision

Questions such as those below were described as typically being brought to supervision and illustrate the varied factors that clinicians present.

Skills-based development

My service user says that she 'hates mindfulness and body scans re-traumatize her'—what should I do?

We're approaching the mentalizing attachment sections of work, but I missed the mentalizing awareness training.

Alliance and relational factors

I'm intimidated by my service user's hostility when I'm advising on her poly-pharmacy, I sometimes 'give in' even though I believe she is over-medicated as I worry about our relationship.

My service user has asked if I can attend a family court hearing with her—am I 'leaning in' too much if I go, or is this in my advocacy role?

Model adherence

My service user has asked for a 2-hour session fortnightly rather than a weekly 1 hour session—is that drifting from model?

My service user was in A&E today after self-harming and missed our planned session, can I offer her another at short notice?

Survey respondents noted the role of supervision in helping them identify and address these multi-factorial aspects. The majority of supervisees stated that SCM supervision differed from their previous supervision in its focus in regard to reflection (66%), the therapeutic alliance (74%), and their own reactions to the work (67%).

When asked about specific aspects of SCM supervision they found helpful, 100% of respondents identified that it supported their risk management, with other factors such as addressing clinical stuckness (83%), identifying obstacles to change (83%), retaining focus and having a clear treatment pathway (78%) also receiving high response levels.

Expanding on this, supervisees fed back that within SCM supervision:

'There is lots of reflective practice, exploring difficult dynamics and reflection on how I am managing my own wellbeing whilst working with this service user group', and that they felt that they benefited from the 'structure of the interventions and ability to look out for drift.'

Despite this, both supervisees and supervisors noted that at times supervision still felt 'very full' and on occasion, especially if a service user is experiencing a crisis, that extra ad hoc supervision is required. This prompted the reflection that often, cases that provoke greater anxiety are brought to supervision, with the potential that other cases may 'drift away from supervision and therefore reflection and planning'.

Model Adherence and Drift

SCM is an emerging treatment approach that is effective when adopted by generic mental health practitioners and teams and delivered with attention to model adherence. As noted, there will always be tensions between adherence and practical and resource constraints of typical UK NHS community services. Attention to model adherence whilst accepting the pressure faced by community teams is an important consideration for SCM clinical leaders and those in supervisory roles. In order to foster confidence and competencies, an SCM Competencies Checklist has been developed. This reduces the pressure on supervisees and supervisors and facilitates the flexible implementation of the model. An example of how model adherence was managed by one service is shown in Box 18.6.

Group Dynamics

Whilst SCM groups provide many benefits and opportunities for service users (normalization of experiences, collectively working together to resolve problems, and a relatively safe training ground for attachment patterns and trying out different ways of relating), there are also potential pitfalls which the group facilitators and individual practitioners should monitor and address. Linehan (1993, 2014) provides a comprehensive overview of the dynamics and dialectics that can occur in DBT groups. Fonagy, Bateman, and Campbell (2017) outline issues relating to epistemic trust in group work. Many such processes are also likely to occur in SCM groups and require skilful management by the practitioner, alongside frequent, high-quality communication between individual practitioners and group facilitators.

Supervision of group facilitators will therefore need to provide restorative space for reflection and processing of group dynamics alongside the formative functions of supervision in terms of skills acquisition. Such skills might include how to manage a range of clinical problems such as hostile or disruptive group members; those who don't contribute; the creation of cliques within the group; breaking of group rules by members; the formation of relationships within the group that

Box 18.6 In Practice: Model Adherence—The SCM Implementation Checklist

Within one of the contributing Trusts an SCM Implementation Checklist was developed. The aims of the tool are to assist model adherence and to help clinicians develop competency and confidence in the delivery and sequencing of SCM.

The scale shares similarities with other psychological model adherence scales (e.g. Cognitive Therapy Rating Scale—Revised, Blackburn, et al., 2001; MBT Adherence Scale, Anna Freud Centre, 2017), and was developed either to assist reflection on an individual session or sessions (potentially with an audio or video recording to aid this, if appropriate) or to help more general reflection of the service user's progress through the programme.

To aid the structure of the tool, the SCM process was considered as phasic with an introductory phase, an active interventions phase, and an endings or transitions phase when the individual approached the end of therapy. In addition to the three sequential phases, there are 'cross-sectional' or ongoing features such as continued attendance to alliance, risk management, and family and carer involvement.

The tool therefore provides a way for both supervisor and supervisee to reflect on the course and timescales of treatments and identify and explore obstacles to progress (e.g. do these obstacles arise from the service user, therapist, or system?), and the practitioner can then signpost the service user to learning and CPD needs, if areas of difficulty or lower confidence levels are identified.

may undermine treatment; or disclosure of information in the group that activates emotion or trauma memories in others.

The SCM supervisor will therefore need to be skilled in managing group processes themselves. Techniques such as triangulation, siding, 'good guy/bad guy', devil's advocate, parking, modelling, 'foot in the door; door in the face', and empty chair can all be useful skills for the group practitioner to acquire. Supervisees might also need to consider dynamics relevant to the individual which might impact on interventions for them in the group. For example, public praise might not be a positive reinforcement for some service users and can lead to feelings of shame which then impact on their experience in the group. Hence, whilst SCM groups are skills-based rather than process groups, there is still a need for practitioners to receive appropriate reflective and formative supervision sessions.

Conclusion

Supervision is an integral part of the successful delivery of SCM and so it needs to be given due care and attention in the implementation of this approach in UK NHS Trusts. The frequency of supervision is likely to depend on a number of factors, including experience of the practitioners, whether they are practising individual or group SCM therapy, the complexity and risk shown by the service users in the treatment programme, and the time available to the teams. Ideally, the higher the complexity and risk level of presenting problems experienced by the service user, the more frequent the supervision needs to be.

Feedback from supervisees was clear in highlighting that initial training is necessary but not adequate to equip practitioners to begin SCM work without significant support and supervision from more experienced staff. In working with service users who tend to present with complex issues, significant attachment-related difficulties, and high-risk behaviours, there is a need for thorough assessment, formulation, and crisis planning in the initial stages of treatment. Such work is likely to go beyond the level of training most generalist care coordinators receive and so support and clinical supervision is necessary in these initial stages to ensure effective engagement of service users. As therapy progresses and the treatment frame is established, regular supervision and support is required to ensure flexible model adherence and therapeutic ruptures are well managed. Knowledge of attachment and psychodynamic theory by supervisors is useful but not essential in supervision to help practitioners step back from the therapy relationship and to see the wider relational patterns occurring within the service between different practitioners involved in service users' care and between the service user and practitioner themselves. This ideally requires supervisors to be trained in a range of psychological interventions and/or be experienced in MBT or psychodynamic approaches but could equally be delivered by senior supervisors trained in other models who understand the relational patterns being re-enacted in the group situation. Finally, an awareness of basic group processes and techniques for managing group dynamics is needed for those supervising SCM groups. This can be facilitated by setting up of supervision of supervision whereby those practitioners trained and experienced to a more senior level can provide supervision to the SCM supervisors.

Initial training is best followed by a period of closely supervised practice in which staff are supervised frequently in order to embed their SCM practice in the clinical workplace. Refresher days, practice groups, use of adherence (checklist) scales, and extra training may also be employed to enhance practice and ensure there is continued professional development when delivering SCM.

Allocation and protection of time for supervision to take place at a frequency greater than the minimum monthly period must be agreed with team leads and managers. It is therefore imperative that 'buy in' from those in leadership roles is sought. Given that the majority of managers and team leads in most health services will not have undertaken any training in SCM, it is not surprising that there will be variation in the implementation of the approach across services unless they are fully involved. The training of team leads and managers in SCM, as well as practitioners and supervisors, is likely to be critical to its successful roll out in mental health services. This training, though not required to be as thorough as practitioner training, should include the rationale for the approach, the structure of the individual sessions and group work and the requirement for supervision to ensure model fidelity, effective outcomes, and practitioner health and well-being. Combining these recommendations would ensure the formative, normative, and restorative functions of supervision are all appropriately addressed.

References

Anna Freud Centre. (2017). *Mentalization-based treatment: adherence and competence scale*. London: Anna Freud National Centre for Children and Families. Retrieved from https://www.annafreud.org/training/mentalization-based-treatment-training/mbt-adherence-scale/.

Anna Freud Centre. (2018). *A quality manual for MBT*. London: Anna Freud National Centre for Children and Families.

Bateman, A., & Fonagy, P. (2016). *Mentalization-based treatment for personality disorders: a practical guide*. Oxford: Oxford University Press.

Bateman, A., & Krawitz, R. (2013). *Borderline personality disorder: an evidence-based guide for generalist mental health professionals*. Oxford: Oxford University Press.

Blackburn, I., James, I., Milne, D., Baker, C., Standart, S., Garland, A., & Reichelt, K. (2001). The revised cognitive therapy scale (CTS-R): psychometric properties. *Behavioural and Cognitive Psychotherapy, 29*, 431–446.

Boorman, S. (2009). *NHS health and wellbeing*. London: Department of Health.

Care Quality Commission. (2013). *Supporting information and guidance: supporting effective clinical supervision*.

Fonagy, P., Campbell, C., & Bateman, A. (2017). Mentalizing, attachment, and epistemic trust in group therapy. *International Journal of Group Psychotherapy, 67*(2), 176–20.

Fuertes, J. N. (2019). *Working alliance skills for mental health professionals*. Oxford: Oxford University Press.

Harrison, J., & Mitchell, S. (2018). *SCM adherence checklist*. Cumbria, Northumberland, Tyne & Wear NHS Foundation Trust.

Horvath, A. O., & Symonds, B. D. (1991). Relation between working alliance and outcome in psychotherapy: a meta-analysis. *Journal of Counselling Psychology, 38*(2), 139–149.

Linehan, M. M. (2003a). *Cognitive behavioural treatment of borderline personality disorder*. London: Guilford Press.

Linehan, M. M. (2003b). *Skills training manual for treating borderline personality disorder*. London: Guilford Press.

Linehan, M. (2014). *DBT skills training manual* (2nd Ed.). London: Guilford Press.

Linehan, M. M., & Korslund, K. E. (2003). *Dialectical behavior therapy adherence manual*. Seattle, WA: University of Washington.

Mitchell, S. (2018). *SCM therapist manual.* Cumbria, Northumberland, Tyne & Wear NHS Foundation Trust.

NICE. (2009). *Borderline personality disorder: recognition and management.* London: NICE.

Proctor, B. (1986). Supervision: a co-operative exercise in accountability. In M. Marken & M. Payne (Eds.), Enabling *and ensuring. Leicester National Youth Bureau and Council for Education and Training in Youth and Community Work, Leicester*, pp. 21–23.

Swales, M. (2010). Implementing DBT: selecting, training and supervising a team. *The Cognitive Behaviour Therapist, 3*, 71–79.

19

Reflections, Synthesis, and Future Directions

Stuart Mitchell, Mark Sampson, and Anthony Bateman

Introduction

Writing this book has been an eminently practical undertaking. It has involved gathering the collective wisdom of many practitioners, supervisors, trainers, service users, and carers delivering, supporting, or participating in SCM as a generalist treatment approach in the United Kingdom and Europe and integrating this into a coherent whole. This chapter provides reflections on this process, a synthesis and summary of our collective learning, and suggests areas where SCM may usefully be developed and applied further.

Reflections

The inspiration for this book came from the collective wisdom of the contributing authors. They are all involved in leading and implementing treatment pathways for personality disorder, training and supervising practitioners, providing expert guidance on or developing the research or evidence base and improving the way in which health and social care systems provide care and treatment for people diagnosed with personality disorder. Since the original manual was published in 2013 (Bateman & Krawitz, 2013), generalist treatments, including SCM, have helped to improve the generalist care for people diagnosed with borderline personality disorder (BPD). The approach has broad applicability to many more service users than would be possible to treat with specialist psychosocial therapies alone. Over time, generalist treatments have improved, as resource efficient strategies have been included in the overall programme of care, such as mindfulness, mentalizing, and distress tolerance skills. Overall, SCM is not technique or theory-driven but high-quality, organized, active, relationally focused clinical care.

Practitioners seek and require supervision and guidance on how to implement SCM across complex mental health systems and how to incorporate the newer elements of SCM into their programmes. Additional clinical workbooks and practical guidance have been developed with this in mind which accompany the training programme. These aim to foster greater confidence and building of practitioners' existing skills and knowledge of implementing good clinical care provided by SCM. Mental health services implementing SCM inevitably grapple with organizational challenges and service dilemmas particularly if they have no current pathway in place for the treatment of service users diagnosed with personality disorder, including both generalist and specialist treatments, such as mentalization-based therapy (MBT) and dialectical behaviour therapy (DBT). There are many examples of good practice in the United Kingdom, Europe, Australia, and the United States where generalist approaches have been implemented successfully, plus areas where further development is urgently needed, such as with older people and people with autistic spectrum conditions (see later in this chapter). We will touch on some of the more complex areas where adaptations to the standard SCM model are needed and have been partially implemented.

Synthesis and Summary

Implementing SCM requires practitioners to follow key principles in all their work with service users, as outlined in Chapter 1. These are the core principles, four Cs of collaboration (stance), consistency, coherence, and continuity to which a fifth C has been proposed, namely communication. A SCM programme has structure, flexibility, and predictability. Practitioners follow a structure to guide their practice which builds interventions, all of which are tailored to the needs of service users, around problem-solving. Within the programme as a whole the different components have a different emphasis at any given point on the pathway for the service user. For example, assessment and alliance building is central to the structure of the programme and to adapting this to the attachment style and personal problems of the service user. This aspect is also central to the clinical stance or SCM-CV adopted by the practitioner treating the service user as a person with agency and autonomy. This helps build epistemic trust between service user and practitioner. Establishing an initial diagnosis (if used in the organization) with sensitivity and formulating the problems to be worked on (goals) in SCM is tailored to the individual. In addition, the focus of SCM and goals of the service user becomes part of the programme design, so that a high level of consistency and coherence is achieved. Agreement on safety plans is essential between the service user and practitioner, within the team as a whole, and between the team and other services the service user might access. This ensures continuity across the programme as a whole.

Treatment and session planning, based on the formulation and SCM problem domains, is emphasized when setting up the agreements with service users, so everyone involved knows who is responsible for what, and who does what at any given time. This ensures continuity and predictability of the programme over the treatment period, including at points of transition within treatment, and at treatment's ending. Individual and group sessions are components where both the general and specific core treatment strategies are used. They centre around an individualized approach focusing on the problems identified between the service user and practitioner, and emphasize consistency and coherence of the treatment programme, as well as self-agency. There is an emphasis on promoting self-agency and responsibility so that teams or services do not become either too anxious or too avoidant about helping the service user manage their own risk. For some service users, this will usually include specific guidance on what services should and should not do at times of crisis, so that, for example, decisions about admission or prescribing are integrated in the SCM programme as a whole.

It is helpful to distil the whole SCM programme down to some essential activities (inputs), processes, and tasks (where to focus and what to do), and outcomes expected from the model of care (outputs). In terms of inputs, the work may be focused on direct work with the service users or indirect work with the system of care supporting the person. Each has a different but related focus and process. With direct service user work, therapeutic processes and tasks are provided by individual and group work, supporting transition between services and making appropriate adaptations where needed, such as if the person has autism or a learning disability. There are different processes and tasks within each component. With indirect work, the practitioner is focused on scaffolding or supporting the system so all services act consistently, including at times of transition or change. This may include helping a shared and positive approach to risk and safety and avoiding iatrogenic harm where this has or is likely to occur. Should this require further support, the practitioner may call upon senior practitioners or SCM supervisors to support them at this systemic level, such as with prescribing or admission to hospital. Finally, there are aims and outcomes intended by SCM, which are helpful for the practitioner to monitor over time, regularly assessing progress against these. These include improved problem-solving ability, social and occupational functioning, and better use of mental health services. These processes, tasks, and outputs are summarized in Table 19.1.

Services and teams will inevitably have various difficulties they will need to overcome in order to implement SCM as a generalist treatment model. These may include a number of areas where their clinical pathway is unclear or where other models are more dominant, or where operational pressures are great.

Key principles, pathways, and strategy

Implementation of SCM requires integrating a range of different organizational perspectives and overcoming a number of challenges. At the heart of SCM are the SCM core principles, as described above, around which all aspects of the programme need to be configured if implementation is to succeed. Any mental health service requires an organized approach or well-defined pathway for people

Table 19.1 SCM Components: Inputs, Processes, and Outputs

Inputs	Processes/Tasks	Outputs
Direct service user interventions	• Individual sessions • Group sessions • Managing and adapting to attachment style • Facilitating transitions between services and pathways • Adapting for additional problems	• Solving social, emotional, and interpersonal problems more effectively • Managing crises and safety more effectively • Using mental health and other services more effectively
Indirect systemic interventions	• Supervision of practitioners • Scaffolding/consulting the system interfaces • Managing transitions and joint working between services • Managing iatrogenic harm and inconsistency or disagreement • Changing cultures	• Services avoiding iatrogenic harm and responding more consistently, in accordance with the evidence base and best practice • Implementing SCM consistently and fully

diagnosed with personality disorder and/or complex trauma. This helps provide the structure required for service users and practitioners working in the service. People diagnosed with personality disorder or with complex relational and emotional needs experience significant meta-cognitive and attachment disorganization, which worsens if it is matched by a complex and disorganized care system. Without structure, everybody can feel lost and without a clear focus. A co-governed strategic group (governed by experts by experience and occupation) to help guide and oversee the programme's structure will ensure service users', carers', and care providers' experiences and needs are considered.

Theory, nosology, and research

Significant research and theoretical developments have occurred in the field of personality disorder classification, assessment, and treatment over the last decade or more, particularly in the area of trait-based dimensional approaches to classification and implications of these for clinical practice (Lejuez & Gratz, 2020). Both DSM-5 and ICD-11 have moved towards trait-dimensional approaches to personality disorder which have been replicated across different cultures and for which there is much research support (Bach & Presnall-Shvorin, 2020; McCabe & Widiger, 2019; Ofrat, Krueger, & Clark, 2018;). Clinical assessment using this approach may now focus on assessing severity of functional impairment along with distress experienced, which may then be followed up by assessment of five to six trait-domain specifiers which illustrate how the person expresses their traits which cause them difficulty (Bach & First, 2018). This, in principle, should help reduce the stigma of personality disorder diagnosis in that functional impairment and trait expression become the issues of most concern for formulation and treatment planning, rather than a binary approach to either 'having a personality disorder' or not. New assessment tools have been developed with good psychometric properties which support trait-based clinical assessments of service users (Bach & Presnall-Shvorin, 2020; Clarkin, Livesley, & Meehan, 2018; Oltmanns & Widiger, 2018;).

In addition, there has been research which indicates there is considerable overlap between personality disorder, complex trauma, psychosis, dissociation, and other attachment difficulties (Berry, Bucci, & Danquah, 2020; Ford & Courtois, 2014). These issues are complex for practitioners to disentangle and may indicate the need for expert consultation before deciding on treatment priorities. Often, personality disorder is the primary problem and treatment to ameliorate its negative consequences will lead to improvements in many areas of interpersonal and self-functioning. However, where there is a psychosis, bipolar, or dissociative disorder present then separate or concurrent treatment for this may be indicated (Steele, Boon, & Van Der Hart, 2017). It is important that these research findings and implications are incorporated into the understanding of personality disorder pathways, strategies, and understanding of SCM. They have already been incorporated into SCM training in the United Kingdom, General Psychiatric Management (GPM) in the United States, and Good Clinical Care (GCC) in Australia. It remains the case that service users report being misunderstood or misdiagnosed for many years before an accurate diagnosis, formulation, and treatment plan are developed. It is incumbent on services to develop assessment services further and refine their approaches to diagnosis and formulation. In terms of treatment approaches, SCM and GPM/GCC have always taken a pragmatic approach to using whatever strategies are effective within a flexible but firmly structured supportive treatment focused on problem-solving.

Therapeutic interventions and adaptations

A further aspect of implementing SCM is deciding on the range of interventions to be used and how these may be adapted to the problems of the service user but which remain consistent with the SCM model. Many of the therapeutic processes and strategies used by practitioners aim to generate a trusting attachment relationship and alliance so that the interpersonal, emotional, and self-functioning problems brought by the service can be worked on using problem solving. They also help to 'stabilize the system' so all services and practitioners agree on the shared tasks and take the same stance/approach consistent with the model of SCM. Other interventions are more specific and are used to address particular symptoms or behaviours. Here SCM is permissive and pluralistic, recommending that practitioners choose interventions with which they are familiar. For example, if a practitioner is comfortable with delivering relaxation exercises to help patients manage anxiety, these are used, whereas if they are more familiar with using distress tolerance skills these are delivered.

System supports

Supporting the system and service is a final area worthy of attention to increase the likelihood of SCM being implemented effectively. This includes clinical supervision provided to SCM practitioners, and the scaffolding and consultation received locally to address issues of complexity when they arise. If there is insufficient supervision or this is eroded to minimal contact time, say 1 hour per month, then practitioners can lose clinical focus with their clinical stance drifting away from the 'therapeutic' position, The clinical team delivering SCM need to be aware of the model, understand how it works, and act in ways that have continuity, consistency, and are certainly not contradictory to the treatment plan. For example, prescribing must be integrated into the overall SCM programme and not outside it. Joint working with other services needs to be considered, with additional bespoke training in the model for those clinicians if required. It is important that all services involved work together in an integrated reflective way to ensure continuity and consistency across services, and each service owns their role and responsibilities without taking over the care plan, or, if the plan needs to change, they engage in joint planning with the other services and the service user rather than acting unilaterally or devolving it automatically to other services.

It is vital that operational management are supportive of the SCM implementation plan and know the requirements in terms of resources (time, venues, equipment, cost, etc.) and the benefits of its implementation within the local service. It is helpful to stress that this is an evidence-based intervention, aligned to the organization's strategy (if it is), and it will build on and improve clinical outcomes for service users receiving treatment as usual, such as 'care coordination' in the United Kingdom or 'treatment as usual' elsewhere. It will help with flow through pathways, ensure better and more efficient use of resources, and improve the service user experience so that they are not drifting in services receiving ineffective and at times harmful care and treatments which go on for too long. Service managers and clinical leads will be considering the overall demand on the clinical team, and the staff and other resources they have to meet that need. There may be an emphasis on 'never saying no' to a referral, and treating all practitioners in the same way, with little distinction between roles. SCM provides a foundation that allows for careful negotiation with service managers enabling reduced case load sizes (to, say, around 15–20 for a full-time generalist SCM practitioner) on the rationale that this will help service users access services and achieve better clinical outcomes whilst saving money on unnecessary contacts with other services. Some services limit their interventions to, say, a maximum of 20 sessions per service user. This is too short for those service users with severe impairment or with high comorbidity. At the moment, 12–18 months is the commonest length of treatment. For those with moderate impairment, they may be able to benefit from a briefer SCM intervention of up to 6 months. However, shorter interventions should be part of and not the 'whole' service offer.

A systemic overview of all these factors when planning implementation of SCM is shown in Figure 19.1.

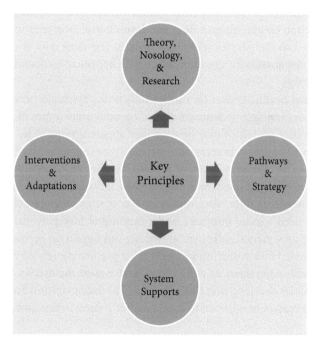

Figure 19.1 Systemic Overview of SCM Components, Pathway, and Processes to Guide Implementation

Future Directions

SCM and other generalist treatment, are gaining in popularity as they are applied to more service users who are diagnosed with personality disorder and related problems. More research on the various application of SCM as a generalist treatment is needed. This is most likely to emerge not only in controlled trial comparisons to other specialist treatments but as specific pre-post evaluations of specific adaptations in clinical practice across different service user groups in different health care settings. General Psychiatric Management (GPM) has already been adapted for adolescents in the United States (GPM-A), as has its equivalent in Australia in Good Clinical Care (GCC) within an early intervention pathway offering more specialist brief therapy to those who need this (Kongerslev, Chanen, & Simonsen, 2015; Llagan & Choi-Kain, 2020). Within the United Kingdom and Europe, this has yet to be developed and any adaptations for adolescents and young people will require further research and evaluation.

Within the learning disability and autism field, there are some developments in the United Kingdom. These need further evaluation to see what effects SCM may have in the treatment of people with complex needs who have difficulty with learning. Of interest will be the overlap and interactions between the problems of autistic spectrum conditions and BPD and how clinical interventions like SCM can be adapted so that service users may benefit. The same may also be true of those people diagnosed with attention-deficit with hyperactivity disorder (ADHD; Calvo et al., 2019).

Some mental health services for older adults now implement personality disorder-awareness training. Practitioners have become more aware of personality difficulties in later life which may be especially apparent when older people lose close attachment figures or become more physically or cognitively frail and feel insecure. There is increasing evidence of personality disorder occurring later in life (Beatson et al., 2016), although there may be a reluctance to embrace the concept of personality disorder or difficulties, due to the fear of stigmatizing an older person. Practitioners need a more informed understanding of how personality changes over time and how mental and physical changes can impact on personality. More research is needed into staff attitudes to later-life personality-related changes and the factors influencing them, as well as how service users themselves think about their personalities changing over time. This could be used to inform how interventions like SCM might be adjusted to increase effectiveness in this group of service users.

Further research into different programmes for carers and families is another area where development of the SCM model would be useful. There has been good progress made with regard to brief interventions for carers and families, which offer psycho-education, support, and skills to be used in everyday interaction with service users with personality disorder. It would be useful to investigate further how to train families and carers to become more involved in treatment itself, improving outcomes further. Co-producing new family and carer interventions would be key. Finally, exploring the domain of systemic therapy and SCM would certainly be interesting.

The 2020/21 COVID-19 pandemic introduced SCM service delivery challenges. Many practitioners around the world have had to adapt rapidly to using online/telephone approaches as face-to-face contact was not deemed safe or possible. This has advantages and disadvantages and may work for some service users, but not for others. There may be a loss of personal 'felt connection' when online, and for service users who experience anxious or disorganized attachment, this may trigger high levels of anxiety as it feels like a dramatic loss of personal contact with their practitioner (see Box 19.1). For other service users, working online feels a

---

Box 19.1 Adapting SCM to Online: Clinical Practice Guidance

1. **Maintain the model** as you would do in face-to-face contact
2. **Adapt to the remote environment** by:
   - Mentalizing the effects of the virtual technology.
   - Mentalizing the effects of the pandemic.
   - Work more on making mentalizing and problem-solving explicit rather than implicit.
   - Focus on the interactional processes between you and your client(s).
   - Help the client de-role from being a client so they can make the mental transition back to their home environment.
3. **SCM Group work online**
   - You can have several members in any group, up to eight maximum, with two facilitators.
   - You may convert a current group that has already met in person to an online format or start with an entirely new group of clients.
   - With a new group, if there are severe problems with developing safety and trust, you may want to have the first one to two sessions in person.
   - Agree the ground rules for running the group online, including camera, sound, lighting, privacy, and confidentiality, wearing of headsets, distractions, turn-taking etiquette, and group difficulties that may arise.
   - It may help to discuss early on how you would not expect everyone to look directly at the camera on the screen all the time, but to look away, and vary their gaze from time to time.
   - Aim to send out worksheets and handouts by secure email to clients before the group so you can work on them as documents in the group.

- Agree in each session the work of the group and which theme or topic you will focus on, as you would do face to face, but using different methods for discussion and feedback.
- Work out how you will manage silent, dominant, or distressed group members.
- Facilitators may need to be more explicit, active, and work a little harder to mentalize each group member and foster collaboration and trust between group members within the online situation.
- Consider when/if you may need to meet individual group members remotely or face to face in situations of high risk or suicidality.
- Maintain the boundaries of the group, starting and finishing on time as you would do if face to face, and mention every member's name before you finish so they feel you are mentalizing them.
- Help each group member mentalize the transition to joining the SCM group, and then their de-rolling from this when they leave the group session within their home environment.

4. IT (and relational) considerations
- Lighting—ensure you have your PC/tablet/laptop facing a window with good lighting.
- Background—ensure you have a clutter free neutral background or use a plain virtual background.
- Distractions—ensure you and your clients put up a 'do not disturb' or 'engaged' sign on the door to the room.
- Quality of sound and picture—consider using, and suggesting your clients use, a headset with mic (or earbuds) as this enhances the quality of the call and reduces mental and physical strain.
- Internet connection—use a wired Ethernet cable wherever possible.
- Intensity—agree with individual clients how close or distant to the camera you will be that feels most comfortable for them.
- Attention—be mindful at all times of where your effort and attention are directed. Switch off any distractions from emails, etc.
- Body language—check your facial expression in the camera box from time to time and adjust your expression as needed to indicate your intended 'marked mirroring' of clients' mental states.

safer and even a preferred choice. In the future, there may well be a formulation-informed blended approach to how care is delivered with online and face to face being offered depending on the needs of the service users.

References

Bach, B., & Presnall-Shvorin, J. (2020) Using DSM-5 and ICD-11 personality traits in clinical treatment. In C. W. Lejuez & K. L. Gratz (Eds.), *The Cambridge handbook of personality disorders*. Cambridge: Cambridge University Press.

Bach, B., & First, M.B. (2018). Application of the ICD-11 classification of personality disorders. *BMC Psychiatry, 18*, 351. https://doi.org/10.1186/s12888-018-1908-3

Bateman, A., & Krawitz, R. (2013). *Borderline personality disorder: an evidence based guide for generalist mental health professionals.* Oxford: Oxford University Press.

Beatson, J., Broadbear, J. H., Sivakumaran, H., George, K., Kotler, E., Moss, F., & Sathya Rao, S. (2016). Missed diagnosis: the emerging crisis of borderline personality disorder in older people. *Australian & New Zealand Journal of Psychiatry,* 1–7 doi: 10.1177/0004867416640100

Berry, K., Bucci, S., & Danquah, N. (Eds.) (2020). *Attachment theory and psychosis: current perspectives and future directions.* London: Routledge.

Calvo, N., Lara, B., Serrat, L., Perez-Rodriguez, V., Andion, O., Ramos-Quiroga, J. A., & Ferrer, M. (2019). The role of environmental influences in the complex relationship between borderline personality disorder and attention-deficit/hyperactivity disorder: review of recent findings. *Borderline Personality Disorder and Emotion Dysregulation, 7*, 2.

Choi-Kain, L., & Gunderson, J. G. (Eds.) (2019). *Applications of good psychiatric management for borderline personality disorder: a practical guide.* Washington, DC: American Psychiatric Association.

Clarkin, J. F., Livesley, W. J., & Meehan, K. B. (2018). Clinical Assessment. In W. J. Livesley. & R. Larstone (Eds.), *Handbook of personality disorders: theory, research and treatment* (2nd Ed.). London: Guilford Press.

Dudas, Rob., Lovejoy, C., Cassidy, S., Allison, C., Smith, P., & Baron-Cohen, S. (2017). The overlap between autistic spectrum conditions and borderline personality disorder. *PLoS One, 12*(9), e018447. https://journals.plos.org/plosone/article?id=10.1371/journal.pone.0184447

Ford, J. D., & Courtois, C. A. (2014). Complex PTSD, affect dysregulation, and borderline personality disorder. *Borderline Personality Disorder and Emotion Dysregulation, 1*, 9.

Kongerslev, M. T., Chanen, A. M., & Simonsen, E. (2015). Personality disorder in childhood and adolescence comes of age: a review of the current evidence and prospects for future research. *Scandinavian Journal of Child and Adolescent Psychiatry and Psychology, 3*(1), 31–48.

Llagan, G., & Choi-Kain, L. (2020). General psychiatric management for adolescents (GPM-A) with borderline personality disorder. *Current Opinion in Psychology, 37.* doi:10.1016/j.copsyc.2020.05.006

Lejuez, C. W., & Gratz, K. L. (Eds.) (2020). *The Cambridge handbook of personality disorders.* Cambridge: Cambridge University Press.

McCabe, G. A., & Widiger, T. A. (2020). A comprehensive comparison of the ICD-11 and DSM-5 Section III personality disorder models. *Psychological Assessment, 32*(1), 72–84. doi:10.1037/pas0000772

Ofrat, S., Krueger, F., & Clark, L. A. (2018). Dimensional approaches to personality disorder classification. In W. J. Livesley & R. Larstone (Eds.), *Handbook of personality disorders: theory, research and treatment* (2nd Ed.). London: Guilford Press.

Oltmanns, J. R., & Widiger. T. A. (2018). A self-report measure for the ICD-11 dimensional trait model proposal: the personality inventory for ICD-11. *Psychological Assessment, 30*(2), 154–169. doi:10.1037/pas0000459

Paris, J. (2013). *The intelligent clinician's guide to the DSM-5.* Oxford: Oxford University Press.

Steele, K., Boon, S., & Van Der Hart, O. (2017). *Treating trauma-related dissociation: a practical integrative approach.* London: Norton & Co.

Index